Stuttering and Related Disorders of Fluency

Second Edition

Stuttering and Related Disorders of Fluency

Second Edition

Richard F. Curlee, Ph.D.

Professor
Department of Speech and Hearing Sciences
The University of Arizona
Tucson, Arizona

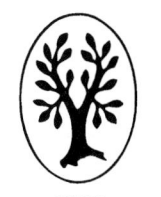

1999
Thieme
New York • Stuttgart

midtown

Thieme New York
333 Seventh Avenue
New York, NY 10001

STUTTERING AND RELATED DISORDERS OF FLUENCY, Second edition
Richard F. Curlee

Library of Congress Cataloging-in-Publication Data

Stuttering and related disordes of fluency / editor, Richard F. Curlee.—2nd ed.
    p.   cm.
  Includes bibliographical references and index.
  ISBN 0-86577-764-0 (Thieme Medical Publishers).—ISBN
3-13-783402-3 G. Thieme, Verlag)
    1. Stuttering. I. Curlee, Richard F. (Richard Frederick), 1935–
  [CNLM: 1. Stuttering—therapy. 2. Speech Therapy—methods. WM
475 S9372 1998]
RC424.S768 1998
616.85′54—dc21
DNLM/DLC
For Library of Congress   98-22183
                                    CIP

Important note: Medical knowledge is ever-changing. As new research and clinical experience broaden our knowledge, changes in treatment and drug therapy may be required. The authors and editors of the material herein have consulted sources believed to be reliable in their efforts to provide information that is complete and in accord with the standards accepted at the time of publication. However, in view of the possibility of human error by the authors, editors, or publisher of the work herein, or changes in medical knowledge, neither the authors, editors, publisher, nor any other party who has been involved in the preparation of this work, warrants that the information contained herein is in every respect accurate or complete, and they are not responsible for any errors or omissions or for the results obtained from use of such information. Readers are encouraged to confirm the information contained herein with other sources. For example, readers are advised to check the product information sheet included in the package of each drug they plan to administer to be certain that the information contained in this publication is accurate and that changes have not been made in the recommended dose or in the contraindications for administration. This recommendation is of particular importance in connection with new or infrequently used drugs.

Some of the product names, patents, and registered designs referred to in this book are in fact registered trademarks or proprietary names even though specific reference to this fact is not always made in the text. Therefore, the appearance of a name without designation as proprietary is not to be construed as a representation by the publisher that it is in the public domain.

Printed in the United States of America
Compositor: Professional Composition   Printer: Hamilton Printing Co.

5   4   3   2   1

TNY ISBN 0-86577-764-0
GTV ISBN 3-13-783402-3

5/11/2000 Graduate School of Ed & Psych

Contents

Contributors

John M. Baumgartner, Ph.D.
Department of Communicative
    Disorders
University of Northern Colorado
Greeley, Colorado

Michelle L. Burnett, M.A.
Department of Physical Medicine and
    Rehabilitation
St. Joseph Mercy Hospital
Ann Arbor, Michigan

Edward G. Conture, Ph.D.
Department of Hearing and Speech
    Sciences
Vanderbilt University
Nashville, Tennessee

Richard F. Curlee, Ph.D.
Department of Speech and Hearing
    Sciences
The University of Arizona
Tucson, Arizona

David A. Daly, Ed.D.
Department of Speech-Language
    Pathology and Special Education
School of Education
University of Michigan
Ann Arbor, Michigan

Mary Louise Edwards, Ph.D.
Department of Communication Sciences
    and Disorders
Syracuse University
Syracuse, New York

Conrad Gold, M.A.
Educational Speech-Language
    Pathologist
Minneapolis Public Schools
Minneapolis, Minnesota

Carolyn B. Gregory, M.A.
Private Practice
Evanston, Illinois

Hugo H. Gregory, Ph.D.
Professor Emeritus
Department of Communication Sciences
    and Disorders
Northwestern University
Evanston, Illinois

Elisabeth Harrison, B.App.Sc.
Stuttering Unit
Bankstown Health Service
Bankstown
Australia

Nancy Helm-Estabrooks, Sc.D.
Department of Neurology
Boston University School of Medicine
East Sandwich, Massachusetts
    and
National Center for Neurogenic
    Communication Disorders
The University of Arizona
Tucson, Arizona

Diane Hill, M.A.
Department of Communication Sciences
     and Disorders
Northwestern University
Evanston, Illinois

Janis Costello Ingham, Ph.D.
Department of Speech and Hearing
     Sciences
University of California, Santa Barbara
Santa Barbara, California

Roger J. Ingham, Ph.D.
Department of Speech and Hearing
     Sciences
University of California, Santa Barbara
Santa Barbara, California

Deborah Kully, M.Sc.
Institute for Stuttering Treatment and
     Research
Edmonton
Canada

Marilyn J. Langevin, M.Sc.
Institute for Stuttering Treatment and
     Research
Edmonton
Canada

Linda J. Louko, Ph.D.
Department of Communicative
     Disorders
University of Central Florida
Orlando, Florida

Walter H. Manning, Ph.D.
School of Audiology and
     Speech-Language Pathology
The University of Memphis
Memphis, Tennessee

Megan D. Neilson, Ph.D.
Neuroengineering Unit
School of Electrical Engineering
University of New South Wales
Sydney
     and
Cerebral Palsy Research Unit
Institute of Neurological Sciences
Prince Henry Hospital
Little Bay
Australia

Mark Onslow, Ph.D.
Australian Stuttering Research Centre
The University of Sydney
Sydney
Australia

Charles M. Runyan, Ph.D.
Department of Communication Sciences
     and Disorders
James Madison University
Harrisonburg, Virginia

Sara Elizabeth Runyan, M.Sc.
Department of Communication Sciences
     and Disorders
James Madison University
Harrisonburg, Virginia

Gerald M. Siegel, Ph.D.
Professor Emeritus
Department of Communication
     Disorders
University of Minnesota
Minneapolis, Minnesota

Preface

I hated it. That inescapable
moment each day my turn would come
and I would have no choice except to read
what David, Karen, Jimmy and Suzanne
read as if they were sliding on glass,
not crashing through it, lurching, stumbling,
every step a public demonstration
of stupidity, each sentence hours,
the teacher's cardboard smile and tapping foot,
rustling in the chairs around me, giggles
of the other kids. Miss Connie used
to punish me, pretending not to hear.

                                    W. D. Ehrhart[1]

The pain and anger expressed in this poem seem to ooze from a still open wound, deeply etched in the author's memories of stuttering while "reading out loud." Such wounds are not uncommon among adults who have spent much of their lives submitting their stuttering and themselves to an incredibly diverse selection of therapies that have been devised, seeking without success to free themselves from stuttering. Sadly, the festering of these wounds can be much more disabling than the speech disability from which such emotions spring. Despite the claims of "cures" or that stuttering has been "solved" that are announced periodically, none have survived the personal experiences of those who tried them. This text offers no such claims and, like its predecessor, includes a broad but selective range of current clinical strategies and practices that have been used successfully with children and adults who stutter. Three similar disorders of fluency are also covered in separate chapters.

This edition has been expanded to fifteen chapters, the first seven of which are devoted to the evaluation and treatment of children who stutter. It is generally agreed that stuttering is best managed in childhood, because children usually respond to treatment faster, become more fluent, and maintain their improvements longer than do most adults. Many, in fact, stop stuttering completely while in therapy and are apparently "cured." This section begins with an updated chapter detailing how I conduct initial evaluations of young preschoolers who are suspected of stuttering and try to identify those who do and do not require treatment. The next chapter is a reprise of the differential diagnostic and therapy procedures that Hugo Gregory and Diane Hill employ with preschool and early elementary school-age children, which is followed by Hugo and Carolyn Gregory's chapter on the integral role that counseling plays in their work with children who stutter and with their families. Then, another new chapter by Elisabeth Harrison and Mark Onslow describes the operant-based therapy procedures that parents are trained to use at home and that have been highly successful in a series of therapy trials conducted in Sydney, Australia. It is followed by updates of two chapters that were included in the first edition—Janis Ingham's extended length of utterance and Charles and Sara Runyan's fluency rules programs—both of which are recommended for kindergarten through elementary school-age children. The chapter by Linda Louko, Edward Conture, and Mary Louise Edwards concludes this section's focus on children's therapy by reviewing the additional challenges that co-occurring phonological disorders present for clinicians and how they can be handled.

Four chapters, all of which are new to this volume, deal with the more challenging task of providing significant, lasting decreases in the stuttering of adolescents and adults. Even though treatment permits most to achieve significant decreases in stuttering in many speaking and conversational situations, complete, permanent recoveries become increasingly rare after adolescence. As a result, how persons adapt to their residual stuttering may often determine how handicapping such persistent difficulties may be. The chapter by Deborah Kully and Marilyn Langevin describes an intensive treatment program for adolescents that they and Einer Boberg developed and refined during annual clinical trials at the Institute for Stuttering Treatment and Research in Edmonton, Canada. It is followed by Walter Manning's chapter on the importance of clinical relationships in helping adults who stutter gain control of their stuttering as well as their avoidance reactions. The next chapter, by Megan Neilson, presents the cognitive training components that were integrated into the behaviorally oriented, intensive fluency-training program that was developed at Prince Henry Hospital in Sydney, Australia. The adult section concludes with a chapter by Roger Ingham that synthesizes the operant management procedures he has used successfully with chronic stuttering disorders.

Three chapters are devoted to the evaluation and treatment of clients who present different but related disorders of fluency—cluttering, stuttering acquired following neurological damage, and acquired psychogenic stuttering. The extent to which the interruptions in fluency that characterize these disorders reflect the same sorts of disruptions in normal function that cause childhood stuttering is still uncertain. Clearly, these disorders, their assessment, and management differ sufficiently from those described in previous chapters, and from one another, to warrant coverage in separate chapters. David Daly and Michelle Burnett offer a new perspective for one of these complex and perplexing disorders in their chapter on cluttering. The following two chapters deal with disorders whose disruptions in fluency are sufficiently similar to those of adults who have stuttered since childhood that they are commonly called stuttering. First, Nancy Helm-Estabrooks has revised her chapter on stuttering associated with acquired neurological damage that appeared in the first edition. Then, John Baumgartner focuses on a clinical population that was not included in the first edition—acquired, psychogenic stuttering—and describes the diagnostic challenges posed by those clients presenting neurological diagnoses as well.

The final chapter reviews the management strategies and procedures of the preceding chapters and places them in their historical and philosophical context. Gerald Siegel and Conrad Gold identify some of the assumptions and principles that appear to guide the diverse clinical practices presently used with these disorders and discuss how they extend or diverge from those of the past.

The preface to the preceding edition of this text noted that stuttering must have predated its mention in the early writings of human civilizations, and that an extraordinary variety of remedies and treatments have been suggested during the 2400 years that have elapsed from the time of the Greek historian, Herodotus, to the present. Substantial advances have been made in achieving a better scientific understanding of the etiology of stuttering and of the disruptions of normal function that result in stuttered speech during this period, but much more remains to be learned. Current therapies for children who stutter appear to be highly successful, and those for adults usually result in their being able to talk without significant stuttering difficulties most of the time. No cure is in sight, however, and the centuries-old search for a solution to stuttering and to other, related disorders of fluency continues. Thus, this text may best be viewed as a report of the progress made to date, near the end of the 20th century.

Richard F. Curlee, Ph.D.

Reference

1. Ehrhart WD. Reading Out Loud. In: Goldberg B, ed. *The First Yes: Poems about Communicating*, Takoma Park, MD, Dyad Press, 1997, p. 20.

Stuttering and Related Disorders of Fluency, 2nd edition.
Edited by Richard F. Curlee, Ph.D.
Thieme Medical Publishers, Inc., New York © 1999.

1

Identification and Case Selection Guidelines for Early Childhood Stuttering

RICHARD F. CURLEE

Incidence of childhood stuttering is highest between a child's second and fourth birthdays, then decreases gradually, ultimately affecting nearly 5.0% of the population.[1] Early childhood stuttering is often episodic at first, varying from day to day and one situation to another, so that the child's speech sounds very much like that of other children much of the time.[2] Onset is usually insidious, gradually emerging from the background of repetitious spoken language often observed in children in this age group;[2,3] however, abrupt onsets of stuttering have been described by approximately one-third of the parents in several studies.[4,5] After stuttering has been present for a few years, most children who stutter can be readily distinguished from those who do not, even if they are highly disfluent.[6,7] Thus, accurate identification of early childhood stuttering, though challenging at times, seldom poses serious difficulties for experienced clinicians.[8–12]

It is widely believed that early identification and treatment of children's developmental disorders, including stuttering, is the most efficient and effective strategy for preventing such disorders from becoming chronic, long-term disabilities.[8,9,11,12] Although a variety of different treatments have been reported to be successful with many young children who stutter,[13,14] many young preschoolers who begin to stutter stop within the first year or two of onset without receiving any professional help.[1,13,15,16] Nevertheless, a substantial percentage, 20%–25% or so, will continue to stutter,[1,16] and if stuttering persists past puberty, it may become a lifelong disability,[13] significantly restricting the educational, vocational, and personal–social activities of some adults.[1] Consequently, even experienced clinicians may feel uncertain when deciding whether to defer treatment a while for a young preschooler, to either see if stuttering is just a transient problem, or to begin therapy without delay.

I believe that the clinical management of these children should be based, as much as possible, on empirical information about childhood stuttering, its onset, and remission. Such information has been expanded recently as a result of an ongoing longitudinal study at the University of Illinois of young children who stutter.[16] Findings from this study suggest that treatment may be unnecessary for most young preschoolers who begin to stutter and are strikingly consistent with findings from a longitudinal study completed in Great Britain some 50 years ago[1] as well as those from a smaller, contemporaneous study.[17] In addition, systematic monitoring of such children's speech has been able to identify most of those who do stop stuttering without receiving therapy.[16] This kind of information is used to support the clinical evaluation procedures and decision-making processes described in this chapter for identifying early childhood stuttering and determining which children are having transient fluency difficulties.

Clinical Evaluation

Identification of childhood stuttering relies on observing clusters of signs and symptoms that distinguish children who are stuttering from their nonstuttering peers. These signs and symptoms include qualitative and quantitative features of disfluent speech and a child's reactions to it, which vary widely in this clinical population. There is no single sign or symptom that must be present, except for stuttered speech, and some children who stutter, won't, during their clinical examination. Thus, findings obtained in a single evaluation session may be inconclusive. Diagnostic signs and symptoms must occur sufficiently often for there to be a problem; therefore, ongoing, follow-up evaluations of a child suspected of stuttering will result, in time, with findings that either do or do not support a diagnosis of childhood stuttering. It has been my experience, however, that the clinical examinations of most of these children confirm the information I gleaned from an earlier case history interview.

Medical diagnoses rely on the symptoms reported by patients, clinical signs observed by physicians, and test findings to differentiate the etiology of patients' medical conditions or disease. A diagnosis of childhood stuttering, in contrast, relies on observations of children's speech to differentiate the early signs of stuttering from the disfluencies of nonstuttering children and to determine what kinds of treatment, follow-up evaluations, or referrals may be needed. Thus, evaluations of young children suspected of stuttering should provide clinicians with the information needed to support one of the following diagnostic conclusions:

1. Few, if any, signs of childhood stuttering are present, and the child's spoken language is age-appropriate.
2. Inconsistent signs of childhood stuttering are present, and further observation and testing are needed.
3. Signs of childhood stuttering have been present less than 1 year, and few behavioral and affective reactions are apparent.
4. Signs of childhood stuttering are present as are one or more other speech–language problems.
5. Stuttering has been present consistently for 1 year or more with no signs of remitting.

I prefer to obtain this information in a series of diagnostic sessions across several days so that there is sufficient time to make additional observations of the child if needed, analyze recordings that have been made, and prepare for subsequent sessions with the child and family. Thus, the first step is to obtain a detailed case history from parents or other caregivers. Next, I schedule sessions to observe and record the child's speech and complete appropriate screening and testing of other speech–language skills. Then I analyze the data obtained, making sure that there is sufficient support for at least a tentative diagnosis. Finally, I meet with the parents to summarize my findings and discuss their implications.

Case History Interview

Interviews with parents who suspect that a child may be beginning to stutter should include a review of the child's overall development, especially speech and language acquisition, as well as a careful exploration of parents' fluency concerns. A substantial percentage of children whose stuttering continues into their school years also have other speech, language, or learning difficulties, especially immature articulatory or phonological skills.[14,18] In some cases, these co-occurring difficulties may constitute a much more significant problem for a child than does stuttering, and any such suspected difficulties should be confirmed or ruled out as part of the child's examination.

The importance of the information obtained from a thorough case history interview cannot be overemphasized. Parents are able to observe their children in a variety of circumstances that are not available to clinicians. Their repeated observations of the child in real-life situations have a validity that observations made in a clinical setting can never achieve, and the interview provides access to recollections of key events in the child's and family's life and descriptions of the child's speech that are often critical in making a diagnosis of childhood stuttering. While the clinician is getting to know a child through the eyes of parents, they are learning what kinds of behaviors and reactions are important for them to observe as a result of the topics covered and the questions asked during the interview. Even more important, however, this interview marks the beginning of a relationship between clinician and parents that can significantly affect the ultimate success of any professional intervention that may later be needed.

Parents' descriptions of a child's speech disruptions are seldom sufficiently specific to be diagnostically useful in my experience. Most simply express concern about "stuttering," then seem somewhat perplexed or frustrated if asked to describe the child's "stuttering" in more detail. Nevertheless, they have little difficulty identifying the kinds of disfluencies that are bothering them (e.g., monosyllable whole- and part-word repetitions, sound prolongations, and tense pauses) if I simulate them. Some may even recall specific examples they have observed, which I feel strengthens the credibility of a report. In addition, simulating specific qualitative features of stuttering helps parents to estimate how many units of repetition they usually observe, their tempo, and whether or not increases in pitch or loudness or accessory behaviors accompany their child's speech disfluencies. When detailed descriptions of a child's speech can be obtained, it is much easier to plan the observations that need to be made in deciding if a child is beginning to stutter, and, if so, which management options are appropriate or if parents are overreacting to normal, age-appropriate disfluencies. The latter possibility seldom occurs, in my experience; I can recall only a handful of parental misdiagnoses of stuttering in over 25 years of clinical practice.

The signs and symptoms that I rely on for identifying childhood stuttering and determining when to initiate treatment can be organized in two groups of questions. Answers to the first group help me to distinguish early childhood stuttering from the disfluencies of nonstuttering children. The second group helps me to distinguish those children who are likely to stop stuttering without treatment from those who appear to need treatment because their stuttering seems likely to persist or worsen without professional intervention or because of the need to treat co-occurring speech–language problems. Many children, even those whose stuttering is severe, often appear to be unconcerned and continue to communicate normally in spite of stuttering, and many stop stuttering without treatment as well.[1,16,17] In contrast, if stuttering is consistently present or worsens over a period of a few months, remission is less likely, at least in the short term, and direct professional intervention should be discussed with parents. A brief rationale and selected supporting references accompany each question.

Indicators of Early Childhood Stuttering

1. *What kinds of speech disruptions are eliciting parental concern?*

   Children who stutter are substantially more disfluent than are nonstuttering children, and there is extensive overlap in the types of speech disruptions observed in both groups.[14,16,19] Among those who stutter, however, monosyllable whole- and part-word repetitions are much more frequent and are often the first signs of early childhood stuttering.[16,20,21] Occasional sound prolongations and tense pauses, which are characterized by fixed articulatory positions, also occur much more frequently in the speech of children who stutter, and together with single-syllable repetitions comprise a cluster of stutter-like disfluencies (SLDs) which are obligatory signs of childhood stuttering.[8,16,19,20,22] Single-syllable repetitions occur frequently in the speech of most young children, but only infrequently are they repeated more than twice.[16,23] On the other hand, if parents are concerned primarily about revisions, interjections, and repetitions of multisyllable words and phrases—interruptions of speech that often reflect linguistic encoding processes[24]—it is likely they are worried about the disfluencies of a child who does not stutter.[21]

2. *Have the child's speech disruptions changed since parents first became concerned?*

   Beginning stuttering is often episodic, with the frequency and severity of a child's disfluent speech varying from one day to the next and situation to situation; several days may pass with no problems being observed.[14,24,25] It is important to find out if a child's stuttering has changed since it began; whether it still seems to be limited to only a few situations, such as display talking at home or when excited at preschool, or whether it has begun to occur throughout many of the child's conversational interactions.[8,10,11] A child whose stuttering initially consisted only of effortless repetitions may begin prolonging sounds much of the time, for example.[9] The longer that a child stutters, the more likely that stuttering will become consistent from one situation to another, that extended periods of fluent speech will occur less often, and that disfluencies will occur in clusters of three or more.[26]

3. *How long have parents been concerned about the child's fluency?*

   Remission of stuttering can occur at any age,[27] but at least one-half of these remissions occur within the first 2 years of the onset of stuttering.[1,16] In addition, early remissions occur more often among young girls than boys[28] and for mild rather than severe stuttering among later remissions.[27,28] Thus, if a child's stuttering persists beyond a year, especially if increases in stuttering frequency and severity occurred in that period, then the likelihood of an untreated remission within 2 years has decreased, and the need to initiate some form of treatment should be carefully reevaluated.

4. *How valid do parents' concerns about stuttering appear to be?*

   When parents are able to describe their child's speech disruptions in detail and document its patterns of occurrence with specific examples of signs that are commonly reported when children are beginning to stutter, it is highly unlikely that their fears are ill-founded. I think that such details reflect careful, purposeful observations, which I believe lends credibility to their concerns that their child has begun to stutter. Sometimes parents/caregivers report that a child's fluency difficulties have been noticed and commented on by friends or relatives. Such reactions to a child's speech by different observers is strong documentation that a child's speech is deviant and that a fluency problem likely exists.

Indicators of Need for Treatment

1. *Is there a family history of persistent stuttering?*

It has been known for a number of years that the incidence of stuttering is much higher in some families, extending across generations and affecting more males than females.[1,29,30,31] This incidence pattern is best explained by models of genetic transmission, even though environmental factors must be included to account for some onsets.[30,31] Only recently, however, has evidence been presented that family histories of either persistence or recovery from stuttering are related to the persistence and remission of childhood stuttering during early postonset years.[31] This study also found that preschool-age girls have early remissions of stuttering much more often than do boys, which may account for the increase in the 2:1 ratio of boys to girls among young preschoolers who stutter to a 4 or 5:1 ratio among adult males and females.[31] It is important, therefore, to have family members conduct a thorough search of the family tree, through third-degree biological relatives, for kin having current or prior stuttering problems. A child from a family having a history of persistent stuttering is much more likely to continue to stutter for at least 3 years post onset. In contrast, a family history of stuttering remissions increases the likelihood that a child from that family may have only transient stuttering difficulties. Thus, in my own clinical work, I usually discuss direct intervention options with parents sooner for boys than for girls and for those children having family histories of persistent stuttering than for those with histories of recoveries, even when their postonset periods and stuttering severity are quite similar.

2. *Are the child's speech and language abilities age-appropriate?*

There is a considerable body of evidence that school-age children who stutter also have other speech, language, or learning disabilities much more often than do peers who do not stutter.[14,18,32,33] Most of these children, of course, have continued to stutter through the post-onset period when remissions of stuttering are highest.[1,16] Clearly their stuttering cannot be considered a transient difficulty, even if they do recover sometime later. I have long suspected that these children have a much higher risk for persistent stuttering than if they only stuttered. Only recently, however, has empirical support for my clinical impression been reported.[34] Segregation analyses by Ambrose, Cox, and Yairi[30] suggest that persistent stuttering does not result from the genetic transmission of a more severe form of stuttering but may be due to the transmission of additional genetic factors. If so, then these additional genetic factors may contribute to the increased incidence of these other disabilities, especially phonological disorders, among those children whose stuttering persists. It is important to keep in mind, however, that the nature of the relationship between stuttering and these co-occurring disorders, other than a statistical correlation, is yet to be determined. I always screen preschool children's speech–language development and sometimes find problems that parents/caregivers have not noticed. Their presence, of course, necessitates further testing and becomes another issue I need to discuss with parents.

3. *Has the child's speech disruptions changed from predominantly two- or three-unit, seemingly effortless repetitions, to sound prolongations, tense pauses, and lengthy repetitions that are often accompanied by muscle tension and ancillary facial and body movements?*

Although childhood stuttering most often begins insidiously, a substantial proportion of children evidence signs of severe stuttering from the very beginning.[10,24,30] Indeed, systematic study of a group of preschoolers soon after stuttering onset found all of these signs,[19] and a follow-up study[30] reported that more than one-third of a larger group of preschoolers had abrupt onsets of stuttering. No differences were found, however, in the untreated remission rates of children who have either gradual or abrupt stuttering onsets. Nevertheless, if a child's disfluencies are accompanied increasingly by muscle tension and interruptions or cessation of articulator movement, airflow, and phonation over a period of several months, then the risk that stuttering will persist, perhaps for life, has increased.[8,11,13,16]

4. *Does the child often react emotionally or express concern about his or her disfluent speech?*

It is not unusual for parents of young preschoolers who stutter to comment that their child seems unaware of being disfluent and has shown no signs of concern. As a child grows older, however, a number of emotional and cognitive reactions are likely to emerge,[8,14] especially if other children have begun to react to his or her stuttering. Common, early reactions of young children include frequent blinking and breaking of eye contact during stuttering,[9,35] and the appearance of frustration, especially when stuttering is unusually severe.[10] These kinds of emotional reactions ordinarily precede a child commenting about his or her disfluencies (e.g., "Mommy, I can't talk right" or "Daddy, I can't say that word") or trying to avoid talking or saying specific words, all of which are common among older children and adults who stutter. When these signs begin to appear, after a child has been stuttering for several months, this expanding constellation of affective and cognitive reactions indicates to me that childhood stuttering is evolving into a more severe, complex problem that may be considerably more challenging to treat successfully.[10]

A thorough case history interview should provide a clear impression of the kinds of fluency difficulties likely to be observed when the child is evaluated. I usually conclude the case history portion of the interview by asking parents if there is anything else I should know about the child that hasn't been discussed or if there are other concerns that haven't been mentioned. If not, I then summarize my impressions of their concerns about the child and ask if there is anything I have left out or misunderstood. After acknowledging any corrections or additions that are made and responding to any questions or further concerns that have arisen, I give them a booklet on childhood stuttering that has been prepared specifically for parents,[36,37] ask them to read it and jot down any questions they have which we need to discuss at our next meeting. I often comment at this point that the more they can learn about stuttering, the better able they will be to assist in its remission. Finally, just before they leave, I review the tests and observations planned for their child and ask them to bring a recording from home, preferably a video-recording, of the kinds of speech difficulties problems that are causing them concern. This is especially important if they have described the child's stuttering as highly variable and episodic.

Because I schedule the child's evaluation for a subsequent day, I will have ample time to develop a diagnostic plan for screening or assessing other speech–language–learning skills and selecting activities that should permit me to observe the child's speech disfluencies when talking with different partners and performing tasks that involve different spoken language skills.

Clinical Observations and Testing

Evaluations of children who are suspected of stuttering should include observations of the child conversing with a parent/caregiver and the clinician while engaged in speaking tasks that vary in structure, complexity, and communicative stress. Videotape recordings of these conversations and tasks are used for subsequent analyses of the child's fluency and language. They may be used also to illustrate some of the child's specific problem behaviors when discussing the evaluation's findings during the follow-up meeting with parents. My "typical" diagnostic plan for a preschooler who may be stuttering includes the following:

- I usually begin an evaluation by observing and recording the child and parents interacting together, often with a favorite game, puzzle, or book brought from home. This allows a young preschooler to become familiar with the clinic environment with familiar people and favorite play material and provides an opportunity to record a speech sample under relatively unstressful circumstances. It also allows me to observe how they communicate with one another and how parents/caregivers respond to the child's speech difficulties.

- After 5–10 minutes, I (or another clinician) join the child and parent and begin to interact with them. In a minute or two, the child is asked to help find another toy or game from a box or cabinet prepared for that purpose. If the child seems comfortable interacting and talking, then the parents can move to an adjoining observation room while the evaluation proceeds. If a child seems apprehensive, however, then I think it is best to have the parents remain as long as that appears to be important to the child. Having a clinician in the observation room to respond to parents' questions and discuss diagnostically significant behaviors that occur is ideal. Also, I find that subsequent discussions of diagnostic findings are much easier when parents have observed an evaluation.

- I like to alternate the administration of speech–language tests with games and play throughout the diagnostic session but usually assess receptive language abilities first, before the child begins to tire. I also include tests having items requiring the repetition of words, phrases, or sentences to see if disfluencies increase as the length and complexity of responses increase or decrease if such items are presented with slow speech models. For example, I elicit responses for phonological or articulatory analyses with auditory models if a child's responses to picture stimuli are frequently disfluent. If such modifications in test administration are likely to invalidate a test's results, then I complete additional testing during another diagnostic session if I suspect a child may have problems in these areas.

- Video-recordings of the child's speech talking with the clinician during unstructured play activities need to be analyzed and compared with those recorded with parents at home and during the diagnostic session to assess the consistency of the child's disfluencies across different speaking partners and settings under relatively unstressful circumstances. These same recordings can be used, of course, for language sample analyses which, along with findings from standardized tests of spoken language, will determine if further assessment of the child's expressive abilities is indicated. If a child is obviously stuttering, I want to see if modifying the speaking task or how the child speaks will reduce its frequency. For example, speaking tasks that require short, descriptive, concrete responses usually elicit less stuttering than do those requiring longer, less-representative, informational, narratives. Similarly, whispering, speaking slowly with exaggerated pitch inflections or in unison with the clinician often results in reduced stuttering. In contrast, if a child has not stuttered during an evaluation, or very infrequently, I want to see if stuttering will increase if: 1. the child is asked to describe some past event or future plan or re-tell a familiar story like "The Three Bears" or; 2. I interrupt or disagree with him or rush his speech, saying we need to hurry or; 3. use any other tactic that increases the difficulty or communicative stress of the task. I am hoping, of course, that these tactics will allow me to observe the kinds of disfluencies that are causing concern but have yet to occur during the diagnostic session as well as see if they increase substantially when the child is stimulated emotionally or is excited.

• The clinical examination should also include a routine audiometric screening of hearing and a peroral screening of the speech mechanism, including speech diadochokinetic tasks, which often seem to trigger unambiguous instances of stuttering. These examinations seldom provide diagnostically significant findings in evaluations of children suspected of stuttering, so I usually save them for the end of the session, when a child's active cooperation is most difficult to obtain but is less critical in obtaining reliable results.

A major goal of this portion of the diagnostic evaluation is to observe the kinds of speech problems that were described by the parents during the case history interview. Thus, I make sure to ask them if the child's speech was typically fluent or disfluent during the evaluation. If I am confident that the child is stuttering, I want to know if I have seen examples of the child's best, typical, or worst speech. In contrast, if I am uncertain that a child is beginning to stutter and parents report that what I observed was atypically fluent, which happens much more often than the reverse, then I will schedule at least one more diagnostic session. Usually, however, parents' concerns are confirmed through observations of the child's speech, and the focus of the evaluation shifts from problem identification to assessing the variability and severity of the child's problem and, ultimately, deciding if professional intervention is needed.

The disfluencies of preschool-age children near the onset of stuttering can vary substantially. Consequently, it is important to obtain samples on different days as the child talks with different conversation partners and is engaged in different speaking tasks when assessing the consistency and severity of stuttering of early childhood stuttering.[38] Ideally, each of these samples should approximate 500 syllables in length, and parents/caregivers should confirm that a sample includes the kinds of disfluencies that are causing concern. Unless samples are representative of a child's speech, they are of limited value in assessing the consistency and severity of a child's problem.

Samples should include the consecutive conversational turns of a child until 500 or more syllables are included, after echoes of utterances and one-word conversational responses have been excluded, unless they contain disfluencies. After identifying the initial and final words of the sample, I count the number of words or syllables it contains. Words may yield satisfactory measures for two- and three-year-old children, but syllable measures are better for children whose utterances include a sizable percentage (e.g., >25%) of multisyllable words. I count the number of syllables or words in the sample twice. If the counts agree, then I use that count for subsequent calculations of the percent words or syllables disfluent. If not, then I count a third time and use either the modal or median count for future calculations.

There is no standardized or widely agreed upon procedure for either counting children's disfluencies or calculating percentages of occurrence. The two that are described count all types of disfluencies and those that are designated as SLDs; however, their definitions of SLDs, counting protocols, and calculation procedures differ. The first procedure is one that I have used for a number of years, the second is based on procedures described by Yairi.[16]

Procedure A: Count each syllable or word as either fluent or disfluent. Each syllable or word should be counted only once, regardless of the type or number of disfluencies that accompany its production. Thus, if disfluent words are counted, no more than one disfluency should be counted for each multisyllable word. If disfluent syllables are counted, a multisyllable word can have as many disfluencies as there are syllables. I count the number of words or syllables disfluent twice. If these counts agree, I use that count to calculate the percentage of words or syllables disfluent. If the counts do not agree, I count the disfluent syllables or words in the sample again and use the modal or median count in my calculations. Next, I count the number of SLDs in the sample, again counting each word or syllable as either fluent or involving a within-word repetition, monosyllabic word repetition having two or more iterations, dysrhythmic phonation, tense pause, or any other type of disfluency that I perceive to involve excessive muscle tension or effort in its production. As before, I count the number of syllables or words that include one or more SLDs twice. If these counts agree, I use this number to calculate the percent syllables or words with SLDs or stutterings. If they disagree, I count a third time and use the modal or median count for calculations.

Procedure B: Only syllables are used in assessing a sample's disfluencies, and each sample is a multiple of 100 syllables (but includes a minimum of 500 syllables), because disfluency counts are converted to the number occurring per 100 syllables. First, every disfluency is counted, regardless of type or how many were produced on a syllable. Thus, syllables may have a multiple number of disfluencies. Two counts of the number of disfluencies in the sample are made. If the counts agree, then that number is used to calculate the total disfluencies per 100 syllables. If the counts disagree, then I count again to obtain a mode or median count for these calculations. Next, every SLD is counted, which includes as many as occur on each syllable. In this procedure, SLDs comprise part-word and monosyllabic word repetitions, dysrhythmic phonations, and tense pauses. As before, two counts are made, and if they do not agree, a third count is made to obtain a mode or median before calculating the number of SLDs per 100 syllables.

Regardless of which of these two procedures is used, a number of other measures will need to be obtained if I am uncertain about a child's diagnosis or if I plan to systematically monitor a child's speech before deciding if treatment appears to be necessary. These supplementary measures may include the following:

- The percentage of total disfluencies that were SLDs.
- The percentage of stutter-like repetitions (SLRs) having two or more iterations; the average number of iterations in 10, randomly selected, SLRs; and the largest number in one SLR.
- The percentage of disfluencies clustering on the same or adjacent syllables or words and the average number of disfluencies per cluster.
- The percentage of SLDs that were accompanied by accessory behaviors in 10, randomly selected, SLDs.
- If appropriate instrumentation is available, the mean duration of 10, randomly selected, dysrhythmic phonations and of 10 tense pauses may be obtained.

As was noted earlier, a substantial number of children who begin to stutter stop without receiving any professional treatment. Although it is not possible to distinguish, with absolute certainty, between those children whose stuttering is transient and do not require therapy and those whose stuttering seems unlikely to remit in the absence of direct clinical intervention, Yairi and his colleagues[16] have been successful in making this differentiation by systematically monitoring a young child's fluency. They have found that those children who stop stuttering without receiving treatment within the first 2 years of onset evidence decreases in SLDs within the first 15 months of onset. These preliminary finding are highly promising and may resolve this difficult prognostic task if they can be replicated in larger samples of childhood stuttering at different clinical centers. Sometimes, however, it may be apparent during a child's initial diagnostic evaluation that professional intervention should begin. Ordinarily, three concerns are involved in such decisions: the extent to which the child's speech presents a communication handicap, the distress experienced by the child or family as a result of the problem, and the child's risk of continuing to stutter unless effective intervention is begun. As before, two groups of indicators, expressed as questions, are presented. Each question should be answered on the basis of findings from observations of the child's speech and reactions to disfluencies during the diagnostic evaluation and subsequent analyses of video recordings of the session. The answers to these questions serve as guidelines for deciding if a child's chance for untreated remission is high or if professional intervention is warranted.

Indicators of Early Childhood Stuttering

1. *Does the frequency of the speech disruptions observed place the child at-risk for, or support a diagnosis of, childhood stuttering or some other fluency disorder?*

Children who stutter, on average, are two to three times more disfluent than their nonstuttering peers.[16] If a child's percentage of total disfluencies exceeds 10% of the words or syllables uttered, I believe the child is at risk for a fluency disorder.[8,9] The frequency of SLDs, however, is even more discriminating, with children who stutter averaging five to six times more than children who do not stutter. Like a number of clinicians,[8–10,12] I use 3.0% or more words or syllables with SLDs as a guideline for diagnosing childhood stuttering. If this guideline is exceeded substantially and consistently across samples, the child clearly is stuttering. It should be noted, also, that even if only a few speech disfluencies appear to be unequivocal instances of stuttering, that is sufficient evidence to conclude that a child has begun to stutter.

2. *Do the type, duration, and prosodic characteristics of the disfluencies observed place the child at-risk for, or support a diagnosis of, childhood stuttering?*

A child whose speech disruptions consist predominantly of revisions, interjections, or multisyllable word and phrase repetitions, whose SLDs comprise fewer than half of all disfluencies, and whose disfluencies usually sound smooth, evenly paced, and effortless, probably is not beginning to stutter. In contrast, SLRs having two or more iterations occur three times as often among children who stutter,[16] and if 25% or more of all SLRs have two or more iterations, then I use this finding to support a diagnosis of childhood stuttering. The disfluencies of children who stutter cluster much more often and are longer.[16] As a guideline, I use findings of one-third or more of all disfluencies forming clusters of three or more disfluencies on more than one-fourth of the clusters as strong evidence of stuttering.[16] Of course, several qualitative features of disfluencies are often used to support diagnoses of stuttering, also. They include unevenly paced and stressed SLRs which may sound faster in tempo, SLDs marked by increases in loudness or pitch or interruptions in air flow or voicing, and averting the eyes and unusual postures or movements of the face and neck suggestive of muscle tension or struggle.[10,22,35] If it is apparent that speech disruptions are becoming more conspicuous and are occurring more frequently and consistently across settings, such changes must be monitored carefully to determine whether the child's stuttering will require direct treatment.

3. *Do observations of the child and parents in conversational interactions indicate a need for parent training or counseling?*

Findings from empirical studies of parent/child conversational interactions and stuttering are inconsistent.[39–43] The only prospective study of childhood stuttering involved families with children who have a high-risk of beginning to stutter because one or both parents stuttered. No reliable differences were found in the communicative styles or speaking rates of those mothers whose children began to stutter prior to onset, although the mean length of utterance of these mothers was shorter than that of mothers whose children continued to be fluent.[44] The receptive and expressive language abilities of the children who did and did not begin to stutter did not differ prior to onset; however, the articulation rates of those who began to stutter was significantly faster.[45] Thus, no support was found for the suspicion that mothers' communicative behaviors contribute to stuttering onsets. Several clinical trials and a number of case studies have reported positive clinical outcomes from manipulating parents' conversational behaviors with children who stutter;[46–48] however, none have controlled for the high rate of untreated remissions of stuttering expected among these children. Parent behaviors believed to be of importance include speaking rate, length and complexity of utterances, interruptions, and turn-switching pauses, although the evidence used to support such beliefs would also support the conclusion that these behaviors are reactions to a child's stuttering rather than precipitating factors. Nevertheless, it is reasonable to expect that some parents may interact with a child who stutters in ways that warrant attention. I can recall observing one mother, for example, who responded angrily whenever her son stuttered, even slapping his face once.

Remission of untreated childhood stuttering is common,[1] with more than two-thirds occurring within the first 24 months of onset.[16] If stuttering persists beyond 1 year without showing some signs of improving, clinical intervention should be discussed with parents, because the child's chances of an untreated remission may be decreasing.[16] If stuttering persists and speech disruptions become longer, more complex and effortful, it is increasingly likely that a child will begin to voice concern and evidence frustration, apprehension, and avoidance reactions about stuttering and speaking, which can become significant handicaps in time.[14,25] If such signs are consistently present without sign of amelioration a year after onset, then I think that direct clinical intervention has to be initiated for that child to have a reasonable chance of stopping stuttering. Consequently, indicators of persistent stuttering focus on those signs that have been found in empirical research to be related to childhood stuttering continuing for three years postonset.

Indicators of Persistent Stuttering

1. *What changes have occurred in the child's disfluencies since onset?*

Although a large proportion of the children who begin stuttering between their 2nd and 4th birthdays and do not receive treatment begin showing decreases in their SLDs within 12–15 months of onset and eventually stop,[16] if SLDs have continued unabated or have worsened a year postonset, it is likely that a child will continue to stutter for at least 2 more years if treatment continues to be deferred.[16] In such cases I meet with parents and suggest that they reconsider initiating treatment with the child. If a child's speech has been monitored systematically at 2- to 3-month intervals in speech samples recorded in and outside the clinic, the stability or increase in the child's SLDs on these recordings can be used to support the need for beginning treatment. It should be kept in mind, also, that stuttering can worsen even when SLDs are decreasing in frequency if they increase in duration, occur in more and longer clusters, or are associated with muscle tension and struggle more consistently.

2. *Were other speech-language skills developmentally appropriate?*

Often, diagnostic evaluations of a child suspected of childhood stuttering will find that speech–language skills other than fluency test substantially below age expectation.[18,32,33] In my experience, such difficulties most often involve failure to use age-appropriate language forms, especially phonology. Language-learning disabilities are present relatively often, also, among school-age children who stutter. Because the prevalence of these speech–language-learning problems is much higher among school-age children who stutter than those who do not, it is plausible that such "other" speech–language problems may contribute to a child's fluency problem or hamper its remission in some way.[34,49,50] If treatment for such "other" problems is initiated, then some attention to the child's fluency problems may be needed to ensure that stuttering does not worsen.

3. *Are the child's disfluencies frequently accompanied by signs of tension or struggle?*

Such signs are often referred to as accessory behaviors[22] and are thought to result from efforts to escape or avoid involuntary disruptions of speech, and may be acquired as self-reinforcing behaviors if escape or avoidance is successful.[51] For example, if a child's sound prolongations begin to extend beyond a second in duration, fluctuate in loudness or pitch, or terminate abruptly, the child's efforts to "escape" from prolonging a sound—an understandable reaction or adaptation to such difficulty—exacerbates the disfluency instead. Even worse, termination of the prolongation reinforces all of the preceding tension and struggle that occurred. Similarly, tense pauses preceding the effortful initiation of words appear to involve increases in muscle tension and effort to initiate a word, which usually results in longer, more anomalous appearing speech[8,10,25] and increases in their frequency of occurrence.[51] Other commonly observed accessory behaviors include extraneous articulatory postures, eye blinks, turning of the head, and curling of the upper lip during stutters.[8,10,22,35] Other adaptations to stuttering include substituting words, whispering, tapping a finger rhythmically to "get started," and slowing portions of utterances prior to an anticipated stutter.[14,25] All of these behaviors indicate that stuttering is becoming more complex and severe, that a child's fluency difficulties are worsening and will become increasingly difficult to treat successfully if allowed to become habitual.[8,10,27,51] As tense postures and movements of the speech mechanism come to characterize a child's stuttering, and embarrassment, apprehension, frustration, and avoidance his or her reactions to speaking and stuttering, it becomes more likely the child will continue stuttering. I suspect that these motor, emotional, and cognitive signs and symptoms are largely self-reinforcing responses that hinder the production of speech that is free of stuttering and which, in time, can be modified only partially in most adults.[10] Thus, the frequent, consistent occurrence of these motor, emotional, and cognitive responses ultimately produces a relatively irreversible syndrome of chronic stuttering.

4. *Does the child display negative emotional reactions or express concern about disfluent speech?*

It is not uncommon for even young preschoolers to seem embarrassed or frustrated about their fluency disruptions and to leave the impression that they often feel apprehensive about their speech. Some may exclaim, with evident emotion, "What's wrong with me?" when an especially severe stutter disrupts their efforts to communicate. When asked about their speech, some may simply state that they stutter or comment that talking is difficult or that words get "stuck" sometimes. A Communication Attitude Test appropriate for school-age children has been developed to quantify how stuttering and nonstuttering children's beliefs about speech differ.[52] Although Wingate[22] views these cognitive/emotional reactions as associated features that commonly accompany persistent stuttering but that are not obligatory symptoms, a substantial percentage of young preschoolers are reported to display such reactions at stuttering onset.[16] If stuttering persists into adulthood, however, reacting to speaking and stuttering with apprehension and fear, holding negative attitudes about speech, and seeing oneself as being disabled by stuttering are viewed by many clinicians[53] as obligatory components in a cluster of symptoms that are always present to some extent among adults who stutter. This view is consistent with my own clinical experience, and I believe that these affective and cognitive symptoms are much more likely to result in severe educational, vocational, or psychosocial handicaps than are the disruptions in communication produced by stuttering.

Case Selection Criteria

Following initial observations and testing of the child, clinicians need to integrate the information obtained from their examination of the child with that from the parent interview. Most often the information from these two sources is complementary and provides a sound basis for drawing a diagnostic conclusion. Occasionally, there are substantial discrepancies, and these discrepancies need to be resolved through further interviews, observations, or testing. In my experience, however, substantial differences between parents' descriptions of a child's stuttering and what I observed during the clinical examination are the result of the child's inconsistent stuttering rather than inaccurate descriptions. Thus, I ordinarily assume that parents' descriptions are accurate and will be confirmed in time by direct or taped observations.

As noted earlier, evaluations of children suspected of childhood stuttering result in one of five diagnostic conclusions. Each is listed below and is followed by a brief sketch of the patterns of signs and symptoms that often characterize each conclusion.

1. *Few, if any, signs of childhood stuttering are present and the child's spoken language is age-appropriate.*

These children often are highly disfluent, but their interjections and repetitions of words and phrases seem to reflect efforts to maintain speaking turns while engaged in linguistic encoding processes. Speech disfluencies of all types may exceed 10% of the syllables or words uttered, but the frequency of SLDs, which seem free of excessive muscle tension and effort, ordinarily falls below 2%–3% of the words or syllables uttered. Their performance on speech–language and hearing screening tests falls within the normal range.

2. *Inconsistent signs of childhood stuttering are present, and further observation and testing are needed.*

Some of these children may be described by parents as having stuttered severely initially, but few, if any, SLDs are present in the recorded speech samples that have been analyzed. This suggests that stuttering is not a consistent problem, which I feel is a positive prognostic sign. Nevertheless, there has to be some concern that even infrequent episodes of severe stuttering may be a forerunner of a significant fluency problem in the future. Some preschoolers may seldom speak during their evaluation, answering questions with short utterances or a shrug of the shoulders. The result, of course, is that little stuttering is likely to occur. In such cases, video recordings from home and during follow-up evaluations at the clinic will determine in time whether or not the child is beginning to stutter and, if so, what clinical management approaches should be considered. It has been my experience that most of these children stop stuttering without receiving any treatment.

3. *Signs of childhood stuttering have been present for less than 1 year, and behavioral and affective reactions are seldom observed.*

These children's speech samples evidence varying levels of SLDs, usually from 3% to 10%. Their speech may seldom be completely free of such disruptions for extended periods of time. They may avert their eyes during disfluencies, some of which may be characterized also by increases in pitch, loudness, or tempo, as if excessive muscle tension were involved. If asked why he or she came to the clinic, many are likely to answer "Because of my speech" or "Because I stutter." Some seem irritated or frustrated when they are having unusual difficulty speaking but are likely to show little concern otherwise. If these signs continue unabated across multiple speech sample environments in follow-up, monitoring evaluations for a year post-onset, I believe that direct clinical intervention should begin.

4. *Signs of childhood stuttering are present as well as one or more other speech-language problems.*

These children show early signs of stuttering and either do not pass or do not comply with instructions for the speech–language screening tests that were administered. Thus, the child's speech–language skills may not be age-appropriate. Treatment decisions, of course, should be determined largely by follow-up assessments, and if management of a phonological disorder or some other expressive language problem is needed, then treatment procedures may need to incorporate fluency-enhancing manners of speaking (e.g., speaking slowly, rhythmically, whispering) so that the child's stuttering does not worsen as a result of therapy. Chapter 7 by Louko, Contour, and Edwards describes their approach to such problems.

5. *Stuttering has been present consistently for a year or more with no signs of remitting.*

Speech is often hard work for these children. Stutters occur frequently, sometimes in excess of 15% SLDs. They often sound effortful and are accompanied by a variety of blinks, facial twitches, lip tremors, or posturing of the articulators. Signs of frustration and avoidance are not uncommon, even among preschoolers, and usually increase with age. Although these signs may be present in some children at or soon after stuttering begins, they frequently decrease substantially within a few weeks. Typically, however, this level of severity is seldom present consistently until a child has been stuttering several years. There are several reasons why these children should be enrolled in treatment without delay. First, stuttering that is this severe constitutes a significant communication handicap for most children. Second, remissions occur less frequently among those whose severe stuttering has persisted for some time.[13,27] Finally, there is reason to believe that treatment outcomes are better and that remission occurs more frequently in young children than in older teens and adults who stutter.[54]

It would, of course, be convenient if every child's signs and symptoms clustered in just one of these diagnostic categories. In actuality, many of these children present signs in more than one category in some samples or in different categories in other samples. If there is substantial uncertainty which diagnostic conclusion is appropriate, further observation and testing are needed. Many clinicians, however, believe that every child who stutters or who is at risk for beginning to stutter should receive some type of professional intervention, and they have advanced a variety of arguments for enrolling them in therapy, and sometimes the parents as well.[11,55] They argue, for example, that early treatment of young children is more efficient and effective, and even if it might be unnecessary, no harm would be done. They are correct when they say that many preschoolers stop stuttering during treatment and appear to be "cured," which seldom occurs among older teens and adults.[13] To date, however, such treatments have not had untreated comparison groups to control for the high rate of remission of stuttering among this age group of young children. Consequently, the percentage of children who stop stuttering as a result of early treatment is uncertain. Even single-subject studies which can demonstrate that decreases in a child's stuttering are related to the treatment employed are unable to determine which of these children would have stopped stuttering at some later time without treatment. Thus, there are a number of reasons why other clinicians believe that therapy is not the only management alternative that should be considered.

First, there is substantial evidence that most children who begin to stutter will stop whether they receive professional intervention or not.[1,14,16,27,56,57] Some of these remissions may reflect a natural growth or maturation process. Others might result from common sense, folk remedies employed by the parents or from an effective compensatory behavioral adjustment discovered by a child in coping with stuttering. Regardless, the majority of these young children, probably three-fourths or more, do not require treatment in order to stop stuttering. In addition, there is no evidence that postponing therapy for 6 months, 1 year or more, results in less efficient, poorer treatment outcomes. Thus, systematic monitoring of a child who stutters during the first year postonset clearly is an alternative for many of these children, especially in light of all of the accompanying fees and time commitments that may be involved in treatment.[58] Still, the uncertainty about the necessity of treatment for a specific child who stutters seems to present a dilemma for some clinicians.

My preference in dealing with such uncertainty is to let parents decide. This places the decision of whether or not to enroll a child in an early intervention program which may not be needed in appropriate hands. It also introduces parents to the type of clinical partnership that I want to establish if direct intervention for the child's fluency difficulties is begun. Consequently, once initial observations and testing of the child are completed, a follow-up meeting is scheduled at a time when both parents can attend. This meeting provides them an opportunity to raise questions that may have arisen since the case history interview or as a result of reading the informational material they have been provided.

I like to begin this session by chatting briefly with parents, to set them at ease, before beginning our discussion of evaluation findings. I may ask how the child's speech has been or if any questions or concerns have arisen since we last met. I usually begin my review of diagnostic findings by saying something like "I think I have good news for you" or "I know you're interested in learning what we found, so let's get started" and then launch into a careful summary of the findings. I try to relate what was observed during the clinical examination to what was reported during the case history interview. Linking the diagnostic signs observed during an examination with the "problems" the parents have described makes it easier for them to understand and accept the conclusions I have drawn. Nevertheless, I always check on parents' reactions to the information I am providing throughout the meeting. If it is apparent that a child is stuttering, I relate this finding to information on the remission of stuttering in young children and to the treatment outcomes expected for a child this age in the clinic. Once this has been accomplished they are prepared for me to review the clinical management alternatives that I believe are appropriate for their child. If more than one alternative seems appropriate, which is often the case, I involve the parents in discussing and deciding what seems best for their child.

A few parents may need be told that their child does not appear to be evidencing age-inappropriate or abnormal fluency problems and that there is no reason for concern on their part. In more than 25 years of clinical practice, I have evaluated only a handful of pre-schoolers suspected of stuttering whose fluency was unequivocally normal, and their family seemed relieved and satisfied when told that the child was not stuttering. Nevertheless, I am aware that some parents may not accept that nothing is wrong with their child's speech in spite of the diagnostic findings; however, I suspect that follow-up monitoring evaluations would likely assure such family members that any developing speech problems that warrant professional attention will not be overlooked.

Most parents whose children are seen within 6 months or so of stuttering onset prefer to have their child's speech systematically monitored for awhile to see if stuttering decreases substantially over the next few months. Many of them indicate that have tried to modify how they interact and converse with their child, in keeping with the informational material they were provided. I suspect that they may feel less apprehensive or concerned if they are actively involved in trying to resolve their child's problem. Another management alternative, initiating therapy without delay, is chosen most often if a child has been stuttering 1 year or more or is obviously upset about it. Naturally, parents who are highly concerned themselves about the child's speech usually want to begin therapy sooner than do those who are less alarmed. I also ask parents to choose between having their child seen two or three times per week in the clinic or learning how to implement a home management program for the child themselves. Chapter 4 by Harrison and Onslow describes response-contingency training procedures which they have used successfully with young children.

Only a few parents, in my experience, decline to initiate therapy when no other management alternatives are suggested. Under such circumstances I see if they will agree to monitoring the child's speech for awhile and try to understand their reluctance to begin therapy. Perhaps they need additional time in order to accept the possibility that their child's "problem" is unlikely to be a passing phase of speech development and that professional intervention is needed. Perhaps there are financial or transportation difficulties. Regardless, if parents feel supported and that their decision is respected rather than rejected, it is usually only a few weeks until they begin to ask questions about therapy if the child continues to have significant stuttering problems. Although monitoring may have only delayed the inevitable, there is no evidence that such delays are harmful in the long run and may, in fact, result in beginning treatment sooner than would otherwise occur in such families.

Thus, the concluding interview of a diagnostic evaluation often is an initial clinical management session. It should educate parents about stuttering and enlist them as partners in the clinical management of their child. They need to know that there are no guarantees, that the odds strongly favor their child stopping stuttering regardless of what they decide to do initially, but that some children who receive treatment continue to stutter. Some sessions may be filled with questions, long pauses, and much uncertainty; but if parents have confidence in the clinician, they are likely to leave the session feeling that they have made the right decision for their child and that their child's fluency difficulties will not become a severe, lifelong handicap. Thus, a successful session results in the parents feeling that, with the support and assistance of the clinician, their child's stuttering will be managed successfully.

Clinical Management Decisions

As has been noted in several previous sections, a variety of treatment strategies have been used with apparent success with young children who are beginning to stutter.[11,13,42,46–48,55,59,60] Indirect strategies are those that try to improve the child's speech by targeting the environment or some aspect of the child's behavior other than stuttering for change. At present, most indirect strategies rely on general parenting instruction, and counseling in some cases, to accomplish their goals. Parent counseling, in particular, is frequently used as an adjunct to other treatment procedures employed in childhood stuttering,[11,45,46,59,60] and a diverse range of procedures and goals have been described. Chapter 3 by Hugo and Carolyn Gregory presents their views. In contrast, direct strategies largely rely on response-contingent conditioning programs, fluency training, and other programmed learning procedures to decrease stuttering. Many clinicians, of course, use several different procedures, often in combination, in working with young children who stutter.[59] Subsequent chapters in this text describe a variety of procedures that are suitable for preschool through school-age children.

Systematic monitoring of a child's stuttering, both at home and in the clinic, is necessary to determine if satisfactory improvement is occurring with or without treatment. The parents need to be enlisted as active participants in monitoring the child's stuttering. There are many ways in which monitoring can be accomplished satisfactorily. What follows is one such way. Audio or video recordings of the child's speech during unstructured play with parents, siblings, or friends should be analyzed and reviewed monthly. Monitoring at the clinic should be scheduled at 2- to 3-month intervals. However, for those children whose stuttering is steadily decreasing on at-home recordings and elsewhere by parent report, I may delay follow-up visits until 6 months has passed. In contrast, children whose stuttering worsens substantially between scheduled follow-up visits should be seen during this period of heightened stuttering, if possible. During each clinic visit, samples of the child conversing with a parent and with a clinician during play or other unstructured activities should be obtained. When no stuttering is apparent in these samples, other recordings should be made of such tasks as an extended narrative or retelling of a familiar story or of the clinician speaking rapidly, frequently interrupting, and hurrying the child's speech. I use such stressful conversational interchanges to evaluate the sensitivity of a child's stuttering to stress and emotional arousal and as an indicator that in-clinic monitoring can be reduced or terminated.

When untreated remission of stuttering occurs, frequency and duration measures of SLDs gradually decrease; however, consistent, continuous decreases in stuttering across samples and time rarely occur in my experience. Typically, stuttering continues to wax and wane in frequency from one day to another and situation to situation but becomes more intermittent and less noticeable across monthly intervals. In time, the at-home and in-clinic recordings are free of stuttering and parents report that no stuttering has been observed elsewhere.

Expected Outcomes

Clinical records are subject to a number of biases. The data from these records apply only to those families who chose to obtain assistance for a child's stuttering at a specific clinic, a university speech–language training clinic in this case. The data are always incomplete because clients stop treatment for a variety of reasons; the child begins school, the family moves, loss of employment, divorce, or illness disrupts the family's contact with the clinic, or parents decide to "stop therapy for awhile," apparently satisfied, although the child still stutters occasionally. Even those whose treatment ends only after there is no evidence of stuttering for a number of months may not return to the clinic if stuttering should happen to recur. For these and other reasons, clinical records are anecdotal reports at best, and their validity is always open to question. The expected outcomes summarized below are based on such records and should be interpreted accordingly.

Well over half of the children whose parents choose to defer active intervention and monitor the child's speech through recorded speaking samples at home and the clinic, supplemented by their own observations, can be expected to stop stuttering. As a group, these children have not been stuttering as long and probably evidence less frequent and less consistent stuttering at the time of their initial evaluation than do those whose parents decide to initiate therapy. Those who do not stop or show substantial decreases in stuttering in their monitored samples within 12–15 months of onset are enrolled in therapy, if parents permit. Children with concomitant speech–language problems are enrolled in therapy without delay as are most of those who have been stuttering 1 year or longer and whose stuttering appears likely to persist. Over half of these children are dismissed with little if any residual stuttering remaining within a year. Of those remaining, many will continue to evidence below average skills in phonology or other areas of language after a year of therapy. They may continue to stutter also, even though some improvement usually has occurred. A few show little progress at first, and alternative treatment procedures should be tried or referral to another clinic considered.

Conclusion

Diagnostic evaluation procedures and guidelines for identifying childhood stuttering and deciding which children may have transient difficulties and which appear to require treatment have been described. Such decisions, at present, rely heavily on the experience and judgment of clinicians because sufficient data from adequately controlled clinical research are not yet available. Based on the data that are available, and some 25 years of clinical experience, I have suggested that most children who begin to stutter do not require treatment and will stop stuttering within 2 years of onset. Although I believe that treatment can be deferred without harming these children or adversely affecting their later treatment, I also believe that a child's parents should make the decision of whether to defer or begin treatment without delay. In addition, systematic monitoring of a child's speech should be maintained until stuttering has stopped or it seems likely that stuttering will persist unless treated. Such monitoring provides empirical support for the decisions to be made and should also reduce errors of human judgment.

Deferring treatment in favor of systematic monitoring should be considered for children who are not yet 5 years of age and have been stuttering less than a year. Deferring treatment after this period or with older children may entail greater risks. When there are other issues to consider, however, such as other speech–language problems, stuttering sufficiently severe to handicap communication, apprehension and concern about stuttering by parents or child, or parental decisions that the child should be helped without delay, treatment should be scheduled as soon as possible. Thus, the decision to defer treatment ordinarily arises for only two of the five diagnostic conclusions: when only inconsistent signs of childhood stuttering are present or when signs have been present less than a year and other problems or complicating factors are absent.

Suggested Readings

Ambrose NG, Cox NJ, Yairi E: The genetic basis of persistence and recovery in stuttering. *J Speech Hearing Res* 1997; 40:567–580.

This article is the first to provide empirical support which suggests that family histories of chronicity and remission of stuttering are significantly related to the recovery or persistence of stuttering among children in later generations of the families.

Conture EG: Evaluating Childhood Stuttering, in Curlee RF, Siegel GM (eds): *Nature and Treatment of Stuttering: New Directions, ed 2.* Boston, Allyn & Bacon, 1997.

This chapter describes the tactics, procedures, and assessment criteria that another clinician employs to achieve many of the same goals and objectives which guided the evaluation protocols detailed in this chapter.

Conture EG, Fraser J (eds): *Stuttering and Your Child: Questions and Answers*, Memphis, Speech Foundation of America, 1989.

This short publication provides information and advice about stuttering for parents in a question and answer format by a panel of clinicians having substantial experience working with children who stutter.

Curlee RF, Yairi E: Early intervention with early childhood stuttering: A critical examination of the data. *American J Speech-Language Pathology* 1997; 6:8–18.

This article provides a more detailed examination of the data on the efficacy of early intervention for young preschoolers who stutter, discusses some of the implications of providing therapy for every young child who begins to stutter, and concludes that the current database is insufficient to support informed treatment decisions at present.

Yairi E: Disfluency Characteristics of Childhood Stuttering, in Curlee RF, Siegel GM (eds): *Nature and Treatment of Stuttering: New Directions, ed 2.* Boston, Allyn & Bacon, 1997.

This chapter presents a critical assessment of the information on childhood stuttering, its onset, and progression or remission, and summarizes the findings obtained to date from the University of Illinois longitudinal study of preschool-age children who stutter. These findings are a major source of support for monitoring the disfluent speech of such children during the first year postonset.

References

1. Andrews G: The Epidemiology of Stuttering, in Curlee RF, Perkins WH (eds): *Nature and Treatment of Stuttering: New Directions.* San Diego, College-Hill Press, 1984.
2. Yairi E: Disfluencies of normally speaking two-year-old children. *J Speech Hearing Res* 1981; 24:490–495.
3. Winitz H: Repetitions in the vocalizations of children in the first two years of life. *J Speech Hearing Dis, Monograph Supplement No. 7* 1961; 26:55–62.
4. Yairi E: The onset of stuttering in two- and three-year-old children. *J Speech Hearing Dis* 1983; 48:171–177.
5. Yairi E, Ambrose N: Onset of stuttering in preschool children: Selected factors. *J Speech Hearing Res* 1992; 35:782–788.
6. Westby CE: Language performance of stuttering and nonstuttering children. *J Commun Dis* 1979; 12:133–145.
7. St. Louis KO, Hinzman AR, Hull FM: Studies of cluttering: Disfluency and language measures in young possible clutterers and stutterers. *J Fluency Disord* 1985; 10:151–172.
8. Adams MR: The Young Stutterer: Diagnosis, Treatment, and Assessment of Progress, in Perkins WH (ed): *Stuttering Disorders.* New York, Thieme-Stratton Inc, 1984.
9. Conture EG: Evaluating Childhood Stuttering, in Curlee RF, Siegel GM (eds): *Nature and Treatment of Stuttering: New Directions, ed 2.* Boston, Allyn and Bacon, 1997.
10. Curlee RF: A Case Selection Strategy for Young Disfluent Children, in Perkins WH (ed): *Stuttering Disorders.* New York, Thieme-Stratton Inc, 1984.
11. Gregory HH, Hill D: Stuttering Therapy for Children, in Perkins WH (ed): *Stuttering Disorders.* New York, Thieme-Stratton Inc, 1984.
12. Pindzola RH, White DT: A protocol for differentiating the incipient stutterer. *Language, Speech & Hearing Services in Schools* 1986; 17:2–15.

13. Curlee RF: Stuttering Disorders: An Overview, in Costello JM (ed): *Speech Disorders in Children*. San Diego, College-Hill Press, 1984.
14. Bloodstein O: *A Handbook on Stuttering*, 4 ed. Chicago, National Easter Seal Society, 1987.
15. Glasner PJ, Rosenthal D: Parental diagnosis of stuttering in young children. *J Speech Hearing Dis* 1957; 22:288–295.
16. Yairi E: Disfluency Characteristics of Childhood Stuttering, in Curlee RF, Siegel GM (eds): *Nature and Treatment of Stuttering: New Directions*, 2 ed. Boston, Allyn and Bacon, 1997.
17. Ryan B: Development of Stuttering, a Longitudinal Study, Report 4. A paper presented at the annual convention of the American Speech-Language-Hearing Association, Seattle. Abstract published in *ASHA* 1990; 32:144.
18. Blood GW, Seider R: The concomitant problems of young stutterers. *J Speech Hearing Dis* 1981; 46:31–33.
19. Johnson W, Associates: *The Onset of Stuttering*. Minneapolis, University of Minnesota Press, 1959.
20. Yairi E, Lewis B: Disfluencies at the onset of stuttering. *J Speech Hearing Res* 1984; 27:154–159.
21. McDearmon JR: Primary stuttering at the onset of stuttering: A re-examination of data. *J Speech Hearing Res* 1968; 11:631–637.
22. Wingate ME: A standard definition of stuttering. *J Speech Hearing Dis* 1964; 29:484–489.
23. Zebrowski PM: Duration of the speech disfluencies of beginning stutterers. *J Speech Hearing Res* 1991; 34:483–491.
24. Wexler K, Mysak E: Disfluency characteristics of 2-, 4-, and 6-year-old males. *J Fluency Disord* 1982; 7:37–46.
25. Van Riper C: *The Nature of Stuttering*, 2 ed. Englewood Cliffs, Prentice Hall, 1982.
26. Hubbard C, Yairi E: Clustering in the speech of stuttering and nonstuttering preschool children. *J Speech Hearing Res* 1988; 31:228–233.
27. Sheehan JG, Martyn MM: Stuttering and its disappearance. *J Speech Hearing Res* 1970; 13:279–289.
28. Yairi E, Am Ambrose NG: Onset of stuttering: Age, sex, onset type, and other factors. *ASHA* 1990; 32:144.
29. Kidd K: Stuttering as a Genetic Disorder, in Curlee RF, Perkins WH (eds): *Nature and Treatment of Stuttering: New Directions*. San Diego, College-Hill Press, 1984.
30. Ambrose NG, Cox NJ, Yairi E: The genetic basis of persistence and recovery in stuttering. *J Speech Hearing Res* 1997; 40:567–580.
31. Felsenfeld S: Epidemiology and Genetics of Stuttering, in Curlee RF, Siegel GM (eds): *Nature and Treatment of Stuttering: New Directions*, 2 ed. Boston, Allyn and Bacon, 1997.
32. St. Louis KO, Hinzman A, Mason N: A descriptive study of speech, language and hearing characteristics of school-age stutterers. *J Fluency Disord* 1988; 13:331–356.
33. Louko LJ, Edwards ML, Conture EG: Phonological characteristics of young stutterers and their normally fluent peers. *J Fluency Disord* 1990; 15:191–210.
34. Yairi E, Ambrose N, Paden E, Throneburg R: Predictive factors of persistence and recovery: Pathways of childhood stuttering. *J Commun Dis* 1996; 29:51–77.
35. Conture EG, Kelly EM: Young stutterers' nonspeech behavior during stuttering. *J Speech Hearing Res* 1991; 34:1041–1056.
36. Conture EG, Fraser J (eds): *Stuttering and Your Child: Questions and Answers*, Memphis, Speech Foundation of America, 1989.
37. Cooper EB: *Understanding Stuttering*, Chicago, National Easter Seal Society, 1990.
38. Costello JM, Inghan RJ: Assessment strategies for stuttering, in Curlee RF, Perkins WH (eds): *Nature and Treatment of Stuttering: New Directions*. San Diego, College-Hill Press, 1984.
39. Meyers SC, Freeman FJ: Mother and child speech rates as a variable in stuttering and disfluency. *J Speech Hearing Res* 1985; 28:436–444.
40. Meyers SC, Freeman FJ: Interruptions as a variable in stuttering and disfluency. *J Speech Hearing Res* 1985; 28:428–435.
41. Meyers SC: Verbal behaviors of preschool stutterers and conversational partners: Observing reciprocal relationships. *J Speech Hearing Dis* 1990; 55:706–712.
42. Egolf D, Shames G, Johnson P, Kasprisin-Burelli A: The use of parent-child interaction patterns in therapy for young stutterers. *J Speech Hearing Dis* 1972; 37:222–232.

43. Wilkenfeld J, Curlee RF: Effects of adult questions and comments on the frequency of stuttering. *Am J Speech-Language Path* 1997; 6:79–89.
44. Kloth SAM, Janssen P, Kraaimaat FW, Brutten GJ: Communicative behavior of mothers of stuttering and nonstuttering high-risk children prior to the onset of stuttering. *J Fluency Dis* 1995; 20:365–377.
45. Kloth SAM, Janssen P, Kraaimaat FW, Brutten GJ: Speech-motor and linguistic skills of young stutterers prior to onset. *J Fluency Dis* 1995; 20:157–170.
46. Rustin L: *Assessment and Therapy Programme for Dysfluent Children*, Tucson, Communication Skill Builders, 1987.
47. Mallard AR: Family intervention in stuttering therapy. *Seminars in Speech and Language* 1991; 12:265–278.
48. Kelly EM, Conture EG: Intervention with school-age stutterers: A parent-child fluency group approach. *Seminars in Speech and Language* 1991; 12:309–321.
49. Starkweather CW: Learning and It's Role in Stuttering Development, in Curlee RF, Siegel GM (eds): *Nature and Treatment of Stuttering: New Directions*, 2 ed. Boston, Allyn and Bacon, 1997.
50. Adams MR: The demands and capacities model I: Theoretical elaborations. *J Fluency Disord* 1990; 15:135–142.
51. Starkweather CW, Gottwald SR: The demands and capacities model II: Clinical applications. *J Fluency Disord* 1990; 15:143–158.
52. Brutten GJ, Dunham: The Communication Attitude Test. *J Fluency Dis* 1989; 14:371–377.
53. Sheehan J: Conflict Theory of Stuttering, in Eisenson J (ed): *Stuttering: A Symposium*. New York, Harper & Row, 1958.
54. Shearer WM, Williams JD: Self-recovery from stuttering. *J Speech Hearing Dis* 1965; 30: 288–290.
55. Starkweather CW, Gottwald SR, Halfond MH: *Stuttering Prevention: A Clinical Method*, Englewood Cliffs, Prentice Hall, 1990.
56. Wingate ME: Recovery from stuttering. *J Speech Hearing Dis* 1964; 29:312–321.
57. Dickson S: Incipient stuttering symptoms and spontaneous remission of stuttered speech. *J Commun Dis* 1971; 4:99–110.
58. Curlee RF, Yairi E: Early intervention with early childhood stuttering: A critical examination of the data. *American J Speech-Language Pathology* 1997; 6:8–18.
59. Peters TJ, Guitar B: *Stuttering: An Integrated Approach to its Nature and Treatment*, Baltimore, Williams & Wilkins, 1991.
60. Van Riper C: *The Treatment of Stuttering*, Englewood Cliffs, Prentice-Hall, 1973.

Stuttering and Related Disorders of Fluency, 2nd edition.
Edited by Richard F. Curlee, Ph.D.
Thieme Medical Publishers, Inc., New York © 1999.

2

Differential Evaluation—Differential Therapy for Stuttering Children

Hugo H. Gregory
Diane Hill

Our frame of reference for evaluation and treatment of stuttering in children takes into consideration characteristics of the child, environmental conditions, and the way in which these factors interact. Support for this approach is derived from research and clinical experience indicating that individuals who stutter are a heterogeneous group and that differing patterns of factors appear important in each child or adult.[1-7]

We will show how a differential evaluation procedure is used to 1. determine the existence of a problem and 2. if there is a problem, to which child and environmental variables it is related. Treatment strategies will be discussed, indicating how each takes into account a child's specific needs. The major emphasis will be on developmental intervention with preschool children, followed by a brief consideration of elementary school-age children who display varying degrees of stuttering behavior and awareness that speech is difficult. The latter discussion will help to show how the decision-making process with children who are showing more obvious stuttering behavior and awareness compares to that with children in the earlier stages of a developing stuttering problem.

Prevention and Management of Stuttering in the Early Stages of Development

Overview of Differential Evaluation Process

The diagram in Fig. 2-1 is an overview of the differential evaluation process employed at Northwestern University and shows, in general, how a clinician chooses appropriate evaluation and treatment strategies. The level of initial evaluation is determined by information received from the parents.

INITIAL CONTACT BY PARENTS

The evaluation process begins with the parent's first contact, usually a telephone call expressing concern. Ample time (20–30 min) is needed, for a telephone interview. It is

22

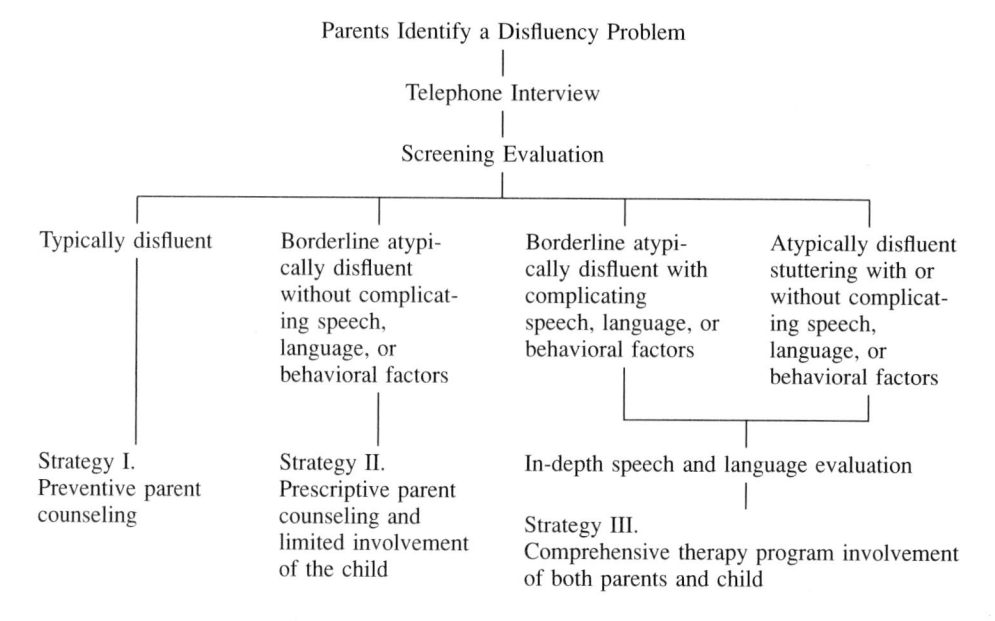

Figure 2-1.   Overview of Differential Evaluation in Therapy. From Gregory HH, Hill D: Stuttering Therapy for Children, in Perkins W (ed.) *Stuttering Disorders*. New York: Thieme-Stratton, Inc., 1984 (ref. 23).

important to listen carefully to parents' descriptions of what they have noticed about the child's speech, their responses to the child's disfluency/stuttering, and their observations about factors that may have precipitated stuttering or are maintaining it.

Open-ended questions are posed to elicit the best parental insights: "Tell me what your child's stuttering is like." "When did you first become concerned?" "Does it seem to be more noticeable at some times than at others?" "Have you noticed situations in which your child has more trouble?" Follow-up questions are asked to clarify statements by the parent. If a mother says that the child "gets stuck" at the beginning of a sentence, then the clinician may give examples of a one-syllable word repetition, a prolongation, or a block to help the parent explain. Once there is some clarification of the fluency pattern, additional questions are asked about the early development of speech and the current status of speech and language skills. It is also important to obtain information about motor development, social development, and health problems. Finally, the parent is asked about advice, evaluation, or treatment that has been received elsewhere. As the telephone interview ends, the first decision is made concerning the need for evaluation and how comprehensive it should be.

FLUENCY SCREENING EVALUATION

As can be seen in Fig. 2-1, a Fluency Screening Evaluation, consisting of 1 hour of observation and testing of the child and 1 hour of feedback to the parents is scheduled if the parents describe a pattern of speech disfluency considered to be more usual for preschool children or signs of beginning stuttering that have been observed for less than 6 months, and there are no concerns about other aspects of the child's speech and language development. The Fluency Screening Evaluation consists of four parts: 1. a brief case history of speech, language, and fluency development and other factors, such as illness, that may be important; 2. an analysis of fluency in monologue, play, play with pressure, and parent–child interaction; 3. an analysis of parent–child interactive behaviors such as interrupting, fast-paced turn-taking, or asking many questions; and 4. a cursory assessment of speech, language and hearing.

Decisions following this evaluation may result in utilizing Treatment Strategy I (Preventive Parent Counseling) or Strategy II (Prescriptive Parent Counseling and Limited Involvement of the Child) or in scheduling an In-depth Speech and Language Evaluation (see Fig. 2-1).*

IN-DEPTH SPEECH AND LANGUAGE EVALUATION

This includes more extensive assessment in each of the four areas mentioned above, with attention given to a more thorough case history; a comprehensive evaluation of speech, language, oral motor, auditory, and visual motor skills; and observation of the child's response to the clinician's modeling of a more easy, relaxed speech pattern. Ordinarily, an in-depth evaluation leads to the child and parents' involvement in Treatment Strategy III (Comprehensive Therapy Program; Involvement of Both Parents and Child; Fig. 2-1). However, on occasion, findings reveal a recent improvement in fluency, and if there are no complicating speech, language, or other concerns, less intensive Strategy II may be followed.

Evaluation Procedures

Since what we do is similar to widely used diagnostic procedures, they are not described in detail. Those features that are of particular importance in making decisions about therapy will be highlighted, and brief case illustrations will be provided.

ANALYSIS OF FLUENCY

Information about the quantitative and qualitative characteristics of disfluency in the speech of nonstuttering and stuttering children has helped us to be more precise in our evaluations of a child's speech fluency.[2,3,8] Breaks in fluency at the word level (sound- and syllable-repetitions and prolongations of sounds) usually occur less frequently than do nonrepetitious disfluencies and one-syllable word disfluencies in the speech of most children. Therefore, in general, clinicians are more concerned about increases in these within-word disfluencies in a child's speech. In addition, we are more concerned about one-syllable word repetitions and part-word repetitions if there is a higher frequency of units of repetition per instances (i.e., two or more) and even more so if increased tension manifests itself in an irregular tempo. Thus, both frequency of types of disfluency and qualitative features are considered in determining whether a problem exists or the nature of a problem.

In clinical evaluations and parental guidance, we have found it useful to refer to a continuum of disfluent speech behaviors from "More Usual" at one end to "More Unusual" at the other (Fig. 2-2). Column 1, Typical Disfluencies, is followed by column 2, Atypical or Stuttering Disfluencies. Note that in keeping with our research knowledge and clinical experience,[9–13] we have labelled the last two types of disfluencies in column 1 and the first two in column 2 as "cross-over behaviors," from "typical" to "atypical."

---

*Treatment strategies are described later in this chapter.

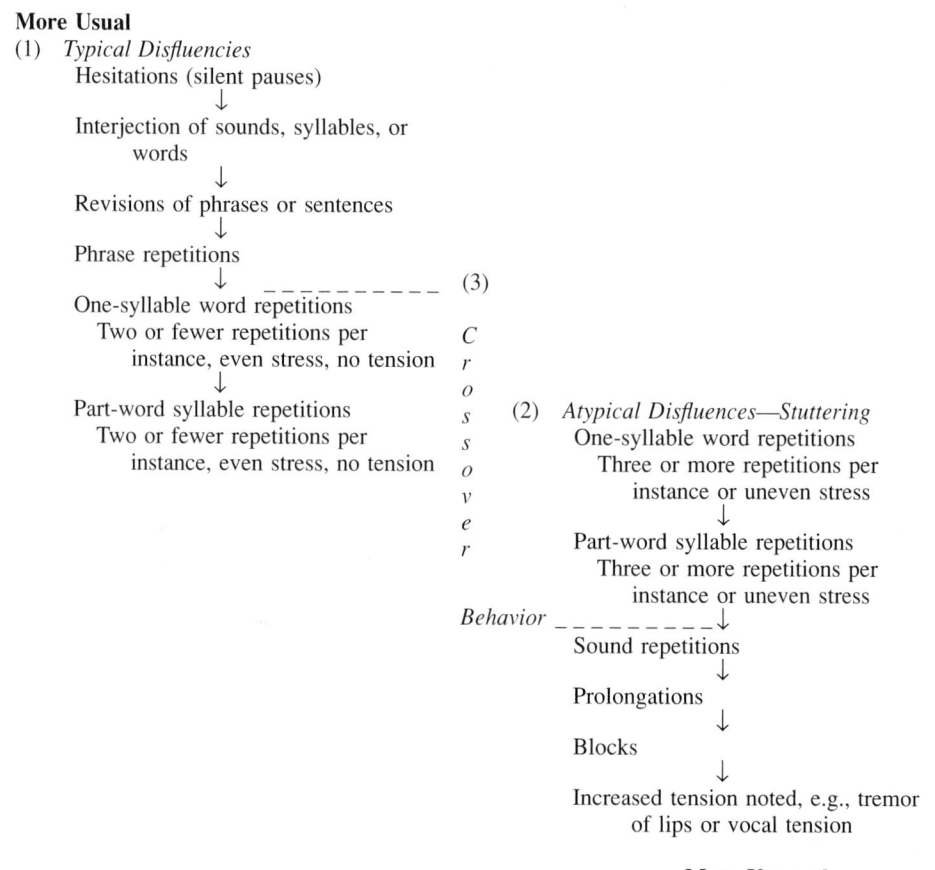

More Usual
(1) *Typical Disfluencies*
Hesitations (silent pauses)
↓
Interjection of sounds, syllables, or
words
↓
Revisions of phrases or sentences
↓
Phrase repetitions
↓ _ _ _ _ _ _ _ _ _ _ (3)
One-syllable word repetitions
Two or fewer repetitions per   C
instance, even stress, no tension   r
↓   o
Part-word syllable repetitions   s   (2) *Atypical Disfluencies—Stuttering*
Two or fewer repetitions per   s   One-syllable word repetitions
instance, even stress, no tension   o   Three or more repetitions per
v   instance or uneven stress
e   ↓
r   Part-word syllable repetitions
Three or more repetitions per
instance or uneven stress
Behavior _ _ _ _ _ _ _ _ _ _ ↓
Sound repetitions
↓
Prolongations
↓
Blocks
↓
Increased tension noted, e.g., tremor
of lips or vocal tension

More Unusual

Figure 2-2.   Continuum of disfluent speech behaviors.[13a]

More usual: Typical disfluencies in preschool children's speech listed in the order of expected frequency (hesitations the most frequent). These disfluencies are relatively relaxed, as, for example, noted by repetitions being even in rhythm and stress; however, if any are noticeably tense, then they are considered atypical.

More Unusual: Atypical disfluencies that are very infrequent in the speech of children. More characteristic of what listeners preceive as stuttering. If in a speech sample of 200 syllables or more, there is more than 2% atypical disfluency (stuttering), this should be a basis for concern, especially if airflow or phonation is disrupted between repetitions (one-syllable word or part-word syllable) or if a schwa-sounding vowel is substituted in the repetition of a syllable (for example, "muhmuhmuhmama"). Blocks and other signs of increased tension and fragmentation of the flow of speech should be a basis for immediate attention.

Cross-over Behaviors: On the continuum, such qualitative features as the number of repetitions per instance, the stress pattern involved, and the presence of tension distinguish typical and atypical disfluencies.

Total Disfluency: More than 10% total disfluency (nonrepetitious and repetitious) should signal a reason for concern. These children are very disfluent. Research indicates that highly disfluent children are also likely to show a higher frequency of atypical disfluency which is more likely to be noticed by a listener.

Summary Statement: Although most typical disfluencies are characterized by the fragmentation of a sentence or a phrase unit, most children show some part-word syllable repetition. Cross-over behaviors include more fragmentation of the word, and finally, atypical disfluencies include more fragmentation of the syllable (the core unit of speech) and increased tension. Experience indicates that increased tension is the principal factor leading to more serious disruption of speech.

Often the stress pattern and number of repetitions per instance of these will mark an evolution into stuttering. Thus, noting the occurrence of these cross-over behaviors helps in identifying early indications of stuttering.

The continuum is also useful in helping clinicians and parents compare a child's disfluencies with what is usual in children's speech and what types of disfluencies are more unusual, or characteristic of stuttering. The more frequently the more unusual or atypical disfluencies occur, the greater the concern about the development of a stuttering problem.

The speaking situations in the Screening Evaluation include 1. a monologue based on picture descriptions (e.g., action picture story sequences), 2. play dialogue (e.g., comfortable conversational interaction with the clinician while playing with a toy village or other objects), 3. play with pressure in which the clinician's responsiveness systematically varies (e.g., loss of eye contact, verbal interruption, challenging or disagreeing, competition in play, hurrying the child), and 4. parent–child interaction (e.g., parents and child interact while exploring a standard set of play materials and games). Storytelling (e.g., guided telling of a familiar story with pictured material such as "The Three Bears") is added in the In-Depth Evaluation to assess the relationship between language formulation and fluency.

Samples are videotaped and analyzed utilizing the Systematic Disfluency Analysis (SDA) procedure.[14] Verbatim transcriptions of 200 syllables in each of the speaking situations are studied. In addition to the identification of disfluency types, such as those listed in the continuum, audible and visible qualitative features and the combining of several disfluency types in one instance of disfluency are also noted. Percentages of typical and atypical (stuttering) disfluency are determined. It has been our clinical experience that if a child has 2% or more atypical disfluencies (stuttering) on any one of the 200 syllable samples, then there is reason to give careful consideration to beginning therapy. Several clinicians have pointed out that total disfluency is another element that enters into the decision-making process, and we consider 10% total disfluency another reason for considerable concern. Even though a child is below criterion (less than 2%) on atypical fluency disruption (stuttering), 10% or greater frequency of total disfluency warrants further evaluation to determine the factors (e.g., some verbal expressive deficit) that may be contributing to such a high occurrence.

We emphasize the importance of scoring verbatim transcriptions and documenting the types of disfluencies, including their audible and visible features, before commenting on the pattern of disfluency. It is difficult for the clinician to focus simultaneously on eliciting a high quality sample and note qualitative features at the same time. In keeping with the continuum concept and data from the SDA we classify the pattern into the following diagnostic categories.

Typically Disfluent—Less than 10% typical disfluency and less than 2% atypical disfluency (stuttering).

Borderline Atypical Disfluent—10% or more typical disfluency and/or 2% to 3% atypical disfluency.

Atypically Disfluent/Stuttering—3% or more atypical disfluency and/or 10% or more total disfluency.

The following example presents a summary of information from the SDA.

Danny, age 3 years, 11 months

	MONOLOGUE	PLAY	PRESSURE PLAY	STORY RETELLING
% Typical disfluency	3.0	5.0	7.5	1.5
% Atypical disfluency	1.5	5.0	11.0	1.5
% Total disfluency	4.5	10.0	18.5	6.7

Danny was considered to be typically fluent in the Monologue and Story Telling situations, but he emitted significantly elevated amounts of stuttering, as well as a sizable increase of more typical disfluency in the play with pressure and particularly in parent–child interaction. The demands placed on him by the clinician and the parent appeared to be cues for speech disruption. An initial hypothesis was that psychosocial factors were of significance in this case and that speech and language developmental factors were not significant.

The following pattern of increased stuttering and typical disfluency is very different.

Christy, age 3 years, 9 months

	MONOLOGUE	PLAY	PRESSURE PLAY	STORY RETELLING
% Typical disfluency	13.5	5.5	6.0	11.5
% Atypical disfluency	1.0	.5	0.0	5.5
% Total disfluency	16.5	6.0	6.0	17.0

Here, it appears that the demands for increased language formulation imposed a disrupting effect on the flow of communication, particularly in retelling "The Three Bears" story. Christy was normally fluent when she was free to choose what to talk about in the play situation. The high amounts of more typical disfluency were of as much concern as the indication of beginning stuttering in terms of her further evaluation and treatment. In ongoing assessment, we would want to assess her receptive and expressive language skills carefully with a specific focus on vocabulary and word finding.

These two examples illustrate the importance of sampling fluency across several speaking situations. Parents sometimes report that their child did not stutter during previous evaluations. If the clinician spoke to the child in a relaxed, accepting manner and made few demands, it is not surprising that stuttering was not elicited. We use the pressure play situation to assess the effect of this kind of demand.

CASE HISTORY

The history includes information such as the informant's statement of the problem, any family history of stuttering, general development and medical factors, speech and language development, and environmental conditions. This background helps to focus the clinical examination on factors that may be contributing to a problem, and, in turn, have a direct bearing on treatment. For example, we need to know how an informant's perception of a child's speech compares to that of the clinician or even the child's own evaluation. It may be that parents are hypersensitive about speech fluency. Knowledge of family history may be important in terms of what it implies about the likelihood of parental sensitivity about disfluency or the possibility of a genetic link. Today's parents have read about stuttering being inherited and they want information about it (see ref. 15). If there is a history of language delay, the present status of language should be evaluated more extensively and carefully.

As an adjunct to the case history, we have used such measures as the Holmes Social Readjustment Scale for Children.[16] This scale, administered to the parents, quantifies the degree of stress for a child based on such life events as moving to a new home, starting a new activity, having a mother who goes to work, staying with a babysitter, or being enrolled in daycare center. A total score designates average, above average, or heavy stress for the child being evaluated. One sees readily how this information may help the clinician and parents understand how the child's need to cope with a situation may be influencing the development of speech and language skills.

PARENT–CHILD INTERACTION ANALYSIS

First explored by Kasprisin-Burrelli, Egolf, and Shames[17] and by Mordecai,[18] these analyses supplement case history reports and begin the process of directly observing the parents and the child and mapping out suggestions for communicative and interpersonal change. It is important in counseling parents not to confuse the information gained from observing them interacting with their children with the idea that parents are causing stuttering. Rather, styles of interacting may be contributing to the growth and maintenance of stuttering, or on the other hand, may show a potential for supporting the development of increased fluency.

The analysis of a 10- to 15-min interaction is based on the verbatim transcription of a parent's and child's utterances and can be used as a baseline to assess change. The following examples of parental interactive behaviors, if identified, are targeted for intervention: verbal interruption, asking many questions, asking a second question before an initial one has been answered, filling in words, guessing what the child is about to say, constant correction of the child's verbal and nonverbal behavior, verbal or nonverbal reactions to disfluency in the child's speech, and rapidly paced conversation involving poor turn-taking.

The clinician should look at the ratios of a parent's questions versus comments, questions and statements of demand versus instances of praise and support (e.g., recall Sheehan's demand/support ratio[19]), and parent utterances versus those of the child. The parent's speech rates and the adequacy of pauses for providing time for the child to initiate an utterance should be observed also. Finally, a parent's negative interpersonal patterns such as annoyance, bribery, and threats to elicit behavior in contrast to more positive patterns such as offering choices, rewarding, encouraging, and sharing should be noted as well.

It is even more significant to document the occurrence of stuttering when related to certain parental behaviors. One 3-year-old we saw recently reacted with increased stuttering when he was verbally interrupted in the parent–child interaction situation. These interruptions were a frequent characteristic of the mother and became one of the principal targets of change for her. A final comment is that we should make sure that we know how both parents, mother and father, may be interacting in ways that increase stuttering.

EVALUATION OF SPEECH, LANGUAGE, AND OTHER BEHAVIOR

Based on clinical observations, surveys, and research reports,[2,20,21] a strong belief has developed that stuttering children have a higher prevalence of language and articulation problems. However, Nippold[22] has questioned this belief, stating that due to the variations in criteria used to judge the presence of a related problem, it is difficult to draw conclusions from these studies. Still, we agree with Nippold's advice that since some children who stutter do have additional speech and language problems, all aspects of communication should be evaluated carefully. It has been our observation that the potential impact of these deficits, when present, vary not only in terms of the severity of the problem but also in relation to the child's awareness level, frustration tolerance, and reactions from individuals in the environment.

Here is an illustration of what we mean:

Joey, by his parents' report, had been noticeably disfluent since he began to speak. He was delayed in speech and language development and was difficult to understand. At age 3, while enrolled in therapy for a phonological disorder, the parents observed that he was stuttering and became very anxious about it. They were confused, because he had made great progress and his speech was much more intelligible, for which they were thankful, but now he was stuttering. The parents observed that Joey was more fluent in structured utterances but that there were frequent disruptions in the flow of speech during his more spontaneous, connected speech. During stuttering, he seemed to increase speech loudness, "widen" his mouth, and show more variability in pitch. Observation of parent–child–sibling interactions revealed a pattern of rapidly paced conversations and poor turn-taking. Frequently, more than one person spoke at the same time. Joey had to talk louder and louder and faster and faster to be heard. His older brother spoke rapidly and often interrupted Joey.

In this case, it is clear that both child factors (i.e., delay in speech and language development and an existing stuttering problem) and environmental factors (i.e., communicative stress in the family) should receive attention. Thus, both Joey and his family were involved in therapy.

Children who have attentional problems, those who are passive and withdrawn, or those who are fearful or perfectionistic, may require therapy directed to these problems while we give attention to speech. Also, either before therapy or during treatment, we may solicit the consultation of a clinical psychologist or educational specialist about problems such as these.

Differential Therapy

In keeping with the thesis of this chapter, differential therapy, what is stressed in treatment, is based on the findings of a differential evaluation.[4,6,23] Commonalities exist in intervention strategies, but procedures are modified, to some extent, for each child. In general, most clinicians intervene first to reduce communicative stress in the environment. More in-depth evaluation and intervention may or may not be necessary.

TREATMENT STRATEGY I. PREVENTIVE PARENT COUNSELING: CHILD TYPICALLY DISFLUENT

1. *Parent Feedback*. We describe how speech develops and include information about the occurrence of disfluency, perhaps by using the continuum depicted in Fig. 2-2. Using the results of the SDA, we help parents to understand the basis for our judgement that their child's disfluency at the present time is typical for his or her age. We encourage the parents to agree or disagree that the samples we have gathered are representative of the speech pattern about which they are concerned. If they say, "He usually repeats words five or six times and sometimes covers his mouth," and if only a screening evaluation has been done, a more extensive evaluation should be conducted, or Strategy II, Prescriptive Parent Counseling, may be undertaken.

2. *Discuss Interactive Styles*. Some communicative and interpersonal situations that have been related to increased disfluency and stuttering, such as those covered in the previous section on parent–child interaction analysis, are described for parents. We reinforce the appropriate and positive behaviors that they report, and then discuss possible parent–child interactions that may require further monitoring. For example, it is usually helpful for all

parents if we mention the value of commenting more and questioning less to encourage more conversation and impose fewer verbal demands, during this critical period of the child's speech and language development. It is also useful to describe Sheehan's demand/support ratio.[19] In general, we encourage parents to give attention and time to their children, express appreciation for what they do in the way of childhood tasks, and be reasonable in their demands, basing them on the child's age and readiness.

3. *Increase Understanding of Communicative Stress.* The concept of time pressure in communication is discussed. We give such concrete examples as an adult beginning to talk just before or immediately after a child speaks, or asking a second question before a child has finished answering the first. We emphasize how children during their preschool years, when speech and language are developing and important emotional and social development is taking place, may show increased disfluency as they attempt to compete.

4. *Increase Understanding of Speech and Language Development.* Findings of the speech and language evaluation are given, and suggestions are provided for monitoring and supporting development in any area that is only marginally within normal limits on formal testing. Normative guidelines are provided.

5. *Provide Information Through Reading.* Parents read sections on speech interaction and nonverbal communication in such books as *If Your Child Stutters: A Guide for Parents*[24] and *Stuttering and Your Child: Questions and Answers.*[25] These publications reinforce the information given in counseling sessions and serve as future references for the parents.

One counseling session, or possibly two, are usually sufficient to complete these tasks. A schedule of monthly phone contacts is planned to confirm continued normal fluency development. The parents are encouraged to call whenever they are concerned. Normally, follow-up contacts continue for 3–6 months, with a fluency recheck at the end to assess formally the child's disfluency across speaking situations.

TREATMENT STRATEGY II. PRESCRIPTIVE PARENT COUNSELING, BRIEF
THERAPY WITH THE CHILD: CHILD BORDERLINE ATYPICALLY DISFLUENT
WITHOUT COMPLICATING SPEECH OR LANGUAGE FACTORS

1. *Parent Feedback.* Based on observations made and information obtained during the screening evaluation, feedback is given to the parents regarding the clinician's judgments that their child is showing some borderline stuttering behaviors. The parents and the child are then scheduled to attend four biweekly sessions that are 1 hour in length. At these sessions, the child is involved in fluency-enhancing activities. Parents participate in discussions, observations of their child, activities with the child and clinician, and finally with their child alone.

2. *Charting Disfluent Episodes.* The parents are instructed how to identify disfluencies and chart episodes of unusual disfluency using a form shown in Table 2-1. These charts are used to discuss patterns of child factors and environmental factors that parents observe to be related to increases in their child's disfluency. Parents are asked to choose one at a time to problem solve. For example, one mother discovered that her daughter stuttered more in the morning while dressing. As she analyzed the reason why, she realized that the two of them were "battling" about the choice of what to wear. The solution that the mother chose was to lay out two clothing choices, then leave it to her 3½-year-old to decide. The result was a decrease in conflict and in the child's disfluency, and a mom who was pleased with her successful management of the situation.

3. *Modeling Positive Communicative Styles Conducive to Increased Fluency.* During each

Table 2-1. Chart of Disfluent Episodes

Person	Message	Type of Disfluency	Child Awareness	Listener Reaction	Fluency Disruptors
Mother talking on the phone	Child interrupted his mother and wanted her attention	Irregular rhythm on syllable repetitions in the first word of the sentence	Overall tense, but not aware of disfluencies	Mother said she would talk as soon as she finished	Getting listener attention, not tolerant of delay

session, the child is involved in activities that promote fluency. While the child is with the clinician, the parents and another clinician watch from an observation room, as the clinician with the child models communicative behaviors that are supportive to fluency development. Such behaviors include speaking in a more easy, relaxed manner; giving the child time to respond to comments, questions, or instructions; reducing direct questioning and increasing commenting; allowing a short pause before replying to the child's statement; and reinforcing the child when appropriate. While parents are watching, the clinician observing with them comments about the conversational interaction between the child, and the other clinician and highlights these fluency-enhancing behaviors. In this way, the parents learn vicariously, before they enter the situation and participate with the child and clinician. Then, parents have the opportunity to begin practicing the behaviors they saw modeled. Gradually, in successive sessions, parents take over more of the clinician's role. The clinician who is observing provides written feedback, and in addition, comments are made following the session, about the parent's responding by saying, for example, "Good commenting today. Did you notice how much more conversation you had with Julie? You were also successful in increasing the time you allowed for her to answer your questions. Great!"

4. *Reassessment of Child and Parent–Child Interaction.* At the conclusion of four sessions, follow-up fluency analyses and parent–child interaction analyses are done to evaluate progress. If the child's fluency is within normal limits, plans are made for monthly telephone contacts for 3–6 months. In some cases, additional prescriptive parent–child sessions are recommended. In a few cases, more intensive and more direct treatment of a child is carried out as parent counseling continues. If, at any time after dismissal, parents have concerns about increases in disfluency, the clinician can advise by telephone or see the family as soon as possible.

TREATMENT STRATEGY III. COMPREHENSIVE THERAPY PROGRAM: CHILD BORDERLINE ATYPICALLY DISFLUENT WITH COMPLICATING SPEECH OR LANGUAGE FACTORS OR ATYPICALLY DISFLUENT (DEMONSTRATING MORE DEFINITE STUTTERING BEHAVIORS) WITH OR WITHOUT COMPLICATING SPEECH, LANGUAGE OR BEHAVIORAL FACTORS

Children are involved in the Comprehensive Therapy Program when they are judged to be demonstrating atypical patterns of disfluency. Generally, these patterns have persisted for 6 months or longer. Oftentimes, parents report that there has been a decrease in the cyclic variation. We assume that greater cyclic variation means a less well-established problem. In addition, the observed differences in speech fluency have not resolved with maturation, the parents attempts to use the information provided them on communication interaction, or the family's involvement in a less intensive therapy program such as prescriptive parent counseling. The majority of children in this program are 3 or 4 years old.

The child is seen for at least two 30- to 50-minute therapy sessions a week, and the parents participate in a parent group session and a portion of their child's therapy session once a week. Depending on the severity of the problem, more frequent sessions may be necessary. Typically, the child and parents take part in this format for from two to four 10-week sessions, and, if needed, children continue to receive individual therapy with parent participation until treatment goals are met. Clinicians should organize their programs as they think best, but fewer than two individual sessions each week for a child with this kind of problem is not likely to succeed.

The following procedures are more specific to Strategy III.

1. *Facilitating the Child's Fluency.* For more than 25 years, we have based our approach to fluency development in children on the principles of modeling (i.e., observational learning), counterconditioning, and modified programmed instruction. Children develop more fluent speech by observing first the clinician, and then the mother and/or father, speak in a pattern that we call "slower, more easy, relaxed speech." This speech pattern counters the tension that may exist, and it is taught beginning with shorter utterances and progressing to those of increasing length and complexity. An analysis of the literature on early intervention indicates a trend toward the increased use of such fluency-enhancing procedures[26–29] with preschool children who have fluency problems.

The desired result is for a young preschool child to speak in a slower, easy, relaxed manner with adequate loudness and appropriate inflection. Because children of 2–5 years of age are still developing perceptual, speech–motor, and vocal skills, the clinician's model must be quite obvious at first. Speech rate is slow and smooth, which enables the child to perceive the model's easy approach when initiating speech, followed by smooth movements. Rate of speech is normalized as instruction in easy relaxed speech moves from words to phrases and longer utterances, and as these modifications become more stable in the child's speech. Thus, slow speech is not the goal! More relaxed speech with easy approaches to its initiation, smooth movements, normal rate, and natural inflection are the desired outcomes. We are shaping an ongoing, developmental process.

Initially, instructions to the child should be general and encourage close attention to the clinician's model through listening and watching. The clinician might say: "We're going to play a game and I'm going to show you how to play. Watch me and listen. I want you to name this just like I do." While engaging the child's interest, the clinician not only verbally models slower and more easy, relaxed speech, but also moves in a relaxed manner providing such visual, rhythmic cues as moving cards or pieces of a game smoothly and slowly across a table or rolling a ball gently. Listening to and watching the model is reinforced: "I like the way you listened and waited for your turn"

When the child's learns to attend and evidences some understanding of this more relaxed speech pattern, he or she is asked to imitate a word or phrase "doing it just like I did." Whenever possible we begin at the phrase level, because these are more meaningful speech units and more natural inflection is possible. However, some children must begin at the word level in order to produce good-quality, easy, relaxed speech responses. At first, reinforcement is more general, for example, "Good listening, you remembered to tell me the name and the color—blue ball. You said that like I did." As the child is more successful, reinforcement becomes more specific. "You said that smoothly, good!" or "That was smooth and easy." As target responses becomes longer and include several sentences, models emphasize an easy approach more and the normalizing of transitions throughout phrases. Again, reinforcement becomes more specific. "I like the way you said that. You had an easy beginning." Later, "I like the way you said that. You had an easy beginning, and you said it smoothly."

Slower, easy, relaxed speech is learned and stabilized through response imitation and repetition, moving through several hierarchies. These hierarchies involve 1. length and complexity of response (i.e., single words, phrases, etc.), 2. type of model, (i.e., direct model—clinician says "sun," child says "sun;" delayed model—clinician says, "sun, now you tell me," child says "sun;" intervening model—clinician names a picture, child names another picture; no model—child names picture; and question model—clinician says, "What is this?" child says what it is, e.g., "ball"), 3. propositionality (i.e., imitation, recall, stereotyped response, self-formulated, etc.), 4. situational (i.e., at table, on floor, standing, walking, etc.), plus hierarchies of any other variable affecting a child's speech.

The criterion for the stability of slower, easy, relaxed speech responses employing any hierarchy is set at 90% in 15–20 trials for two consecutive treatment sessions with 100% reinforcement, followed by two sessions employing the same criteria for correct speech responses, but with 50% reinforcement. As production of easy, relaxed speech is more successful, variables are introduced that create more real-life situations, for example, walking around a building and asking for objects needed for a project. We manipulate generalization and transfer variables related to topic, location, physical activity, people present, etc., depending on the differential evaluation of factors judged to contribute to increased disfluency and stuttering in a particular child.

2. *Increasing Tolerance to Fluency Disrupting Influences.* As the clinician continues to make observations about factors that tend to disrupt a child's fluency and the parents share their observations, a hierarchy of these factors is developed. A child's hierarchy may include such stimulus conditions as verbal interruption, excitement, competition during a game, noisy environment, asking questions, walking and talking, etc. Before work ends at a given length of utterance (e.g., four-word sentences), desensitization procedures are introduced.[29] Once there is a basal fluency level (i.e., slower, easy, relaxed speech characterized by only typical disfluencies), a stressor, such as increased excitement, is introduced in a mild manner. The next time, excitement is increased. When normal fluency begins to break down, the clinician reduces the stress. Later, in the same session, after normal fluency is reestablished, stress is applied again. This cycle is repeated across sessions until the child is able to maintain normal fluency in the presence of disruptive factors. This procedure is used only by the clinician, not by the parents. Children's environments cannot be made optimal; therefore, this process is important in preparing them to maintain increased fluency in real-life communication situations. Some normal (i.e., typical) disfluency, as occurs in most children, should be expected. Again, the continuum in Fig. 2-2 is used as a guide.

3. *Developing Competence in Skills Having the Potential to Interfere with Fluency.* Children whom we see have needs quite often for therapy focusing on their articulation and expressive language, including word retrieval. In most cases, we work on fluency first, stabilizing it at the four-word length of utterance, before introducing work on other areas of communication. Syntactic structures can be worked on as we go from shorter, less complex utterances to longer, more complex ones in modifying fluency.

Our approach to helping children with word-finding difficulty is twofold: 1. We help them to learn to cope more appropriately with the time pressure related to word lapses, and 2. we improve skills that facilitate word finding. In helping them to feel more comfortable with delays and pauses in the flow of speech, we model delays in our responses to naming objects, commenting, "I couldn't remember the name for that. Sometimes it's hard to think of words. Everyone has some trouble thinking of words." We reward increasing pause time and desensitize feelings to respond rapidly with such games as throwing a ball back and forth more slowly with the clinician. Following this, we may play a game in which the child takes a turn throwing the ball back only after thinking of an animal or a fruit and is prompted to take time thinking. Parents are encouraged to give ample time for the child to converse and not to fill in words or interrupt. Rather, parents are advised to provide word choices, perhaps saying, "Were you thinking of a banana, an apple, or an orange?"

The second goal is to develop strategies that facilitate word finding. One way we have done this is by practicing associations between objects and their attributes, stressing semantic associations such as color, size, shape, and function. We then practice descriptions using various words used in the exercises. For example, to facilitate improved word recall we use activities that accomplish the following: develop word association, categorization, and descriptive skills; build flexibility in word recall by saying, for example, "Think of four things that fly" or "Think of three fruits" or "Think of five green things;" expand vocabulary and word knowledge; and develop specific cues that facilitate the process, for example, we say, "Describe the object;" or "Think of the first sound," or "Think of what group it belongs in."

In this two-part process, children become more confident in their ability to convey messages. They are able to cope more effectively with the demands of conversational interchange, and word-finding difficulties are less of a disrupting influence.

Generalization and Transfer

We have observed success in generalization and transfer when parents, and sometimes other siblings become a part of the therapy process. At first, they observe the clinician and the child and follow the clinician's model. In the usual progression, parents are assigned to do at home what they have already done in the clinic. In this way, both parents and children are experiencing generalization and transfer. Also, in this manner, the process seems very natural to them and is usually quite successful. In some instances, other siblings, depending on our judgment of the probable success of doing so, also become a part of the therapy process, and this can contribute to the effectiveness of transfer.

Summary of Parent Counseling

In describing our three intervention strategies, a variety of parent counseling procedures have been described: such as giving parents information about speech fluency, disfluency, and stuttering; teaching them to chart and discuss episodes of stuttering; helping them to modify communicative and interpersonal stress; and training them to model the behavior we wish their children to acquire. It is important to remember that verbal counseling should always be accompanied by the clinician modeling any changes that are suggested for the parents. This is discussed in more detail in Chapter 3, p. 56.

Parent groups may identify issues that can be particularly troublesome such as appropriate expectations for child behavior, parent–child separation difficulty, and sibling rivalry.

Clinicians should be able to handle this type of discussion while remaining alert to the possible need for family counseling by another specialist. As is emphasized in the following chapter, it is our belief that the success of therapy is, to a great extent, dependent on the relationship we establish with parents and their ability to enter into a problem-solving process with us.

Therapy for School-age Children with More of a Confirmed Problem

DIFFERENTIAL EVALUATION

Whether the referral is from a parent or teacher or, as in some few cases, results from an expression of concern by a child, we attempt to find what the informant views as a possible problem. The child's speech is screened during conversation and, as appropriate, by having the child read. The need for further evaluation is determined, and the parents and/or teachers are given feedback about our initial impressions. If it appears that treatment will be needed, a more in-depth evaluation is done.

As illustrated in Fig. 2-3, evaluation of these children is considered to be a differential process, just as it was in working with preschool children. It includes a case history, a complete speech analysis, other more formal tests and observations, and in some cases, related examinations by another specialist, such as a psychologist.

Gregory[3,29] provides a detailed description of these procedures, and the reader is referred to chapters on evaluation by Riley and Riley[4] and Williams[31] and books on stuttering therapy (by Conture,[5] Cooper,[26] Gregory,[3] Ham,[32] and Peters and Guitar[33] for additional information about evaluations that can be applied to this system.

DIFFERENTIAL THERAPY

A differential evaluation results in initial decisions about therapy, but evaluation continues throughout therapy. The latter point will be illustrated clearly as we describe approaches to speech modification.

The following examples indicate how information gained in evaluation determines the direction of therapy:

1. Understanding how a child's perception of his or her problem compares with that of the parents, teachers, and the speech–language pathologist tells us something about a child's sensitivity and motivation and the sensitivity of the child's parents and teachers. If a child shows little concern or interest in therapy, therapy should begin on a trial basis only, or be postponed until motivation is greater. A discrepancy between the way the parents and teachers perceive the child's speech may tell us either about sensitivity on their part or about differences in the stimulus conditions that are associated with stuttering at home and at school. Directions of counseling are determined by this kind of information.

2. From knowledge about how communicative stress (the way people talk with the child) and interpersonal stress (the way people interact with the child and with each other in the child's environment) influence the child's speech, we begin to consider how such factors as time pressure or rapid family pace may need to be modified. Such information, of course, may also have implications for the school environment.

3. Information about speech and language helps to determine if a deficit in receptive

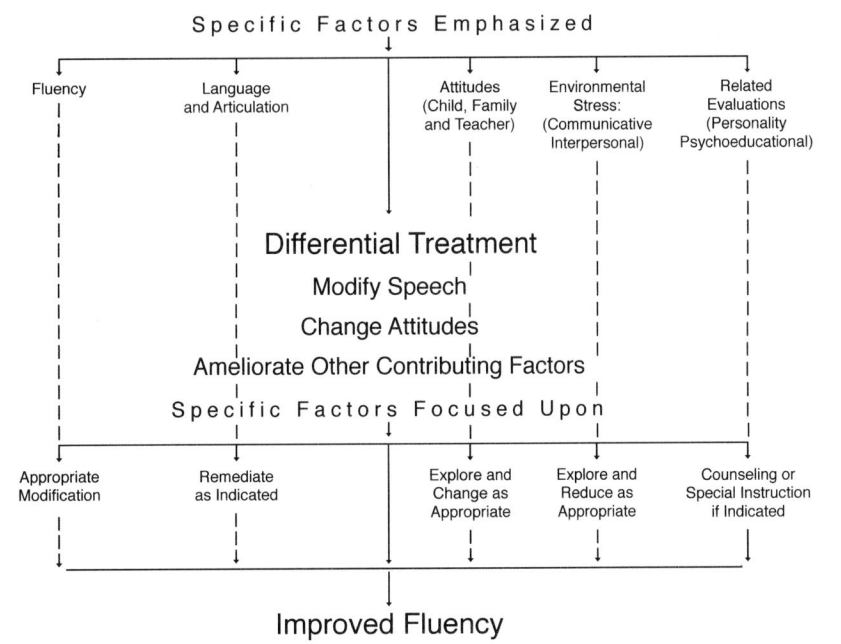

Figure 2-3.   School-age children who stutter—differential evaluation and treatment. Adapted with permission from Gregory and Campbell.[39]

or expressive language is associated with the child's stuttering problem and should be taken into consideration in planning therapy.

4.   Having knowledge of a child's adjustment has implications for how he or she may respond to therapy or may indicate the need for referral to a clinical psychologist. The more we know about a child's personality, the better we can judge how we should relate to him or her.

Speech Modification.   From 6 or 7 to around 11 or 12 years of age, it is difficult to be certain about a child's awareness of his or her problems, the consistency of avoidance behaviors and inhibitory tendencies, and the child's self-image as a person with a speech problem. There is essential agreement among a number of clinical contributors, such as Adams,[34] Bloodstein,[35] Cooper,[26] Costello,[36] Gregory,[3] Shine,[28] Van Riper,[29] and Williams,[37,38] that procedures should be used to enhance elementary school-age children's confidence in their ability to speak easily and enjoy communication. As is true of therapy for a preschool child, analysis of stuttering behavior is, in general, viewed as counterproductive, at least until otherwise indicated, as we will explain later.

Less Specific and More Specific Approaches.   Historically, the terms "direct" and "indirect" have been used to characterize two general approaches to stuttering therapy for children. "Direct" usually refers to modifying a child's speech, and "indirect" means working with the parents. With elementary school-age children, we work directly with the child's speech, but we consider it more appropriate to think of what we do as "less specific" or "more specific."[3,39] A differential evaluation of how to best modify an elementary school-age child's speech is made during the therapy process. In our view, it is best to begin with a *less specific approach* that emphasizes the development of fluency skills. A *more specific approach* that focuses on residual stuttering can be used to the extent necessary. The latter assumes that certain cues associated with speech and stuttering are stronger and specifically associated with sounds, words, and situations.

In the *less specific approach*, the clinician models an easier, more relaxed approach with smooth movements beginning with words, then phrases, and working up to longer, more complex utterances. There is no analysis of stuttering. For example, in practicing words, initial consonant–vowel (CV) or vowel–consonant (VC) combinations are produced with more relaxed, smooth movements that are slightly slower than usual. The remainder of the word, beyond the initial CV or VC, is produced at a normal rate and with normal prosody. Children who stutter often show a tendency to assume anticipatory articulatory positions for sounds (e.g., at the beginning of a word) such as closing the lips for "p," rather than thinking of the "p" *and* the following vowel as a single *smooth movement.*

With phrases, an easier, more relaxed approach with smooth movements is emphasized on the first CV or VC combination of the first word. The remainder of the word and all subsequent words in the phrase are blended together. In connected speech, the child is instructed to focus on monitoring the beginning of each phrase. We say, "Make an easy relaxed approach, and then let it go, making a smooth movement through the phrase." Rate and prosody should be kept as natural and normal sounding as possible.

Pausing, resisting time pressure, and general relaxation are part of the therapy program. We point out to the child that stuttering involves tension that breaks up the smooth flow of speech and that relaxation should be carried over into the coordinated movements involved in talking.

If the cues associated with stuttering on particular sounds and words are of sufficient strength that stuttering is persistent, then a *more specific approach* is employed *as needed.* For example, 1. child A may need the more specific approach on only a few words, 2. child B may need this attention on several sound transitions, 3. child C may need rather extensive work on several aspects of speech production (sounds, words), and 4. child D may be unable to modify speech fluency to any significant degree without using the more specific approach. The last example is rare.

The following steps illustrate the more specific approach.

1.   The clinician feigns the introduction of tension in her or his speech to produce syllable repetitions, sound prolongations, vocal tension, bilabial blocks, etc. The child imitates some of the "clinician's blocks."

2.   The clinician models the modification of this feigned stuttering by, for example, slowing a repetition, shortening a prolongation, or easing the tension in the initiation of a word. The child does the same, imitating the feigned behaviors and modifications modeled by the clinician.

3. Following the clinician's model, the child imitates the actual difficulty he or she is having (e.g., prolonging the /s/ sound at the beginning of words) and then experiments with making the prolongation longer, then shorter, more tense, less tense, etc.

4. Modifying speech is finally evolved into an easier, more relaxed approach with smooth movements.

5. Voluntary disfluency may be modeled and taught if the child is unduly sensitive about disfluency. Children need to understand that some disfluency (e.g., word repetition, phrase repetition, interjections, and revisions) is a normal aspect of speech. Cancellations are used following stutterings that are persistent. Also, time-out contingencies may be employed by the clinician to help children be more effective in carrying out a speech change procedure.

Speech clinicians will recognize that in actual practice elements of the more specific approach can be integrated with the less specific approach. For example, if a child shows particular difficulty being successful with the easier, more relaxed approach with smooth movement on words beginning with /s/, the clinician may include some of the more specific approach by first modeling tension and poor transitions at the beginning of words, and then having the child copy these models and see how approaches to words can vary in tension, length of the /s/ sound, repetition of /s/, repetition of first syllables of words, etc. Then, these productions are contrasted with the easier, more relaxed approach with smooth movements in words and phrases.

Elementary children are very concrete,[40,41] and require considerable repetition to learn well. Repetition is acceptable if the clinician frequently reinforces the child and makes clear what is being learned. Children this age usually generalize more slowly; therefore, transfer activities must be carefully planned and practiced. The school is an excellent environment for planning and practicing carryover to situations of real life. In addition, the child's prognosis will be improved by bringing the parents in at regular intervals to show them what the youngster is learning. In this way, they will be better able to reinforce the child appropriately.

Attitude Change.   Some clinicians use a direct approach to attitude change, bringing up topics for discussion, much like they might do with secondary school-age and adult clients. On the other hand, some feel hesitant to focus on a child's thoughts and feelings. We believe that clinicians should keep discussions of speech on a concrete level, making specific comments about speech being more easy and relaxed or making smooth movements in contrast to tense beginnings or broken movements. It can also be helpful to use pictures or models of the speech mechanism. We encourage the children to describe in their words what they think is occurring when they talk, such as: "Words get trapped in my throat," as the child points to the larynx; "I feel tense here," pointing to the chest, or "I repeat and can't stop it." These descriptions can be discussed with reference to a picture of the speech mechanism and how speech is produced.

Analogies between changing a speech skill and the way in which a person learns to modify swinging a baseball bat or tennis racket have been found useful by many clinicians as one way of making activities meaningful to a child who needs concrete explanations.

In terms of feelings, most children feel better when they realize that speech is a more flexible process that can be changed. Our first approach, and one that requires patience and restraint, is to be a good listener. In most cases we should wait until a child brings up situations such as teasing from peers, advice from parents, or how a teacher makes him or her feel about participating in class. As therapy progresses, questions may be asked, such as "How do you feel about talking?," "Where do you like to talk the most?," etc. Once feelings are expressed and acknowledged, the clinician can suggest some possibilities for handling them. For example, teasing can be discussed as a need of the teaser. Acknowledging a problem and saying that you are in therapy to improve will often stop it.

Almost always a child will resist change to some degree. The clinician should recognize this and be understanding about it. We might say, "It feels and sounds funny because it is different." As children get used to more relaxed speech, for example, and as the speech–language pathologist, teachers, parents, and others reinforce it, attitudes change. We also think that reinforcement is key in motivation. We must be sincere about it, but we should be very proud of progress made by a child. Videotaping is a good approach to attitude change about modifying speech. As youngsters watch themselves on television and as people approve (i.e., give positive reinforcement), change becomes more realistic.

Parent and Teacher Counseling. It is crucial to the success of therapy that parents understand and participate in the therapy process. One of our most successful procedures, as was discussed in early intervention, is for the parents to learn to modify their speech in the same ways that the child is learning to do. The parents need to learn how stresses, such as time pressure in a communication situation, increase stuttering and make it difficult to change. Therefore, training in proper turn-taking in the family can be very important. We have found that most parents can modify this behavior; they simply have not understood the importance of reducing such pressures. One father, who had very high levels of expectation for his 8-year-old son and who talked in a fast, animated way with his son, with little pause time, said, "I thought that was the way to make it interesting." Teachers can also be crucial in helping speech–language pathologists understand how the child responds to classroom activities. Of even more importance, the teacher can support what the clinician is working on with the child in the classroom.

Treatment Results

Most contributors about early intervention[5,6,27,28] have been saying in their formal presentations at professional meetings and through the media that we are highly successful at normalizing speech development and preventing stuttering when proper intervention takes place within 6 months of the observed onset of the problem. In prescriptive parent counseling, which we view as preventive, we are nearly 100% successful after four to six biweekly sessions with parents and children. Only a few of these children show a recurrence that concerns parents or that requires further intervention. As noted before, if parents are concerned, they are urged to telephone immediately, and we give the appropriate counseling or reevaluation. In the comprehensive therapy program, successful intervention may take 8–12 months, but approximately 5% of children have persisting problems that may require referral for family counseling or psychoeducational evaluation and longer-term follow-up. Unfortunately, some parents do not accept recommendations for referral and the needed follow-up. One additional note: Comparing results now with those of 10 years ago,[24] we are seeing children who are younger and sooner after onset, both of which may be contributing to a better outcome.

Comments on the results of therapy for elementary school-age children are based on a philosophy of either succeeding; finding out why we are not succeeding, then taking new steps aimed toward better progress; or deciding that success cannot be expected at the time and discontinuing treatment.[30] One of us (H.H.G.) has been alarmed by the number of teenagers and adults who report that they went to therapy year after year as children and do not feel that they were helped. He now emphasizes that therapy for elementary school-age children that is not producing results that are obvious and rewarding to a child in a period of 3–4 months should probably be discontinued. Therapy is successful for about eight out of 10 of these youngsters who gain confidence sufficient to be comfortable about communication and are able to speak easily in most situations. About one in 10 does not reach this level and will need therapy later, perhaps when there is a greater concern about speaking better. Progress is slow and problematic in another one in 10, due to personal or family problems of adjustment, which leads in many cases to recommending referrals for psychological counseling and guidance.

Suggested Readings

Conture E, Fraser J (eds): *Stuttering and Your Child: Questions and Answers*, Publication no. 22. Memphis, Stuttering Foundation of America, 1989.
Provides answers to questions most often asked by parents who are concerned about stuttering and their child. Represents careful thought by seven authorities who met together to discuss this topic.
Gregory H (ed): *Stuttering Therapy: Prevention and Intervention with Children*. Publication no. 20. Memphis, Stuttering Foundation of America, 1984.
Focuses on the development of speech fluency in children, determining when a problem exists, and if so, what factors (including emotional and environmental, language, and speech motor) may be contributing to the problem. Discusses prevention and early intervention.
Ratner NB (ed): *Stuttering and Parent–Child Interaction, Seminars in Speech and Language*. New York, Thieme Medical Publishers, Inc., 1993.
Examines available information about parent–child interactions and stuttering, a topic always discussed in the evaluation and treatment of stuttering in children.
Wall MJ, Myers FL: *Clinical Management of Childhood Stuttering* (2nd ed.). Austin, TX, Pro-Ed, 1995.
With reference to research and clinical information, this volume provides a three-factor model for the assessment and treatment of stuttering. Factors are psycholinguistic, psychosocial, and physiological. Includes a review of major treatment approaches.
Perkins W (ed): Stuttering: Challenges of therapy. *Semin Speech Lang* 1991; 12(4).
Provides information about school-age children who stutter and treatment approaches as practiced by leading authorities in the United States.

References

1. Andrews G, Craig A, Feyer A, Hoddinott S, Howie P, Neilson M: Stuttering: Review of research findings and theories, circa 1982. *J Speech Hear Disord* 1982; 48:226–246.
2. Bloodstein O: *A Handbook on Stuttering*. San Diego, Singular Publishing Group, 1995.
3. Gregory H: *Stuttering: Differential Evaluation and Therapy*. Austin, TX, Pro-Ed, 1986.
4. Riley G, Riley J: Evaluation as a Basis for Intervention, in Prins D, Ingham R (eds): *Treatment of Stuttering in Early Childhood*. San Diego, College-Hill Press, 1983.
5. Conture E: *Stuttering*. Englewood Cliffs, NJ, Prentice-Hall, 1990.
6. Starkweather C, Gottwald S, Halfond M: *Stuttering Prevention: A Clinical Method*. Englewood Cliffs, NJ, Prentice-Hall, 1990.
7. Van Riper C: *The Nature of Stuttering*. Englewood Cliffs, NJ, Prentice-Hall, 1982.
8. Starkweather CW: *Fluency and Stuttering*. Englewood Cliffs, NJ, Prentice Hall, 1987.
9. Dejoy D, Gregory H: The relationship between age and frequency of disfluency in preschool children. *J Fluency Disord* 1985; 10:107–122.

10. Wexler K, Mysak E: Disfluency characteristics of 2-, 4-, and six year old males. *J Fluency Disorder* 1982; 7:37–46.
11. Yairi E: Disfluencies of normally speaking two-year old children. *J Speech Hear Res* 1981; 24:490–495.
12. Yairi E: Longitudinal studies of disfluencies in two-year old children. *J Speech Hear Res* 1982; 25:155–160.
13. Yairi E, Lewis B: Disfluencies in the onset of stuttering. *J Speech Hear Res* 1984; 27:154–159.
14. Campbell J, Hill D: *Systematic Disfluency Analysis*. Unpublished, Evanston, Northwestern University Dept. of Communicative Disorders, 1987.
15. Felsenfeld S: Epidemiology and Genetics of Stuttering, in Curlee R, Siegel G (eds): *Nature and Treatment of Stuttering*. Boston, Allyn & Bacon, 1997.
16. Holmes T, Masuda M: Life Change and Illness Susceptibility, in Dohrenwend B, Dohrenwend BS (eds): *Stressful Life Events*. New York, John Wiley & Sons, 1974.
17. Kasprisin-Burrelli A, Egolf D, Shames G: A comparison of parental verbal behavior with stuttering and nonstuttering children. *J Commun Disord* 1972; 5:335–346.
18. Mordecai D: *An Investigation of the Communicative Styles of Mothers and Fathers of Stuttering Versus Nonstuttering Preschool Children during a Triadic Interaction*. PhD dissertation. Chicago, Northwestern University, 1980.
19. Sheehan J: Role-conflict Therapy, in Sheehan J (ed): *Stuttering: Research and Therapy*. New York, Harper & Row, 1970.
20. Blood G, Seider R: The concomitant problems of young stutterers. *J Speech Hear Res* 1981; 46:31–33.
21. Wall M, Meyers F: *Clinical Management of Childhood Stuttering*. Austin, TX, Pro-Ed, 1995.
22. Nippold MA: Concomitant speech and language disorders in stuttering children. *J Speech Hear Res* 1990; 33:803–804.
23. Gregory H, Hill D: Stuttering Therapy for Children, in Perkins W (ed): *Strategies in Stuttering Therapy*. New York, Thieme-Stratton, 1980.
24. Ainsworth S, Gruss J: *If Your Child Stutters: A Guide for Parents*. Memphis, Stuttering Foundation of America, 1981.
25. Conture E, Fraser J: *Stuttering and Your Child: Questions and Answers*. Publication no. 22, Memphis, Stuttering Foundation of America, 1989.
26. Cooper E: Intervention Procedures for the Young Stutterer, in Gregory H (ed): *Controversies about Stuttering Therapy*. Baltimore, University Park Press, 1979.
27. Meyers S, Woodford L: *The Fluency Development System for Young Children*. Buffalo, United Educational Services, 1992.
28. Shine R: Direct Management of the Beginning Stutterer, in Perkins W (ed): *Strategies in Stuttering Therapy*. New York, Thieme-Stratton, 1980.
29. Van Riper C: *The Treatment of Stuttering*. Englewood Cliffs, NJ, Prentice-Hall, 1973.
30. Gregory H: Therapy for elementary school age children. *Semin Speech Language* 1991; 12:323–334.
31. Williams D: The Problem of Stuttering, in Darley F, Spriestersbach D (eds): *Diagnostic Methods in Speech Pathology*. New York, Harper & Row, 1978.
32. Ham R: *Therapy for Stuttering: Preschool through Adolescence*. Englewood Cliffs, NJ, Prentice-Hall, 1990.
33. Peters T, Guitar B: *Stuttering: An Integrated Approach to Its Nature and Treatment*. Baltimore, Williams & Wilkins, 1991.
34. Adams M: The Young Stutterer: Diagnosis, Treatment and Assessment of Progress, in Perkins W (ed): *Stuttering Disorders: Current Therapy of Communication Disorders*. New York, Thieme-Stratton, 1984.
35. Bloodstein O: Stuttering as Tension and Fragmentation, in Eisenson J (ed): *Stuttering: A Second Symposium*. New York, Harper & Row, 1975.
36. Costello J: Treatment of the Young Chronic Stutterer: Managing Fluency, in Curlee R, Perkins W (eds): *The Nature and Treatment of Stuttering: New Directions*. San Diego, College-Hill Press, 1984.
37. Williams D: Stuttering Therapy for Children, in Travis L (ed): *Handbook of Speech Pathology*. New York, Appleton-Century-Crofts, 1971.

38. Williams D: A Perspective on Approaches to Stuttering Therapy, in Gregory H (ed): *Controversies about Stuttering Therapy*. Baltimore, University Park Press, 1979.
39. Gregory H, Campbell J: Stuttering in the School Age Child, in Yoder D, Kent R (eds): *Decision Making in Speech-Language Pathology*. Toronto, BC Decker, 1988.
40. Piaget J, Inhelder B: *The Growth of Logical Thinking from Childhood to Adolescence*. New York, Basic Books, 1958.
41. Flavell J: *The Developmental Psychology of Jean Piaget*. Princeton, NJ, Van Nostrand, 1963.

Stuttering and Related Disorders of Fluency, 2nd edition.
Edited by Richard F. Curlee, Ph.D.
Thieme Medical Publishers, Inc., New York © 1999.

3

Counseling Children Who Stutter and Their Parents

Hugo H. Gregory
Carolyn B. Gregory

Counseling and Stuttering Therapy: A Frame of Reference

In making presentations on counseling and stuttering therapy, we have often heard the view that counseling refers to those situations in which clinicians respond to clients' expressions of feeling. Many clinicians feel uncomfortable in such situations, reporting that they have not been trained to deal with feelings. Indeed, most speech–language pathologists seem to be most comfortable when counseling is limited to providing information, such as what is involved in therapy. When they hear discussions of counseling procedures based on Rogers' client-centered approach,[1] of listening and understanding a client's feelings and thoughts, they want to know if and when any information is given. In an ASHA convention program on counseling in 1995, one speaker said that counseling involved giving information sometimes, but another said that it didn't. Only infrequently do speech–language pathologists think of counseling as involving changing behavior, just like speech therapy!

Many speech–language pathologists report never having had a course in counseling or even recalling it being covered in other speech–language pathology courses. Those who have taken a counseling course, usually outside a speech–language pathology program, report seldom being helped to apply the approaches covered to the treatment of stuttering. Partly in response to the confusion that present day-clinicians have about counseling, we developed a frame of reference that clarifies some of the issues about the role of speech–language clinicians as counselors and the treatment of stuttering.

We view counseling as embracing affective, cognitive, and behavioral factors. All types of counselors, as well as all psychotherapists, deal with these variables. Speech–language pathologists who work with people who stutter are concerned with these same cognitive–affective factors, which they often call attitudes, as well as speech characteristics. Counselors, psychotherapists, and speech–language pathologists employ the skills of listening, responding to feelings and beliefs, informing, directing behavioral change, and problem solving; it is the problems they treat that differ. As specialists in communication disorders, no one can counsel in this area as well as speech–language pathologists can without special preparation and experience. Clearly, no other professional group knows as much about stuttering. Marriage counselors may use the same cognitive, affective, and behavioral procedures in working with marital relationships and difficulties, whereas psychotherapists use them with clients whose emotional difficulties and general life problems in home and work relationships may be less well-defined at the onset of treatment. Thus, just as psychotherapists and other specialized counselors employ relaxation, systematic desensitization, and various forms of behavior modification, in addition to traditional verbal (cognitive–affective) interchanges in working with their clients' problems, speech–language pathologists have become more knowledgeable about attending to emotional conflicts related to speech problems, family therapy, social skills training, and stress management techniques. This is another way of emphasizing the point that psychotherapists, counselors of all types, and speech–language pathologists use many of the same procedures and are all learning new skills to improve their therapeutic effectiveness. Again, it is the nature of the problems they treat that differ.

In following our broad frame of reference for counseling, speech–language clinicians need to be aware of their limitations in dealing with some of the problems that people who stutter and their families may have. For example, if a mother whose child stutters begins to express feelings of inadequacy about coping with her home and family or some other type of general conflict, clinicians need to consider the possibility that she may need help which exceeds their expertise. Referral for specialized counseling may be crucial in improving this mother's ability to deal constructively with her family situation and in enhancing her ability to support her child's speech therapy. Sometimes it is the speech–language pathologist who first helps parents to face such concomitant difficulties.

Applying the Frame of Reference

Counselors from various disciplines and speech–language pathologists deal with clients, whether children and their parents or teenagers and adults, whose problems involve cognitive, affective, and behavioral variables. Therefore, counseling and speech therapy focus on the same processes, employ similar procedures, and require similar skills. This frame of reference takes much of the mystery out of counseling and helps speech–language pathologists to view counseling as an integral part of their therapy activities, not a separate type of therapy! For example, speech–language clinicians do not help children to modify their speech without considering their thoughts and feelings. Likewise, parents' beliefs, feelings, and behavior are seen as a fundamental aspect of the treatment of children's speech problems. In planning therapy for a school-age youngster who stutters, the child's attitudes should receive as careful consideration as speech when decisions are made about therapy. The following discussion highlights concepts and procedures representing cognitive, affective, and behavioral treatment concepts and procedures that should be integrated into a clinician's ongoing experience.

Relating to and Understanding Parents

One of the characteristics of a therapeutic relationship, whether at the time of a diagnostic evaluation or later during treatment, is that the clinician recognizes that parents have unique feelings and beliefs which should be understood as well as possible before making decisions about treatment. There are at least three reasons why clients should be understood before information is given and recommendations are made:[2] 1. Clients appreciate the interest we show; seldom, for example, will anyone else have tried to understand parents' experiences and concerns about their child's speech. In addition, it is best to relate the information that is given and therapy goals to the parents' observations and needs. Indeed, clinicians cannot know what information to give or how to proceed until they have begun to gain such understanding. 2. What is done during a diagnostic evaluation and early in treatment establishes some of the basic conditions of a therapeutic relationship. If clinicians are too dominant and directive at the beginning, a client is likely to believe that the relationship is that of a teacher and student. In this case, the clinician is less likely to come to know some of the client's important feelings and beliefs, not only during an evaluation but during therapy as well. We believe that it is easier to move from being more permissive and understanding, at first, to more educational and directive later, than vice-versa. 3. Clients' attempts to describe and explain their concerns initiates a process of self-evaluation and a reorganization of their thinking and feeling, thereby, opening the way to their receiving new information and direction.

This approach is consistent with Rogers' concept of "unconditional positive regard," valuing without judging what a client is saying.[1] In responding empathically, clinicians need to identify with a client's feelings, as best as they can, and communicate their understanding to the client. Presumably, clinicians recall some past experience similar to what the client is discussing, which evokes a memory trace and revives some of the feelings that were involved. For example, the feelings that a clinician experiences when seeing a child frustrated by being unable to do some task may be similar in some ways to the feelings a mother has when she sees her child stutter. When the clinician expresses this empathic understanding to the mother, she or he is communicating, "I think I can understand your feelings. I accept your emotional reactions." In turn, the mother is likely to be saying to herself, "This person seems to know how I feel." In this way, the clinician's accepting and understanding attitude serves as a model for the mother's self-acceptance. We still recall some years ago when we gained the insight into the possibility that when Rogers[1] was being very accepting in manner, he was modeling self-acceptance for his clients.

In addition to his focus on communicating unconditional positive regard and being empathic, Rogers also emphasized the importance of a clinician being honest and genuine.[1] Similarly, Van Riper[3] warned that children and adults seem to be quite sensitive to clinicians who wear a "false face." It is much better for a clinician to say, "I have never encountered this particular situation before with other parents, and I need to think about it" than to pretend to know what should be said or done. Clinicians who do not know every answer immediately, like other "humans," are usually viewed by parents and other clients as honest and trustworthy. If this clinician says at a later session, "I've been thinking about the issue you brought up, and I would like to share several thoughts with you," this shows that she is actively involved with the parents' concerns and cares about them. Moreover, the clinician is modeling genuine self-disclosure for the parents. The more that a clinician and parents solve problems together, the more trust there is likely to be in their relationship. Although a Rogerian approach[1] is not appropriate for all of the cognitive–affective–behavioral goals of stuttering therapy, some of the concepts he described about relationships and interviewing make important contributions in working with parents of children who stutter, especially during the early stages of establishing a positive client–clinician relationship and in gaining an understanding of the nature of a presenting problem.

Interview Behaviors that Facilitate a Clinician's Understanding of Parents and Parents' Self-Understanding

The following discussion highlights some of the verbal and nonverbal behaviors for either taking a case history or counseling sessions with parents which have been described as facilitating insight into clients' behavior and which our own experiences have found useful.

1. *Attention and careful listening*: Clinicians need to clear their minds of distracting thoughts and be relatively calm and relaxed to be able to attend to parents as well as they should. Relaxation training has helped us to focus our attention, which also seems to contribute to parents' relaxation at times. Our experience has been that practicing being calm, using more pauses in our own speech, and accepting of periods of silence during an interview is appreciated by parents and seems to be conducive to their sharing of feelings and thoughts. Some clients' most sensitive issues or best insights emerge following a period of silence.

Clinicians should attend by relating to what a parent has said, not asking a new question until the focus of discussion has been considered carefully and is fairly complete. In responding, we try to refer to what a parent has said, perhaps even using some of the same words or phrases. For example, "I can appreciate that it is hard for you to see Billy having trouble talking when he's telling you something." "These concerns you have about excitement increasing Billy's stuttering are important in telling me about factors that may be related to his problem." As long as parents are talking, disclosing what they are thinking or feeling, we keep listening!

2. *Questioning*: Open-ended questions are best to initiate discussion, giving parents more latitude to respond, but a more direct question may be needed to elicit specific information about the topic being discussed. Examples of an open-ended question are as follows: "Tell me how Billy's speech is of concern to you." "I wonder if you could describe as much as possible how you talk with each other in your home, at dinner or bedtime." These kinds of questions leave it up to parents to choose what is foremost in their minds. If a parent has been describing a child's stuttering, the clinician can focus in specifically, for example, by modeling a particular disfluency, such as a part-word syllable repetition, and asking if the child does that when speaking?

Although it is appropriate during a diagnostic evaluation for clinicians to ask some specific, short answer questions to verify developmental information and the like, we believe it is best to proceed in a discussion format as much as possible. It is important for parents to feel that the clinician is giving them time to express themselves fully.

3. *Continuing remarks*: If a parent is talking about an observation, feeling, or thought in response to an open-ended or more specific question, a clinician's minimal statement, such as "mmm-humm," "I see," "I'd like to hear more about that," or "Could you recall a bit more?" acts as a positive reinforcement and will encourage the speaker to keep going.

4. *Paraphrasing content*: This refers to restating a client's basic message in similar, but fewer words, which allows the clinician to test her understanding and communicate that she is trying to understand. For example, "It sounds like you are concerned about your babysitter's rapid and indistinct speech" or "You seem to be worried about these big family gatherings on the weekends and the pressures involved." If parents agree with a paraphrase, this is the best assurance clinicians can have that they understand correctly. It also

reinforces parents for their effort to communicate. If they should correct or clarify a statement, that is also good; it allows a meeting of minds.

5. *Reflection of feeling*: In responding to a parent's statement that expresses feeling, positive or negative, clinicians should attempt to capture the emotion expressed, verbally or nonverbally. Over the years Rogers[1] has emphasized that a clinician's attempt to understand feelings enriches client–clinician relationships and invites the sharing of other feelings that may involve more emotion, perhaps guilt or shame. However, if a person seems to have extremely strong feelings about the topic being discussed, it may be best to be cautiously conservative when making a reflection, knowing that there will always be time later in a therapeutic relationship to revisit feelings related to a particular topic. Some examples might be the following:

"You seem a little upset about all of this rough-housing that Dad likes to carry on with the boys, thinking that he should understand that this increases excitement and Billy's stuttering."

"You have really been suffering some feelings of guilt about putting off getting advice about Johnnie's stuttering."

Oftentimes, in responding to a clinician's paraphrase or reflection of feeling, a parent will add further descriptions. Sometimes, however, in response to a reflection of feeling, a parent may say, "No, that is not quite it." No harm results from such off-target responses, because most clients will continue to explain, giving the clinician further chances to understand. This may also be a sign that the clinician should have waited until she knew more or asked for clarification rather than attempting a reflection, "I'm not sure I understand. Could you tell me a little more about how you feel?"

There is a natural tendency to want to mollify some feelings with such remarks as "You shouldn't feel bad about that. All parents tend to have disagreements about what to do with their children." A better practice is to simply respect an honest disclosure, "You were disappointed that your husband didn't understand your concern about Billy's stuttering last year when you thought it was time to see a speech–language pathologist." People do enough concealing of feelings, and clinicians should not encourage them.

6. *Counter-question*: Parents often have questions that clinicians need to answer factually, such as, "Is stuttering genetic?" "Is it true that more boys than girls stutter?" But when questions are raised around topics that parents are likely to have opinions or feelings about, it is often wise to say, "What have you thought about that?" Such questions as "Why does he stutter some times and not at others?" and "Can stuttering be increased by bickering at home?" should elicit a clinician's request for more information or the parent's ideas. Some counselors contend that counter-questions give parents, from the beginning of a relationship, a sense that they will maintain or share control, that all authority has not been given to the clinician.

7. *Interpreting or Explaining*: Paraphrasing and reflecting express a clinician's understanding of how a client perceived or felt about a topic. In making an interpretation, the clinician offers a new perspective or frame of reference of the discussion that has taken place. Although there can never be absolute certainty about the degree of correct understanding, clinicians should feel that they have sufficient depth of understanding and that there is mutual trust before an interpretation is made. For example, following several sessions with parents and a grandmother who visited in their home every day, the clinician said: "The level of stress and excitement in your home appears pretty high some of the

time, especially from around five in the evening until bed time." Later in the same session, she said: "You seem ready to begin thinking more about how you can plan to reduce stress and about the possibility that all of you will be happier by making some changes."

One objective of these procedures is for parents to have positive feelings toward the clinician and feel comfortable in evaluating and discussing their experiences. As clinicians believe that they have gained a clear and correct understanding of parents' thoughts and feelings and their descriptions of the child's problem, it is appropriate to begin giving more information about stuttering and about therapy and to begin to formulate treatment objectives. This will be covered later in this chapter in discussing therapy.

Clinicians should proceed, as we have, to review their options when interacting with parents and assess their behaviors. We have found that listening to recordings of our interactions with parents is a very helpful learning experience.

Relating to and Understanding Children

Just as clinicians should be nonjudgmental in initial discussions with parents, they should be permissive in establishing rapport with a child. When seeing a preschool child, we ask parents to bring a few of a child's favorite books and toys to the first meeting. It is a good idea, also, to have a toy village, train, or game such as lotto in readiness, and parents can be asked ahead of time about a child's interest. One preschool child we saw was very interested in trains, so when he saw our toy train and discovered that we liked trains, too, rapport was immediate and lasting. Likewise, a positive relationship is facilitated when school-age children realize that the clinician is interested in TV programs, movies, sports, or computer games that are also of interest to them.

A video or audio recording should be started before the parents and child enter the room. While interacting with the child, the clinician can observe the child's speech and how he or she adjusts to a new situation. We try to speak in a more relaxed fashion, with clearly distinguishable pauses between phrases, and also pause after the child ends a statement before commenting. Periods of silence are not avoided, but accepted. Informal observations are made of a child's enjoyment of communication. Does the child initiate a topic? How assertive is the child? Are there tendencies to withdraw and perhaps cling to a parent? How does the child enter into and enjoy play?

Some clinicians plan ahead with the parents to leave the room at a certain point and ask them to play or converse with their child as they ordinarily would. A video recording is made, although many clinical situations allow clinicians to observe this parent–child interaction from another room through a one-way mirror. The way in which the parents and child relate to each other is noted; for example, the ratio of parents' questions versus comments, the frequency of parental questions and statements of demand compared to statements of praise and support, their "overriding" of the child's utterances by beginning to speak before the child finishes, finishing the child's statements, and speaking rapidly. Thus, during this interaction, clinicians not only obtain a better understanding of the child, but also how parents interact with the child. Gregory, Campbell, and Hill[4] and Chapter 2, p. 28, in this book provide a more complete description of parent–child interaction analysis procedures. Although this may appear to be an artificial situation, we have found that parents and children interact in ways that parents usually say is representative of real life. For either preschool or school-age children, these observations supplement what may have been reported in a case history.

It is important for speech–language pathologists to realize the significant impact that these first interactions may have on both a child and parents. In the previous section, we discussed clinician behaviors that help to establish positive affective and cognitive responses in parents. Here, clinicians need to keep in mind that it is crucial for the child to have positive emotional responses to interactions with the clinician at the beginning of therapy. Optimally, the child should enjoy himself so much during an evaluation that he is disappointed to leave at the end! The relationship being established will have considerable influence on the value of a clinician's positive reinforcement during therapy and how the child responds to behavior modeled by a clinician. The image of the clinical situation in the child's mind should be associated with positive, pleasant feelings, which we believe are prerequisites to successful therapy.

Clinicians' Understanding of Transference

When we talk with colleagues in clinical psychology or psychiatry about counseling, they often ask: "How do you handle the transference?" A general definition of transference is the unconscious transfer of feelings which a client had for a person during infancy or childhood on to someone in a present relationship. The analysis of clients' transference of such feelings onto the therapist is a crucial part of traditional psychoanalysis, and we believe that it is important for speech–language pathologists who work with children to recognize that children may project feelings they have about their parents and other adults onto the clinician. This takes us back to our earlier discussion of being permissive, tentative, and nonjudgmental when establishing a relationship with a child, giving the child time to see that the speech–language pathologist may not be like other adults. Likewise, some parents may transfer the attitudes they have about doctors, teachers, or other professionals onto their child's speech–language clinician.

Sometimes clinicians must also deal with the issue of countertransference when their feelings about a child or a parent are rooted in feelings from the past. By actively seeking to understand the uniqueness of each client and family, clinicians can guard against projecting feelings that originated from previous experiences onto current clinical relationships and distorting their understanding of the present situation. Speech–language pathologists need to maintain an ongoing program of self-study and examination to prevent countertransference from biasing their perceptions.

Timing the Giving of Information and Dealing with Parents' Concerns

Earlier in this chapter we gave a rationale for clinicians to delay giving parents information before they have gained an understanding of how the parents perceive their child's problem and of family situations that might be involved. Of course, some basic information often needs to be given when the case history is taken or feedback is given about the child's evaluation, such as the types of disfluencies observed. If parents ask about stuttering being inherited, then we advise clinicians to summarize the best information available, after clarifying the parents' interest or reasons for concern, and then begin the process of integrating the possibility of this predisposing factor with environmental influences. If parents seem resistant to participating in the child's therapy, we usually discuss how communicative and interpersonal environmental stresses have been found to increase some children's disfluency and stuttering, and the importance of parents' insight into such factors and learning to deal with them.

At a certain point in treatment, clinicians may recognize that it would be helpful to give parents more information about the development of stuttering, what Gregory and Hill call child factors and environmental factors in Chapter 2, p. 29, which appear to contribute to the development of a problem. When giving information, we try to be conversational and provide frequent pauses for parents to interject some of their thoughts or feelings. A favorite strategy is to watch for an opportunity to relate some information to a comment made by a parent. For example, if a parent seems confused about how stuttering develops or what causes stuttering, we may relate information about the development of children's fluency, perhaps emphasizing disfluency differences in children, and describe the development of stuttering from more simple interruptions of speech to the child's more complex overt and covert reactions. This information provides a context for describing preventive steps that need to be taken for a preschool child or in discussing issues that need to be raised about a school-age child who is being treated. It is important, however, to be concise and avoid getting in an extensive discussion all at once. Details can be added later.

Parents commonly bring up several types of topics, and the following brief discussions describe how we like to respond to these topics:

1. *Sibling interaction*: Parents may find that a 3- or 4-year-old child with a stuttering problem seems threatened by the attention they are giving to a new baby or by a rivalry that develops among their children. For example, a 2-year-old's burgeoning language abilities and competitiveness with a 3- or 4-year-old who is beginning to stutter or conflicts with an older and younger sibling when the child who stutters is the one in between, either can increase communicative stress and the child's stuttering. In general, the best advice for parents is for the mother or father to give special time alone to each child. We have been impressed with how children relax when they have their own time with parents. When their need for attention is met in a satisfactory manner, they seem to feel assured that they are valued, which enables them to feel better about themselves. When parents see that a problem is being resolved, they are reinforced for making changes, and many report that they enjoy their children more when they plan special times and activities with each child as well as when all of them are together.

2. *The influence of extended family members such as grandparents*: Sometimes a sister of the mother, or grandparents, may have ideas about how the child's stuttering should be handled. In some instances, a grandparent may live in the home or be a caregiver or visit frequently. It is important that such individuals understand the advice being given to the parents by the speech–language pathologist; therefore, we like to have them accompany the parents for some counseling sessions also. They often seem surprised to learn that it is advisable to do such things as diminish a child's excitement when talking. They may say, "I thought that being excited was a good way to make it interesting!" or "I just thought that was the way to have fun." Clinicians should be understanding, reassuring, and patient when talking with these family members; in most cases, they have been doing what they thought was best for the child and readily change when asked or after seeing the clinician model being enthusiastic in a more relaxed way. One grandmother, who visited her grandson and family every day, found that when she was more relaxed with him it made a difference in his stuttering.

3. *Excitement and tension associated with holidays and big family gatherings*: Excitement is often associated with increased stuttering. In some families, trips or holidays are talked about far in advance, thinking that this increases enjoyment. If a child is beginning to stutter, however, it may be preferable to be calmer about such occasions and forego big

buildups. End-of-the-year holidays are frequently characterized by increases in stuttering by children in therapy or even those who have completed therapy. Parents of such children can be encouraged to relax and follow the rules they are learning in therapy about reducing communicative and interpersonal stress. And if large family gatherings are characterized by increases in a child's stuttering, parents may wish to consider having smaller, more relaxed gatherings.

4. *How disfluency varies over time*: Speech fluency can be a barometer of a child's language development, psychosocial stresses, and other day-to-day environmental differences. There are variations in every child's fluency; thus, variations in fluency are normal. It is often helpful for parents to work with the speech–language clinician in charting increases and decreases in the child's stuttering as they are related to certain circumstances.[4] Together, they can problem solve how to manage family situations better to increase a child's fluency or how to be more accepting of the child's normal disfluencies. Many parents profit from reading such Stuttering Foundation publications as "If Your Child Stutters: A Guide for Parents"[5] or "Stuttering and Your Child",[6] which should be followed up by discussions. Giving parents additional rationales for therapy procedures is another aspect of the information-sharing process that goes on as therapy proceeds. Clinicians must continue to encourage parents to report their observations and feelings so that the partnership between them and parents is reinforced as therapy continues.

5. *Expectations and demands*: Parents are often concerned that if they do not train children appropriately and demand such behaviors as using better table manners and keeping their room straight that they will grow up and never learn. Some seem not to realize that if they and older children in the family model desirable behavior, most children will grow up adhering, in large part, to these modeled behaviors. Parents need to understand the Demand Support Ratio.[7] If they are giving children considerable support by spending time with them and reinforcing desirable behaviors with praise, they are in a better position to obtain their children's cooperation in performing expected behaviors. Parents should be encouraged to think about "How many times in a day am I demanding and how many times in a day do I make encouraging and supportive comments?" Support should always outweigh demands, and most parents profit from discussions of being more consistent in their expectations.

6. *Concern about shyness or aggressiveness*: Shy children are often self-conscious, somewhat fearful, easily embarrassed and are likely to be viewed as being more withdrawn than other children, whereas an aggressive child may be acting out frustration or feelings of conflict. Parents should be urged not to label a child as a "shy" or "aggressive" child, certainly not in ways that are apparent to the child. One parent we worked with, often said in her 9-year-old son's presence, "He's so shy." We suggested that she may be reinforcing this behavior and that he may perceive shy behavior as a way to control her. Gradually she stopped labeling his behavior as shy, and we worked in therapy to reward him for increased cooperation. When a child is showing shy or aggressive tendencies, we ignore them and reward the child for behaviors that are constructive and similar to that of peers.

These comments and suggestions are, of course, introductory. If family interaction problems, questions of what to expect of children, or disruptive emotional–behavioral characteristics of a family member persist during therapy and appear to be contributing to a stuttering problem or disturbing family relationships, then the speech–language pathologists should consider referring the parents, the child, or both for specialized counseling with stuttering therapy continuing as before in most cases.

Building Children's Self-esteem and Supporting Parents

Young children acquire a subjective feeling of self that is appropriate for their level of cognitive development as part of their early psychosocial development. Self-development is discussed briefly at this point, because it is significant in the acquisition of language and the way in which a child responds to speech and language therapy.[8,9] An understanding of children's self-development is important to clinicians in deciding how to relate to a child and how to give parents insight into the way in which self-development relates to the prevention of stuttering during its beginning stages. When a small child is beginning to stutter, clinicians have the opportunity to model behaviors for parents that will enhance the child's positive self-esteem, feelings of security, and confidence. It has been our clinical experience that this appears to be a significant factor contributing to a child's development of normal fluency. In the following paragraphs, several of the significant psychoanalytic studies of the development of self-esteem in children are discussed briefly.

Mahler[10] conducted a landmark observational study of mother–infant pairs, including mothers with a second baby. She identified subphases of infant emotional development and theorized that the unique emotional relationship between a mother and child was responsible for the "hatching of the human personality" at 7–8 months of age. Language developed rapidly during the second year of life, as a child became more mobile and individual, and Mahler described a "reproachment phase" in development, between 16 and 30 months of age, as crucial to the psychological health of a child. After observing young toddlers crawling or walking away from their mothers, then returning again and again for reassurance, she noted that some mothers were usually loving, but others tired rapidly of giving such attention. Those mothers who already had another baby were prone especially to showing only minimal attention. Mahler believed that the children who found their mothers attentive, experienced security, and soon moved on to greater confidence and individuality, which she characterized as better self-esteem. Similarly, Winnicott[11] emphasized the mirroring function of a mother's facial expression. He said:

> What does a baby see when he or she looks at the mother's face? I am suggesting that ordinarily what the baby sees is himself or herself. In other words, the mother is looking at the baby, and what she looks like is related to what she sees there. All this is too easily taken for granted. I am asking that this which is naturally done well by mothers who are caring for their babies shall not be taken for granted. I can make my point by going straight over to the case of the baby whose mother reflects her own mood ... the rigidity of her own defenses.... Of course, nothing can be said about single occasions. All good enough mothers will fail from time to time. Many babies have a long history of not getting back what they are giving. (p. 112).

In keeping with Winnicott's observations, speech–language pathologists may need to help some parents understand the importance of the warmth of their interactions with their child. Most of us have seen the expressions of joy that parents have when relating to their small children. As we said earlier, these basic relationships prepare the way for a child's positive response to clinicians' and parents' positive reinforcement of behavior. Thus, there is the possibility that parents of a child whose behavior is of concern to them, such as stuttering may be, will worry and not be as reinforcing to the child as they would be otherwise.

Kohut and Wolf[12] proposed that there were three aspects of parenting style that were essential to a child's positive self-image: 1. The mirroring parent who applauds the child's behavior (expresses pleasure), as was suggested also by Winnicott.[11] 2. The idealized parent who is a model the child can admire and an image of calmness and relaxation, with whom the child can merge. 3. The parent who is an alter ego, a friend with whom the child feels safe. Kohut and Wolf saw these early parent-child relationships as a period when children learn to feel good about themselves and become able to establish satisfying friendships throughout the course of their lives. Speech–language pathologists should be enthusiastic and positively reinforcing with children who stutter as they model calmness, relaxation, and such speech characteristics as more relaxed initiations, smoother movements, and acceptance of increased pause time. Likewise, models for parents should include attentive facial expression, relaxation, better listening and turn-taking, commenting on what the child says, and reducing the number of questions. Thus, the clinician models not only better communicative behaviors, but also better parental interpersonal behaviors (e. g., playing calmly with the child, spending special time with the child, reducing unrealistic demands, etc.) which nourish the child's self-esteem and identification with parents. In turn, parents' increased understanding of child development and changes in behavior reduce their anxieties about what they should be doing, thereby changing their self-evaluations.*

Clinicians as Models for Children and Parents

Influenced by Bandura's research and behavior modification procedures,[14] clinicians began using modeling procedures in stuttering therapy.[15–18] Learning by observing was described in the earliest speech therapy texts, and it is generally recognized that children acquire much of their behavior in this way; however, Bandura's contributions made clinicians focus on being more systematic in planning procedures for carrying out this natural process. Gregory[15] and Hill and Gregory[16] noted that preschool children respond successfully when rewarded for imitating a clinician's more easy, relaxed speech in a play atmosphere. Clinicians' utterances, which are stimuli to a child, vary along a continuum from shorter to longer and of increasing syntactic complexity, and from less to more meaningful (naming, description, etc.). Desensitization, like Van Riper described,[18] was used after the child's speech had begun to change. In addition to modifying a child's speech, we use modeling procedures for changing the communicative interactions between parents and children, based on findings from the parent–child interaction analysis we discussed earlier in this chapter. This analysis is also used for evaluating the interactions of school-age children and parents and determining modifications to be made. Gregory and Hill[19] recalled some of the statements made at staff meetings at Northwestern University which are pertinent to our use of modeling:

> We will teach the parents everything we teach the child so that they can be better models for the child. We will not talk to the parents so much about what we suggest that they do; we will have them observe our interaction with their children and then modify their behavior in terms of our model. We will not expect our client (child, adult, or parent) to do anything that we cannot model for them. (p. 285)

Discussions with parents, sometime in small groups, have continued, but teaching by example was added in our effort to improve communication and interpersonal interactions

---

*For additional information about self-esteem in very young children, see Mahler MS, Pine F, and Bergman A. *The Psychological Birth of the Human Infant*.[13] See also Bandura's discussion of the way in which self-esteem, self-concept, and related self-evaluative processes can be conceptualized in a learning theory framework.[14] This chapter has emphasized how parents' modeling of behavior and positive reinforcement are related to a child's self-esteem.

between parent and child. Discussions of parental behavior, perhaps including the viewing of videotapes of parent–child interactions, should be done gradually, with a gentle, understanding approach. Just as it is difficult for some people to listen to an audio recording of their own voices, it may be even harder to watch a video recording of one's interaction with a child or spouse.

Parents have responded positively to the modeling approach, saying that they gained more confidence in their ability to change by first observing, then performing and receiving feedback. When clinicians believe that their performance at the clinic is satisfactory, parents are assigned home activities Thus, there is a progression from observation of the clinician, to participation in the clinic, to activity at home. In this way, generalization and transfer of the child's behavior changes are facilitated, also. This more direct work on behavior change with both the child and parents follows a period in which the clinician has established an open, understanding, and supportive relationship with the parents and a similarly positive relationship with the child. Parents understand the rationale for what they are doing and have received guidance about how speech and language development is thought to be related to a child's self-esteem. At this point, clinicians should not become so involved with a child's behavior change that they neglect to check on how the parents are feeling about the changes they are making and their child's progress.

Bandura[14] pointed out that observational learning involves cognitive–affective processes. When a person observes the behavior of another, he or she acquires what can be called a mental "verbal map." Positive reinforcement of parents' behavior changes by the clinician taps their emotional responses, with the objective, of course, that these changes will become self-reinforcing for the parents. The clinician reinforces a child by saying such things as, "I like the way you said that. You said that just like I did." To some extent, the psychological process of identification may be functioning also, so that if the parents and child have positive feelings for the clinician, they will find it more gratifying to do as the clinician does.

Parents learn to problem solve by charting their observations of the child at home and discussing the fluctuations of fluency they charted, how they felt at the time, and what they did. For example, when a child is observed to have an increase of stuttering, the parents should think of modifying their own speech by being more relaxed, pausing more, and slowing their speech and turn-taking. Thus, increases in the child's stuttering become a signal, or in the language of learning, a discriminative stimulus, to the parents to modify their own behavior. Guided practice at the clinic and home assignments are continued until the child's fluency is normalized and the parents feel secure about handling the variations in fluency that occur.

Therapy/Counseling Procedures in Early Intervention

We call these procedures "developmental intervention," because clinicians are taking action to influence a child's speech and language during a period of rapid development. Growth and development favor the child becoming more fluent, and our intervention follows the completion of a careful differential evaluation and is intended to increase the possibility of this occurring. In contrast, our intervention with elementary school-age children, who usually have a more confirmed problem, involves more of a corrective approach, in which a child is helped to make changes in speech that are more directly counter to stuttering. With preschool-age children, parent participation is very important to successful early intervention.

Establishing Rapport: Understanding the Child and Parents

We believe that a key element in the success of therapy is a positive relationship between the parents and the clinician and between the clinician and child. We say to parents of young children, "You have invited us to join with you in planning a strategy that will, hopefully, insure that your child will develop normal speech fluency." We proceed in a calm, unhurried, conversational manner showing our genuine interest in understanding the parents and child and the unique characteristics of their problem. As before, the key idea is to be more permissive with parents at first and to proceed carefully and gradually from listening, to interpreting, making recommendations for change in parents thinking and behavior, and waiting until we feel sufficiently informed to make reasonable judgments about what should be done. We often "delay our response" until we feel more certain about the proper way to proceed.

In establishing rapport with a child who is beginning to stutter, it is best to be more permissive at first, just as we are with parents, with early encounters organized around play. In our opinion, the most important element is for both child and parents to have positive affective responses to the clinician and therapy procedures. Put simply, both must come to like and appreciate the clinician. Periodically during treatment, clinicians should check with parents, asking about their feelings and thoughts. For parents, an atmosphere should be created in which they feel comfortable to communicate their concerns to the clinician and interact naturally with their child. Likewise, the child needs to find it pleasant and fun to come to the clinic and look forward to return visits.

Giving Information to Parents: Discussing the Therapy Process

Parents of children who are thought to be beginning to stutter, or who have been stuttering for several months, may come to the therapy situation with feelings of insecurity, fear, bewilderment. They may have obtained some authoritative information about childhood stuttering which helped to convince them that now is the time for a consultation. Sometimes they are puzzled by some sensational report about research on stuttering or treatment approaches which appeared in a newspaper article or on TV. As parents begin to believe that a clinician has a good understanding of their concerns about the child's speech and the status of the child's difficulty, they will be motivated to know more and begin a program for resolving the child's stuttering problem. Based on information gathered during evaluation and counseling sessions, clinicians can decide upon a general strategy of treatment, such as the ones described in other chapters of this text or in other publications by Adams,[20] Costello-Ingham,[21] Onslow, Andrews, and Lincoln,[22] Starkweather, Gottwald, and Halfond,[23] or Meyers and Woodford.[24] Whatever approach is chosen, parents will usually need further information about speech development, the development of stuttering, and as treatment proceeds, such other issues as sibling interaction, the influence of extended family members, or related problems such as behavioral concerns and language deficits. The clinician's task is to relate such information to an individual child's problem and to the therapeutic process being pursued. For example, in discussing communicative stress factors, parents should be helped to understand the communicative interactions that seem to be particularly relevant in their interaction with their child. Informing parents and clarifying their understanding is a process that is intermingled with behavior modification all along the way.

Building the Preschool-age Child's Self-esteem

An earlier section described how self-esteem develops in preschool-age children and speculated that a developing stuttering problem might influence a parent's interaction at a crucial period in a child's psychosocial development. A parent might show worry and uncertainty, be tentative with positive affect, and not provide a child who is beginning to stutter or has been stuttering for a year or two with much positive reinforcement. It is hoped, of course, that as parents receive guidance from speech–language pathologists, they become more objective and constructive. In being more objective, we mean that they begin to perceive and label events differently and more realistically, and in being constructive, that they are learning how to problem solve with the clinician and will do so later by themselves. As thought is substituted for worry, parents become able to enjoy their child more fully!

When a child is 2 to 3 years of age, the period when parents most often become concerned about stuttering, basic affective patterns are fairly well-established in most children. Still, children are pliable, and shifts in parents' attitudes and behaviors can have significant effects on them. Along with specific communicative changes, some parents may need to consider resolving such interpersonal stresses in the home as disagreements about discipline, spousal conflicts, or a fast-paced family life. They may need to consider the possibility that how relaxed a child is and how fluently he speaks may be related to his feelings of security. Often times, parents have to be encouraged to focus on a child's positive attributes and express pleasure about them. Clinicians can discuss this with parents, but as we describe in the next section, they should also model positive expressions of pleasure and joy for parents. Parents' expressions of approval and pleasure with their preschool child is a form of positive reinforcement that has bidirectional effects. For example, a parent and child having a special time together is conducive to the child feeling better about him/herself and the parent feeling good about having more time with the child. This is what we mean by positive reinforcement having bidirectional effects!

Modeling Behavior Changes for the Child and the Parents

From the beginning of early intervention, we advise clinicians to model relaxation in their speech and general manner, increased pause time, and slower turn-taking when speaking with both parents and child. Over the years, we have been impressed by how readily many preschool children spontaneously begin to follow the clinician's speech model to some extent. The clinician then proceeds to provide more definitive modeling for the child as needed. We invite parents to begin sitting in on therapy sessions, first one at a time, and observing the clinician interact with the child. The clinician should point out what she is doing in the session, such as speaking in a slightly slower, more relaxed way, and explain the procedure. Following some practice of easy relaxed speech alone with the clinician, the parent should try to modify her/his speech during a therapy session, speaking more easy and relaxed with the child. As a parent has success with one procedure, another is added. When the clinician judges that the child is progressing satisfactorily and that a parent has developed adequate proficiency in modeling, home assignments can be given.

As these behavior changes are being learned, discussions of related topics, such as time pressure in communication or how to reinforce the child continue. It is very important to check with the parents routinely, saying for example, "How do you feel about modifying your speech?" or "How do you like having a special time to do something with each child?" and review procedures periodically with them, asking if there are questions.

Generalization, Transfer, and Follow-up

When parents participate in therapy, generalization of the child's improved speech occurs readily in most cases. We have noted, however, that therapy appears to take longer for children who have more severe stuttering or who have been stuttering for a longer period of time, but each case is individual. We believe that the results of therapy are optimal if a child is seen within a year of parents becoming concerned. The frequency of treatment sessions should be tapered gradually as a child's fluency improves. A follow-up program of recheck sessions should be scheduled at appropriate intervals, and parents should be encouraged to telephone if they have questions or concerns. One of the marks of successful counseling for parents is that they learn to cope with their child's fluency variations, in large part, by modifying environmental stresses and their own behavior. Clinicians need to remember, however, that unexpected events do occur on occasion, at which times they may need to be available to listen and understand, then help parents to continue problem solving.

Therapy/Counseling for School-age Children

Intervention with preschool children involves a developmental approach, in which the clinician joins with parents in molding the developmental process and carrying out procedures that are intended to prevent children from experiencing more than minimal feelings that their speech is difficult or different. One teenage youngster, whose speech became normally fluent, referred a friend for stuttering therapy, but said he had only a trace of a memory of seeing us when a preschooler. With elementary school-age children who stutter, however, stuttering behaviors are likely to be more firmly established, together with more complicated feelings and beliefs about their speech and stuttering. Therapy can still aim toward enhancing the development of speech fluency, but clinicians are usually more corrective or direct, in varying degrees, in showing a youngster how speech can be modified, e.g., how initiation can be easier and more relaxed. From age 6 or 7 up to 11 or 12, children's awareness and consistency of stuttering varies a great deal from one another, and in the same child from time to time. Many of these children are likely to develop certain beliefs and feelings that require a clinician's attention. In addition, parents and teachers need to understand the nature of the child's speech problem and how they can cooperate with therapy.

When clinicians see a school-age child who stutters for the first time, they should have ready an age-appropriate game or a book to read. We usually begin by inquiring about a child's interest and indicate that we want to know more about it, whether it is hockey, baseball, or computer games. Sometimes we share one of our own interests with the child, such as skiing, with the hope of stimulating further conversation. An adult, whom we saw as an 11-year-old child, still remembers his first visit in which he told us about his interest in ice hockey. Healey and Scott[25] also emphasize the importance of establishing good relationships with children by getting to know their interests and how they view their world. During these interactions clinicians should be relaxed, pause frequently when speaking as well as a couple of seconds after the child finishes before they begin to speak, just as they would with a preschooler. In this way, clinicians are already beginning to model a way to communicate that reduces time pressure, which some clinicians consider to be a fundamental factor in stuttering.

These first encounters, whether during a diagnostic session or at the beginning of therapy, are crucial in establishing rapport. We saw a 9-year-old child at the beginning of the summer a few years ago who was angry about coming to see us and told us that he had other important plans for the summer. We immediately said, "It's not necessary that you begin now. We can get together this fall if you like?" He said he would like that better, and his parents were relieved to hear that we thought it was OK to wait. We believe that it would have been counterproductive to begin therapy when he felt so negative. Some children do come to therapy with negative feelings which may reflect previous therapy experiences, in some cases. These feelings can be reduced, however, when they find out that therapy can be fun with a clinician who likes them and really wants to get to know them better. We often tell speech–language pathology students, "The clinician must be interested in whatever interests the child." If a child plays hockey, we get interested and may even go to the games! We always begin treatment activities gradually and give considerable positive reinforcement for a child's correct responses. A basic principle of all therapy is that motivation is enhanced by positive reinforcement.[26,27]

With children this age it is appropriate to have them experience some increased fluency early in therapy. This makes therapy concrete and meaningful and clearly shows them that we are going to work on making speech easier and better. Clinicians go about this in various ways,[21,28,29] but we use choral reading, in which the clinician first instructs a child to follow her simultaneous model.[30] In short, a child moves from following a simultaneous model of easy relaxed approaches, smooth movements (ERA-SM) in unison with the instructor, to saying words, phrases, and sentences while imitating the clinician's model, to carry over in descriptions, short-answer questions, and so forth, and finally to spontaneous self-formulated conversation. The clinician should take every opportunity to reinforce the child, not only by saying "good" following target responses, but also such things as "You are learning this very fast. You are good at this!" Sometimes we may say, "I would like to tell your Mother and Dad how well you can modify your speech. Is that O.K.?" Ordinarily, we end each session with a game, which allows us to incorporate the speech changes we are working on in therapy into this activity as soon as it is appropriate. Later, the child may bring a game or a book from home, which will be used in guided practice.

Clinicians should always give youngsters the opportunity to say whatever they wish. As the relationship progresses, most children talk to the clinician about a variety of topics, including what changes they have noticed about their speech or being teased. If such topics do not arise spontaneously, a clinician can use such open-ended comments or questions as, "Tell me what you can about your speech" or "What have you thought is the trouble with your talking." If a child says that "words get stuck in my throat" or "It's like I have glue in my mouth sometime," this can be explored, and ways of modifying speech can be linked to what the child describes. For example, the clinician can help the child make a more easy relaxed approach with smooth movement, showing how this helps to reduce tension in the "voice box" as well as the possibility of words getting stuck. We have found that it is helpful at points such as this to show children a diagram of the speech mechanism and describe how speech is produced as air moves through the vocal folds, which produces sound that is changed further into recognizable speech by movements of the tongue, jaw, and soft palate. Some of the areas where air–voice flow might be blocked by tension in the vocal folds, tongue, or lips can be illustrated and discussed as well. Stuttering is, in many ways, a mystery to these children, as is speech production, and this is one way of taking some of the mystery out of it.

Speech Change and Attitude Change

Modifying speech and attitude change are reciprocally related processes; reductions in stuttering and finding easier ways to talk makes children feel better about talking and about themselves. In addition, a better understanding of speaking, stuttering, and therapy goals and procedures facilitates a child's ability to change. Drawing analogies between learning to change speech and improving skills in a sport is one way of making stuttering therapy more meaningful to a school-age child. Questions such as the following can be discussed: Why does a basketball player take practice shots before a game and again before play resumes at the end of half-time? When you change your tennis swing, why do you have to slow the swing at first? Why does it seem easier to hit a softball when no one is looking than with an audience? Such discussions are aimed at helping children change their perceptions of their problem. Modifications of thoughts about these kinds of activities influence the way a child thinks about therapy.

Therapy provides an opportunity for children to mention experiences, thoughts, and worries that many have not had the chance to talk about before, and listening skills are important here. In a comfortable relationship, a child will usually mention such experiences as being teased, and the clinician can explore such concerns with him or her. Gregory[30] described a 9-year-old child who told the clinician that teasing by a classmate made him "feel sad," and as the child said this, there were obvious signs of emotion. The clinician responded, "You felt bad inside, you felt a little like crying." The child went on to talk about disliking this classmate, and, in fact, feeling angry. Once feelings are out in the open, possibilities for handling situations like teasing can be explored further. For example, teasing can be discussed as a need of the teaser, and the clinician can suggest that if teasing doesn't appear to bother you it will probably stop. The clinician and the child can role play a teasing episode, and the child can choose not to respond at all or to say something like, "I am working on making my speech more easy and relaxed." Chmela and Reardon[31] described how clinicians can bring up a subject, such as teasing, while playing a game with a child just by interjecting during a pause in activity, "How are you feeling about teasing these days?" This somewhat indirect approach seems to be more comfortable for a child and is often successful!

Campbell[32] uses open-ended discussion statements to explore a child's attitudes, such as the following: "The hardest person for me to talk to is …," or "Someone I can talk to about my stuttering is …," or "Sometimes my stuttering makes me mad because …." When working with children, she finds that writing down the child's thoughts helps to make discussions more concrete and meaningful, as well as easier to review for later comment. Campbell[32] also describes procedures for helping children to understand therapy and monitor progress.

Sometimes there may be resistance to change. For example, a clinician might say, "It feels and sounds different because it is new." The child might say, "I don't want to talk slow like that." Then, the clinician could respond, "I don't want you to talk slower, but stuttering does involve increased tension in speech, and when you make easier beginnings and smoother movements and learn to pause better, it may seem to you that you are talking slower. I am teaching you this so you can reduce your stuttering." Later, the clinician might add, "We will practice talking slower, faster, and at your usual rate so that you can do whatever you wish." We have found that videotaping is a good approach to changing attitudes about modifying speech. As children watch and listen to their speech on videotape and as they are reinforced by parents, teachers, and perhaps even schoolmates, speech change becomes more acceptable. Such experiences, over time, help to change attitudes about speech sounding and feeling different, and clinicians should just continue to be reassuring and reinforcing. The clinician's models are important in determining a child's evaluation of changes in speech, but it is especially supportive and rewarding to a child for parents to be changing their speech, too. In addition, it seems to be more and more reinforcing to a child to be relieved of the anxiety from anticipating failure and attempting to conceal stuttering. Better speech becomes self-reinforcing to children as they give successful reports in class, make more telephone calls, and talk without worrying so much about stuttering. Clinicians can help children become more aware of these feelings by saying, "I know how much better you are feeling to be less afraid of talking," or "You are really feeling good about your talking successes."

Some children appear to generalize their sensitivity about stuttering to a desire to avoid all disfluency in their speech. They need to understand that some disfluency, e.g., word repetitions, phrase repetitions, interjections such as "ah," and revisions, is a normal aspect of speech. We advise clinicians to model voluntary disfluencies, beginning with sentences such as "I, I, I would like a hamburger and, and french fries," or "I would, I would like a hamburger and french fries." Then, reinforcing the child playing with fluency by imitating the clinician's models of disfluency counterconditions these children's sensitivity about disfluency and stuttering. Although we remember one 9-year-old who was taught voluntary disfluency said, "This is cool," others may not be so positive about it, but with time and experience, they usually come to think and feel differently. Some find it hard to accept. We assume, in these latter cases, that their avoidance and inhibitory tendencies are very strong. We believe, however, that reinforcement by the clinician and others is a key factor in a child's appreciating voluntary disfluency.

Parent and Teacher Cooperation

It is crucial to the success of treatment that parents understand and participate in the therapy process. We always inform them that therapy will be much more effective if they are supportive and, furthermore, that the child's prognosis is guarded if they do not participate. Following a child's initial evaluation and our analysis of the parent–child interaction, parents are apprised of both child and environmental factors that may be contributing to the child's stuttering, and a tentative treatment plan is outlined. In relating to parents, our objective is for them to have positive feelings toward us and feel comfortable evaluating and discussing their experiences with us. We are also careful, even when feeling the pressure of limited time, not to overload parents by attempting to cover too much information too rapidly.

Some parents experience feelings of guilt about their child's stuttering. They may fear that the child is going to have a lifelong handicap, that they are to blame for a genetic predisposition, or that they did not take appropriate action soon enough. They may be looking far into the future, thinking that their son or daughter will be unable to be a lawyer or successful in some other profession requiring good communication skills. Intense feelings of guilt are counterproductive and may result in parents' avoiding participation. It is not respectful of parents' feelings to say that they shouldn't feel guilty or shouldn't worry; their worry is real. So, we listen and emphasize that they have done the right thing in seeking professional help now and that we are glad to join with them in understanding their child's present difficulty and working out cooperative solutions.

Just as modeling procedures are used when working with a child, the clinician needs to model for parents of elementary school-age children how to change their speech in the same ways that their child is learning to do. Modeling is a powerful technique in working with children and parents, particularly when the child and parents are practicing the same things. Parent participation of this kind is a positive reinforcer for most children. Parents sometimes report that their child is telling them at home to make their speech more easy and relaxed or to take turns talking, indicating a positive attitude of cooperation, parents and child working together.

Clinicians may also need to help parents of elementary school-age children problem solve certain stressful speaking situations. We discuss the importance of building their child's self-esteem by being more expressive of their pleasure about what their child does well and enjoys, such as playing board games, drawing, sports activities, or performing duties at home. Their "being proud" of the child in these areas generalizes to being pleased with the child's improvement in speech and prepares the way for a child to respond more positively to the parents' and clinicians' positive reinforcements for what is being learned in therapy. We think that the more general security and self-confidence that an elementary school-age child feels, the better the prognosis for improved speech.

A large part of a child's communication environment is at school. Thus, it is crucial that teachers help speech–language clinicians to understand how the child responds in the classroom. They also need to be supportive of the child in carrying out such activities as reading aloud, giving a report, or perhaps sharing an experience. Speech–language pathologists should talk with the teacher about classroom procedures, then describe their therapy objectives and discuss ways in which the teacher believes that she can be helpful. Discussions of collaborative models of treatment in speech–language pathology course work seem to have improved clinicians' skills in recent years for working collaboratively with classroom teachers. A key factor in such cooperation is the speech–language clinician's understanding and acceptance of the teacher's obligations in the classroom and expressions of appreciation for the teacher's time and assistance.

Transfer of Speech Change

Attitude and speech change take time, but the process can be facilitated by the clinician and child planning a hierarchy of transfers from the therapy room to outside speaking situations.[33] From the beginning of treatment, changes in speech have progressed by working from shorter to longer utterances and from less meaningful to more meaningful content. Thus, the clinician has been preparing the child to modify his or her speech in situations other than the clinician's office or therapy room at school. When a child is becoming effective in easy-speaking situations with the clinician, it is time for the child and clinician to plan together and draw up a tentative hierarchy of speaking situations in which the child would like to speak better, using procedures such as being more relaxed, ERA-SM, resisting time pressure, that are being practiced in therapy. Role-playing situations in the clinic precedes entering these situations in real life. Oftentimes, the clinician can model an interaction before the child tries it, and the clinician should feel rather certain that the child will experience a substantial measure of success before undertaking the real task or situation. In school situations, the child can practice giving a report in the classroom with the clinician and the teacher before it is presented to the students. This is one example of employing a collaborative model—the clinician and teacher planning with the child and offering support. As a child is more and more successful and is reinforced by the clinician, teachers, and peers, he or she feels increased confidence and motivation.

Dismissal and Follow-up

The clinician should begin talking with the child and parents about phasing out treatment when it is apparent that the child is stuttering less in most real-life situations, is feeling confident about being able to modify speech, understands variations in fluency and what to do, and there appears to be a general feeling of self-confidence about communication. Parents should now have a realistic understanding of the problem, know how to reinforce the child for modifying speech, and are not expecting perfect fluency. They understand that the child's stuttering, even though greatly lessened, is likely to continue to be somewhat cyclic, and they know what they should do to modify their own communicative behavior when the child is having increased difficulty. They also need to work out a home program with the clinician in which they will implement and review the principles and techniques that have been learned in therapy. Both the child and parents should be able to verbalize what they plan to do from one recheck session to the next. At first, therapy sessions become less frequent, for example, once every 2 weeks, then once a month. Intermittent checkups, aimed at problem solving and preventing regression, should be scheduled for a period of 12–18 months, or longer, if needed.

There is one final, but important point to make. If a child is not successful in therapy over a 2- or 3-month period, and the clinician believes that every means to increase improvement have been considered, then dismissal should be discussed with the parents. If unsuccessful therapy continues and is not rewarding to the child, this may damage the prospects for success in therapy at a later date. We believe that, "Nothing succeeds like being successful. Nothing is so punishing as failure." Of course, before a final decision is made, feelings about therapy should be discussed with the child. It has been our experience that many children who leave therapy under these circumstances return when a greater need is realized, sometimes a year later, sometimes in their early teenage years.

Conclusion

Drawing on our experience in evaluating and treating stuttering, preparing student clinicians, and offering continuing education workshops for professionals, we have found it valuable to view counseling and stuttering therapy from the frame of reference that both involve affective, cognitive, and behavioral variables. Moreover, the way in which counselors, psychotherapists, and speech–language pathologists deal with these variables, involves similar skills of listening, responding to feelings and beliefs, informing, directing behavior change, and problem solving. We have emphasized that it is the knowledge that a particular professional has about a problem that differs. It follows from this view, of course, that speech–language pathologists must be aware of their limitations and seek consultation with other specialists for some of the problems that some of their clients may present.

Throughout this chapter we have shown how the affective, cognitive, and behavioral modalities of stuttering treatment and counseling are integrated but in somewhat different ways for preschool and school-age children and their parents. Furthermore, we have brought together the contributions of colleagues in psychology and psychiatry such as Rogers[1] (client-centered counseling), Mahler and Kohut[10,12,13] (self-esteem and personality development), and Bandura[14] (behavior modeling and social learning). In addition, the influence of those clinicians with backgrounds in speech–language pathology and psychology, such as Sheehan[5] and Van Riper,[3,18] who worked in the area of stuttering throughout their careers, has been acknowledged, and their contributions integrated into our beliefs and procedures relating to counseling and the treatment of stuttering.

A priority of this chapter was to show how practical clinical applications are compatible with the point of view that counseling and stuttering therapy involve essentially the same processes. To this end, we have included considerable detail about the specific ways in which clinicians' goals and procedures focus simultaneously on children's and parents' feelings, beliefs and behavior. We hope that this frame of reference will be useful in helping speech–language pathologists understand counseling as an integral aspect of their work in the prevention and treatment of stuttering.

Suggested Readings

Bandura A: *Social Learning Theory*. Englewood Cliffs, NJ: Prentice-Hall, 1977.
  A concise presentation of observational, symbolic, and self-regulatory processes in learning. Describes the scope of modeling influences in behavior development and modification; thus, providing the reader a background for the emphasis of modeling in speech and language therapy.
Kohut H, Wolf E: The disorders of the self and their treatment: An outline. *Int J Psychoanal* 1978; 59:413–425.
  A survey of psychology of the self theory, and applications to therapeutic situations, with a main focus on personality disorders of childhood. Helps the reader to understand the importance of developing self-esteem in children.
Rogers C: *A way of being*. Boston, Houghton Mifflin, 1980.
  Traces Rogers' development of his client-centered approach to counseling with reference to the changing aspects of his life and career in psychology.
Rustin L, Kuhr A: *Social Skills and the Speech Impaired*. London, Taylor and Francis, 1989.
  School-age children can begin to profit from a discussion of social skills. Role playing can include the practice of certain social skills that will improve a child's confidence in communication. This book covers social skills training for all disorders of communication including stuttering.

References

1. Rogers C: *Client-centered therapy*. Boston, Houghton-Miffin, 1951.
2. Gregory, H: Environmental Manipulation and Family Counseling, in Shames G, Rubin H (eds): *Stuttering: Then and Now*. Columbus, OH, Charles Merrill Publishing Co., 1986.
3. Van Riper C: The Stutterer's Clinician, in Eisenson J (ed.): *Stuttering: A Second Symposium*. New York, Harper and Row, 1975.
4. Gregory H, Campbell J, Hill D: Differential Evaluation of Stuttering Problems, in Gregory, H (ed): *Stuttering Therapy: Rationale and Procedures*. San Diego, Singular Publishers, 1999.
5. Ainsworth S, Fraser J: *If Your Child Stutters: A Guide for Parents*. Memphis, TN, Stuttering Foundation of America publication no. 11, Memphis, TN, 1988.

6. Conture E, Fraser, J: *Stuttering and Your Child: Questions and Answers.* Memphis, TN, Stuttering Foundation of America publication no. 22, Memphis, TN, 1989.
7. Sheehan J: *Stuttering: Research and Therapy.* New York, Harper and Row, 1970.
8. Bloom L, Johnson C, Bitler, Christman K: *Facilitating Communication Change: An Interpersonal Approach to Therapy and Counseling*, Rockville, MD, Aspen Publications, 1986.
9. Donahue-Kilburg G: *Family-centered Early Intervention for Communication Disorders: Prevention and Treatment.* Rockville, MD, Aspen Publications, 1992.
10. Mahler M: *On Human Symbiosis and the Vicissitudes of Individuation.* New York, International Universities Press, 1968.
11. Winnicott D: *Playing and Reality.* London, Tavistock, 1971.
12. Kohut H, Wolf E: The disorders of the self: An outline. *Int J Psychoanalysis* 1978; 59:413–423.
13. Mahler M, Pine F, Bergman, A: *The Psychological Birth of the Human Infant.* New York, Basic Books, 1975.
14. Bandura A: *Principles of Behavior Modification.* New York, Holt, Rinehart & Winston, 1969.
15. Gregory H: Modeling procedures in the treatment of elementary school age children who stutter. *J Fluency Dis* 1973; 1:58–63.
16. Hill D, Gregory H: Modeling Speech Change for Children Who Stutter. Unpublished. Chicago. Illinois Speech and Hearing Association Conference, 1975.
17. Gregory H, Hill D: Stuttering Therapy in Children, in Perkins W (ed): *Strategies in Stuttering Therapy.* New York, Thieme-Stratton, 1980.
18. Van Riper C: *The Treatment of Stuttering.* Englewood Cliffs, NJ, Prentice-Hall, 1973.
19. Gregory H, Hill D: Differential Evaluation—Differential Therapy for Stuttering Children, in Curlee R (ed): *Stuttering and Related Disorders of Fluency.* New York, Thieme, 1993.
20. Adams M: The Young Stutterer: Diagnosis, Treatment, and Assessment of Progress, in Perkins, W (ed): *Stuttering Disorders.* New York, Thieme-Stratton, 1984.
21. Costello-Ingham J: Behavioral Treatment of Stuttering, in Curlee R (ed): *Stuttering and Related Disorders of Fluency.* New York, Thieme, 1993.
22. Onslow M, Andrews C, Lincoln M: A control/experimental trial of an operant treatment for early stuttering. *J Speech Hear Res* 1984; 37:1244–1259.
23. Starkweather W, Gottwald S, Halfond M: *Stuttering Prevention: A Clinical Method.* Englewood Cliffs, NJ, Prentice-Hall, 1990.
24. Meyers S, Woodford L: *The Fluency Development System for Young Children.* Buffalo, NY, United Educational Services, 1992.
25. Healey EC, Scott L: Strategies for Treating Elementary School-Age Children Who Stutter. *Language, Speech Hearing Services Schools* 1995; 26:151–161.
26. Gregory H: Analysis and Commentary. *Language, Speech Hearing Services Schools* 1995; 26:196–200.
27. Gregory H (ed): *Stuttering Therapy: Rationale and Procedures.* San Diego, Singular Publishers, 1999.
28. Cooper E, Cooper C: *Personalized Fluency Control Therapy*, revised. New York, DLM Teaching Resources, 1985.
29. Runyan C, Runyan E: Therapy for School-Age Stutterers: An Update on the Fluency Rules Program, in Curlee R (ed): *Stuttering and Related Disorders of Fluency.* New York, Thieme, 1993.
30. Gregory H: Therapy for Elementary School-Age Children, in Perkins W (ed): *Stuttering: Challenges of Therapy (Seminars in Speech and Language).* 1991.
31. Chmela K, Reardon N: The Emotions of Stuttering: Coping Strategies for the School-Age Child. Presentation. Chicago, Illinois Speech–Language and Hearing Association, 1995.
32. Campbell J: Therapy for Elementary School-Age Children Who Stutter, in Gregory H (ed): *Stuttering Therapy: Rationale and Procedures.* San Diego, Singular Publishers, 1999.
33. Boberg E: Behavioral Transfer and Maintenance Programs for Adolescent and Adult Stutterers, in Gregory H (ed): *Stuttering Therapy: Transfer and Maintenance.* Memphis, TN, Stuttering Foundation of America publication no. 19, 1988.

Stuttering and Related Disorders of Fluency, 2nd edition.
Edited by Richard F. Curlee, Ph.D.
Thieme Medical Publishers, Inc., New York © 1999.

Early Intervention for Stuttering: The Lidcombe Program

Elisabeth Harrison
Mark Onslow

The Lidcombe Program has evolved over the past 10 years from a collaboration of academics and clinical speech pathologists in Sydney, Australia. This treatment for early stuttering differs from those in other countries, and one of several reasons for this seems to have been the isolation of Australia from treatment and research centers of the Northern hemisphere.[1] This chapter describes this treatment for preschool-age children who stutter.

The Stuttering Unit is part of the Bankstown Health Service. It is based in a community health center, which is a government-funded public health service. The Stuttering Unit in the Australian health care system is unique, in that its speech pathology staff specializes in treatment of stuttering clients of all ages. The academic input to the development of the Lidcombe Program has come from the Faculty of Health Sciences at The University of Sydney, and specifically, the Australian Stuttering Research Center (ASRC). The ASRC generates research into stuttering and its treatment, which is conducted by academic and clinical staff, and postgraduate students.

Over the last 10 years, this group of clinicians and researchers has focused a considerable amount of their work on the development of the Lidcombe Program. This chapter outlines the treatment with an emphasis on the role of the clinician in the treatment process. The procedures described are based on video recordings of clinic sessions, which have been analyzed for the purpose of gathering detail on the clinician's role. Having conducted the Lidcombe Program for many years, we were surprised at the amount of extra detail that was gleaned from careful observation of assessment and treatment sessions. Many of the events observed by researchers who evaluated these videos had previously been taken for granted. And yet, when all of these details were listed in full, we were surprised at the richness of the interactions that routinely occur in our clinics. On a broader scale, we have also become aware from efforts to teach the Lidcombe Program to other speech pathologists that this degree of detail is necessary. In our outcome research articles, we have given only "bare bones" descriptions of the Lidcombe Program—an overall picture of how it works.[2-5] The purpose of these descriptions has been deemed as an adjunct to the data presented in those articles, and so the descriptions have been oriented toward research rather than clinical practice. In this chapter we seek to redress that balance, and give a detailed picture of how we employ the Lidcombe Program.

Clinical Evaluation

In Australia, information about early treatment of children who stutter is disseminated throughout the community. This information is circulated through the news media, mass-circulation magazines, health publications, and health services. Therefore, referrals to the Stuttering Unit are prompted by many sources of information. The most common referrers are parents of preschool-age children who have become concerned about their child's speech and sought advice from their local doctor, their child's preschool teacher, or a child health clinic. These health and education professionals typically recommend that parents talk to us.

Parents' first contact with the Stuttering Unit is a phone call for information and advice. If parents decide to bring their child to the Unit for assessment, they are given an appointment, usually within 6 weeks. We request that parents bring with them a 10-min audio recording of their child's conversational speech in the home setting and request that both parents accompany the child to the assessment. The main purpose of this initial session is to gather sufficient information about the child and the child's speech to make a diagnosis of stuttering and assist the parents in making informed decisions about whether to undertake treatment. Along the way, parents are given information about stuttering, treatment for stuttering, possible prognoses with and without treatment, and are told about the experience of other parents and children who have been through the Lidcombe Program.

Case History

The first few minutes of the session are spent making introductions, seating the child and parents, and giving the child toys or books to play with. The clinician explains to the child what will happen during the session and that the toys can be played with while the clinician interviews the parents. The child is assured that it is fine to interrupt the adults' conversation at any time. Once the child is settled, the parents are told that the first part of the session will involve getting information from them and answering their questions. Then, the clinician will talk with the child and conclude by making recommendations about treatment and answering any final questions. Case history information is elicited in an unstructured interview, which lasts for one to one and a half hours. The order of the questions varies but the following information is routinely collected:

1. *Onset of Stuttering*: The clinician starts the interview by asking when something unusual was first noticed about the child's fluency. The clinician prompts parents to try to remember who first noted something unusual, and when this occurred. The clinician's interest here is to determine the child's age at onset and, therefore, the time elapsed since onset.

2. *Type of Stutters at Onset*: Parents are asked to describe the type of stutters they noticed at onset. We find that it is helpful to demonstrate the stuttering that is common among preschoolers, particularly rhythmic syllable repetitions, prolongations of sounds, and silent blocks. In most cases, this helps parents to establish the time of onset and describe the type of stuttering that occurred at that time.

3. *Changes Since Onset*: Parents are asked whether or not there have been any changes in their child's stuttering since onset. Two kinds of information are being sought here— changes in types of stuttering, and in frequency of stuttering. The final description that

parents are asked for is whether they have noticed any of the other characteristics often associated with early stuttering. Frequently they report features such as pitch and volume changes during stuttering moments, frequent whispering, a preference for talking with a "play acting" voice, or stamping feet or clapping hands during stutters. Information about these factors and variations in them over time gives a clear picture of the developmental course of the child's stuttering.

The clinician also asks about the child's level of frustration about stuttering. Many parents report that their child is frustrated while stuttering, especially if it is more than moderately severe; however, we find it unusual for parents to report that children under 5 years of age are frustrated about speech, in general. Their frustration usually is short-lived and evident only while they are struggling to speak.

4. *Family History*: Parents are asked if there are any other family members who stutter. Although this is a notoriously inadequate way of eliciting reliable information about family histories, it does allow the topic of genetic factors in stuttering to be discussed. Many parents are aware of other family members who stutter or who used to stutter as children, and they are given information about the increased risk of siblings and cousins to also stutter, and the reasons for early intervention are reiterated.

5. *Previous Speech Therapy*: Parents are asked if their child has had any previous treatment for stuttering or any other speech problem. The clinician is interested in both treatment from a speech pathologist and the more informal treatment that parents may have attempted on their own. Parents are asked to describe this in as much detail as they can, and, in particular, to report when the intervention was started, and whether or not it was continued. The parents are then asked about the child's response to this informally managed intervention. The clinician is particularly interested in any negative responses the child had, and whether they were verbal (e.g., "Mummy don't say that") or nonverbal (e.g. refusing to talk, getting grumpy, or being uncooperative). If the child seems to have responded well to previous formal or informal treatment efforts, the parents are asked to give details about that also.

This section of the assessment session concludes with the clinician giving the parents feedback about the information they have provided. We briefly explain how their information will be used in making decisions about treatment and reassure them that their child's case history is not unusual for a child who stutters.

Observation and Tests

Within-clinic Speech Sample

Attempts are made to elicit a spontaneous speech sample from the child. This can be done by either the parents and/or the clinician during conversation with the child. Because they have been playing with the clinic's toys during the case history interview, most children will have interrupted the interview several times with questions or comments about the toys, and are now feeling at ease in the clinic. In such cases, the clinician simply engages the child in conversation or introduces new activities that are likely to elicit a preschool-age child's interest and conversation. With more reserved children, it can be preferable for one or both parents to play with the child. Parents have the advantage of their child's instant confidence and it is likely that even a shy child will talk, at least a little, with a parent; however, one disadvantage of this approach is that parents may not be skilled in eliciting long passages of spontaneous speech from their children.

The aim of obtaining a speech sample in the clinic is for the clinician to get a first-hand look at the child's speech, gather information about severity of stuttering, and note the presence of any other speech problems. It is very common for this sample to differ from what the parents usually hear at home. Many parents report that, although their child chatted freely in the clinic, their stuttering was much less severe than usual. We often find ourselves telling parents that this is a common occurrence.

A sample of 300 syllables is usually enough to get an impression of the child's speech but some flexibility is needed in determining the length required. For a child with extremely severe stuttering, 20 or 30 syllables would be enough for the clinician to judge the severity of the problem without distressing the child unnecessarily. On the other hand, a child with less severe stuttering may have stuttered only a few times in 300 syllables, and a longer sample is required for the clinician to be confident about diagnosis and make judgments about severity.

The clinician always asks the parents' opinion about this sample of the child's speech. Specifically, the clinician wants to know how this sample compares with the child's usual speech at home both in terms of stuttering and any other characteristics they noticed. Most frequently, parents report that a sample is different from the child's typical speech and are often puzzled by their child's complete fluency, after stuttering severely until they arrived at the clinic. The clinician gives the parents information about the reaction of most young children on their first visit to the clinic, that most preschool-age children, for example, are a little shy, that they may say very little, and that their speech sample frequently is not typical. The parents are also reassured that invalid speech samples will not be used as a basis for clinical decision-making. The clinician tells the parents of any observations made of the child's speech and will comment on the severity of the child's stuttering and any strategies the child seems to be using to control stuttering, such as jaw clenching during speech.

Beyond-clinic Speech Sample

The clinician then listens to the tape that the parents made of their child's speech at home, and analyzes it for the percentage of syllables stuttered. The clinician and parents then discuss the validity of this sample, compare it with the within-clinic sample, and with the child's usual speech at home.

Analysis of Speech Samples

The first analysis made of a child's speech sample is to determine the percentage of syllables that are stuttered (%SS). This is done by the clinician during conversation with the child and when listening to the beyond-clinic tape recording. An electronic, button-press counting and timing device is used by the clinician to count concurrently the total number of syllables spoken by the child and the number of syllables that were stuttered. The device then calculates the percentage of syllables that were stuttered.

During an initial assessment session, the clinician is unfamiliar with the child's speech pattern and type of stuttering, and must make rapid, on-line determinations of what is a stutter in that child's speech and what is normal disfluency. We have found it useful to check with the parents whether or not a particular speech event was what they would usually identify as a stutter. Clinicians at the Stuttering Unit use a consensus definition as the most useful clinical method for identifying moments of stuttering. This means that clinicians use their own perceptual judgment to determine what is normal disfluency and what is an occurrence of stuttering. In the few cases where there is doubt, one or two colleagues also listen to the child's speech, and a consensus is reached about whether or not the disfluencies observed are stuttering.

Speech rate can be calculated easily with the measurement device just described and is used for this purpose with older clients; however, we find that for preschool-age children speech rate information is of little clinical value. We believe that there are neither any useful speech rate norms for this age group, nor acceptable measurement procedures. We have encountered no clinical difficulties as a result of not collecting this speech measure.

Case Selection Criteria

When deciding whether or not to recommend treatment for preschool-age stuttering children, the main issue is finding the optimum time to begin. The effectiveness of the Lidcombe Program in controlling stuttered speech has now been substantiated in numerous clinical reports.[2,4,5] From those studies we know that it takes a median of 10–11 clinical hours for preschoolers to reach the beginning of the maintenance program, at which time their stuttering is essentially zero. At present we are preparing a report of several hundred of the children we have treated in the past few years, and that figure for the median treatment time certainly is correct. We also know that the Lidcombe Program works for older children of school age,[6] but that it takes a few more hours to achieve a less successful outcome with that age group. To add a further dimension to case selection, we know that many children will have a short period of stuttering as preschoolers, and then recover without formal treatment involving a speech pathologist. So, we have a treatment that is maximally effective if applied to preschool-age children, but some of these children will recover without our assistance. Who do we treat? On the one hand, we risk wasting time and money in unnecessary treatment, and, on the other, we risk leaving the child with a lifetime of stuttering which may have been avoided if treatment had begun earlier.

While our research program continues to work on the problem of establishing the optimal time to begin treatment, we have made a series of decisions about timing treatment for clients at the Stuttering Unit. To some extent these are arbitrary decisions, but we have opted for conservative recommendations and prefer to risk overtreatment in the short-term to withholding useful treatment from young children.[7] This is how it works: If it is more than 6 months since the onset of a child's stuttering, we recommend that treatment begins. A more complex judgment is required in cases of children who have been stuttering for less than 6 months. If a child's case history and clinical presentation contains some of the features below, then we may not recommend treatment; however, we do not recommend treatment for children who exhibit all of these following characteristics:

1. Stuttering for less than six months.
2. Stuttering consists only of rhythmic, syllable repetitions.
3. Child and parents are not frustrated by the stuttering.
4. No family history of stuttering.

Children we do not wish to treat immediately are monitored regularly so that treatment can begin if their stuttering continues past the 6 months mark or if other characteristics of their stuttering change our decision to "treatment is recommended."

The clinician's role is to make recommendations regarding treatment to the parents and give them whatever additional information they need to decide whether or not their child will be treated. The decision about whether or not treatment begins belongs to the child's parents and we encourage them to consider their options carefully before making this decision. Parents are told about the overall format of the Lidcombe Program, that most of the treatment is done at home by parents, and that at least half of each clinic session is spent in teaching parents how to conduct treatment, to measure their child's stuttering, and in consulting with them about the child's progress. The clinician also reassures the parents that although this may seem to be a big responsibility, the Program uses small steps in teaching parents how to conduct treatment. We find that parents are reassured to hear that we have successfully treated hundreds of children with the Lidcombe Program at the Stuttering Unit, and in each case have been successful in teaching parents to conduct treatment. Basic "rules" of the Lidcombe Program are that 1. the child's enjoyment of therapy activities is a primary concern of the clinician and the parent; 2. any activity that the child reacts to in a negative manner stops immediately; and 3. all components of the Lidcombe Program are applied by parents with flexibility. Each child and family's circumstances contain unique characteristics, and the Program is adapted by the clinician to each family.

Clinical Management

Treatment Goals

The goals of the Lidcombe Program focus on the three participants in the treatment process: the child, the parent, and the clinician. For the child, the goal of the Lidcombe Program is to eliminate stuttering from all speaking situations and maintain this for at least 12 months. For the parent, the goal of the Program is to learn to conduct treatment and measurement activities effectively enough for the child to eliminate stuttering. The clinician's goal, therefore, is to assist parents' learning of the Program's activities.

Treatment Procedures

The Lidcombe Program is based on weekly visits to the speech pathology clinic by the child and a parent. Most often, the mother accompanies the child to the clinic and carries out the treatment procedures at home. In a number of cases, however, the father is the primary care giver, and occasionally, a relative—for example, a grandparent—may agree to take on responsibility for treatment. In such cases the main issues are 1. that the child spends a substantial amount of time each day with this relative so that regular treatment can occur and 2. that the relative is willing and able to attend each clinic visit with the child and learn the Program's treatment and speech measurement activities. Clinic visits are scheduled for 1 hour, although 45-minute visits are common when treatment is progressing smoothly. We schedule preschoolers' clinic visits in mornings or early afternoons when they are likely to be the most alert and cooperative. The child and parent see the same clinician at each clinic visit.

   Weekly clinic visits and daily therapy at home continue until the child's speech meets discharge criteria on a series of measurements of stuttering. As mentioned above, this occurs in a median of 10–11 clinic visits. The child is then placed in a performance-contingent maintenance program designed to assist the child in consolidating and maintaining speech performance. Children are generally in the maintenance program for 10–12 months.

The components of the Lidcombe Program are not applied in the same way throughout the entire treatment process, because of the changes that occur once the Lidcombe Program begins. Routinely, we begin to see a child's stuttering show signs of decreasing within 4 weeks of starting the Program. Concurrent with this improvement, parents show increases in confidence and competence in carrying out treatment activities. Some components of the Program are more prominent during early stages of treatment, while others are more frequently applied during the maintenance program. What follows is a description of the treatment procedures of the Lidcombe Program. Each section describes the role of that component in the Lidcombe Program and explains how that component is applied differently over the time that the child is engaged in the treatment process.

Fostering a Working Relationship

A sound working relationship between the clinician, parent, and child underpins the Lidcombe Program. The clinician explains this to the parent during the first session and subsequently includes many practical activities which reinforce the importance of this three-way relationship. At the beginning of each session the clinician gives the parent the opportunity to raise any number of important events or observations. This is particularly significant in the first treatment session at our clinic, because there is usually a gap of several months between an initial assessment and the start of treatment. This delay is not ideal and reflects an imbalance between the demand for the Unit's services and the number of staff who work there. A child's stuttering may have changed since the assessment, and this needs to be investigated. Parents are able to report on any other changes in the family's circumstances. The clinician responds to such issues with interest and a simple, positive explanation of how this information will be useful, for example, as background information, as an indication that the child's stuttering is becoming more severe, or as a topic to talk about with the child when eliciting a speech sample.

Sometimes parents raise issues that are not directly related to the child or speech therapy, and it is tempting to deflect such questions or comments and return to treatment activities. A preferable approach is to follow the parent's lead, with the aim of finding out why it is so important. A parent who is preoccupied with another issue, whether of major or minor significance, is not likely to make much progress in learning the Lidcombe Program until the issue has been discussed. Our experience is that approximately half of each session is spent with the child, focusing on treatment activities, and the other half is spent talking with the parent. The time talking with parents is spent on any number of topics, primarily those related to the child's speech therapy program, but the clinician also makes sure that time is available for fostering an effective working relationship with the parent.

The clinician gives the parent and child information at each step of the Program. Some parents are reluctant to ask questions during the first few sessions, but this should not deter the clinician from giving a parent explanations of all activities throughout the clinic session. These include telling the parent what will happen next during the session, the reason for changing activities, what is normal behavior for preschool-age children in a clinic, and reinforcement of the parent's comments and questions. The clinician gives the child information about the toys and books available in the clinic, which toys are available to play with, what will happen next during the session, what the tape recorder and speech rating device used in the clinic do; and allows the child, while supervised, to handle equipment that may be unfamiliar. The clinician also responds to the child's questions, engages in conversation, and in all ways treats the child as a full partner in all the activities and conversations that take place.

Beyond-clinic Speech Measures

Parents are taught to collect two speech measures from settings outside the clinic. One is a stutter-count measure and the other is a perceptual rating of the severity of the child's stuttering.[8] The clinician explains that these measures are necessary in addition to within-clinic measures because they provide a more complete and valid picture of the child's stuttering and are needed for measuring the child's response to treatment.

The first speech measure that parents are taught is the simplest—Severity Ratings (SR). These ratings are made on a 10-point scale, where a rating of "1" means "no stutters" and a rating of "10" means "extremely severe stuttering." A parent's use of the scale is affected by familiarity with stuttering. Those parents whose only knowledge of stuttering is their own child may relate a rating of 10 with the most severe stuttering that they have ever heard from their child. A parent with a wider experience or who can imagine more severe stuttering probably uses the scale differently. Although this is a perplexing problem for researchers, the clinical issue is to establish the reliability between the clinician's and parent's ratings for a particular child. The clinician explains to the parent that their reliability will be established over several weeks and requests the parent to rate their child's speech each day and bring the seven SRs to the next clinic visit. The clinician may ask the parent to assign an SR for each entire day or have the parent rate a 10-minute speech sample every day. If the latter method is used, the clinician will request the parent to choose a variety of times and speaking situations to rate across the week so that a representative range of the child's speech is sampled. All the parent needs to do is choose one situation each day and listen to the child for 10 minutes during that situation.

The clinician advises the parent to expect variations in SR from day to day and not to be surprised if variations, that were not previously obvious, are noticed in the child's speech. We find that learning to rate their child's stuttering each day helps parents notice more nuances in their child's stuttering. The SRs also give parents a language to use in describing their child's stuttering and makes it easier to talk about it in a meaningful way.

Parents are introduced to the concept of SRs in the initial treatment session, asked to collect them each day, and bring them to their next clinic visit. At subsequent sessions, the clinician asks the parent for their SRs early in the session. This serves two purposes: First, it makes it clear to the parent how important their beyond-clinic speech measures are in the treatment process, so important, that they are discussed early in the session, and the information they convey is used by the clinician in making decisions about treatment. Second, the clinician relies on the parent's speech measures to convey information about the child's progress. The speech measures are of such significance that the treatment cannot proceed if they are not available. The within-clinic measures of the child's stuttering, collected by the clinician, have only limited value in comparison to those collected by the parent outside the clinic setting.

With the second speech measure, the parent is trained to tape record a 10-minute conversation at home with the child and to count the number of the child's stutters on the recording. Then, parents are taught to use a cumulative stopwatch to determine the time the child speaks on the recording, and finally, to calculate the child's "stutters per minute of speaking time'' (SMST). Parents are taught this procedure in a series of steps over several weeks. The first step simply is for the parent to make the tape recording and bring it to the clinic. This allows the parent to get used to operating the recorder and using it to record a sample with good sound quality. This may take several weeks, but when parents have successfully mastered recording the child's speech, they are asked to count the number of stutters on the next recording. The clinician listens to the recording during the subsequent clinic visit and counts the number of stutters. While listening to this recording, discussion often occurs between the parent and clinician about identifying various types of stuttering, and the listening is repeated until the clinician's and parent's stutter counts agree for the entire sample. The process of learning to calculate SMST continues in small steps like these until the parent is able to do it reliably, with close agreement with the clinician. As each step is mastered successfully, the clinician reinforces the parent's learning by using their measures to help plan subsequent treatment.

Within-clinic Speech Measures

The clinician elicits a speech sample during each clinic session and obtains a %SS measure as the child is talking. The length of the sample commonly is 300 syllables. In cases of quiet or reserved children, however, we limit the sample to the amount of speech the child offers during 10 minutes of conversation. This sample is collected at the beginning of a session, when any therapeutic effects of being in the clinic are minimized. During the earliest clinic sessions, when the child is becoming used to the clinic and the clinician, this sample is not likely to be valid. Its value in these early sessions lies in focusing discussion between the parent and the clinician regarding 1. the type and frequency of stuttering, 2. its overall severity, and 3. comparison of this sample with the child's speech at home. In later sessions, this sample can be expected to reflect the child's everyday speech and is a useful indicator of the child's progress.

The within-clinic speech sample is assessed for %SS by the clinician while the parent and/or clinician talks with the child. The child is encouraged to select a book or toy that is appealing, while the adult engages the child in conversation about the book or toy and elicits spontaneous speech in natural, sentence-length utterances.

Before commenting on the speech sample, the clinician asks the parent to give it a SR. Concurrently, the clinician also gives a rating. In almost every case, our experience is that parent's and clinician's ratings differ by no more than one point. Repeating this procedure at each clinic session allows interjudge reliability to be maintained; that is, the clinician and parent can be confident that they are talking about the same degree of stuttering when they describe the child's speech with a particular SR.

Intrajudge reliability is established by parents giving SRs to sample tapes of their child's speech, and rating them again after a week or two. Reliability is established if ratings of the same samples differ by no more than one point. The clinician can then be confident that the parent uses the SR scale appropriately to describe varying severity levels of their child's stuttering.

After measuring %SS during the child's conversational speech, the clinician then provides the parent with observations of the speech sample. Along with any other features that the clinician notices, comments would routinely be made on 1. the types of stuttering observed, 2. the validity of the sample, 3. the severity of the stutter, and a comparison of this sample with that from the previous clinic session.

Therapy Activities

The therapeutic activities of the Lidcombe Program are presented in two formats: during structured therapy games and "online." Structured therapy games are used when the child's SRs are high, and online therapy is used when SRs indicate that the child's stuttering is mild. Typically, this means that children receive structured therapy during the first weeks of the Lidcombe Program, then move to online feedback as their stuttering reduces. During both structured and online therapy activities, the focus is on praising and rewarding stutter-free speech. Stuttered speech is corrected at times, but much less frequently than the clinician and parent praise of stutter-free speech.

Praise for stutter-free speech is the paramount therapeutic component of the Lidcombe Program. When a child says an utterance which is free of stuttering, the clinician or parent immediately follows with a reinforcing comment that praises the child's speech. Children respond to a variety of comments, but some that are commonly used are "good talking!", "that was smooth!", "well done, nice smooth talking!", and "that sounds great, no bumps!" The comments are made in a positive tone of voice, with a smiling facial expression and enough enthusiasm to make the message clear to the child. Occasionally, however, we come across children who are particularly sensitive about their speech. Children who stutter severely, or who have become highly sensitive to their stuttering, may respond to praise in a negative way. This may be shown by a scowl, drawing back from the other speaker, or a reduced amount of speech. In behavioral terminology, a comment intended as a reinforcement may in fact be a punishment for these children. The solution is to praise these children sparingly, with occasional, nonspecific comments like "that sounds fine," "you're doing well," or "well done."

Parents are taught that stuttered speech can be dealt with in a variety of ways. For the vast majority of times the child stutters, the clinician simply ignores the stutter and responds to the content of the child's speech. On occasions that parents decide that feedback is warranted, they may choose one of the following forms:

1. The parent can wait until the child has finished the stuttered utterance and then repeat it without the stuttering. The child is not expected to respond and the conversation continues as before.

2. The parent comments on the child's stuttered speech in a neutral tone. For example, comments might be "that sounded like a bump there," or "that was a bumpy one." Again, the child is not expected to respond to the comment, but we sometimes find that the child will repeat their utterance without the stutters.

3. The parent waits until the child finishes the stuttered utterance and then asks the child to repeat the stuttered word. An example of this would be when the child says "W-w-w-what's Tim doing with that one?" and the parent asks "Can you say 'what's'?" If the child says "what's" without stuttering, the parent praises this successful attempt. If the child does not want to say the word again, the parent continues the conversation as before. If more than one word was stuttered, we ask the parent to choose only one word to be corrected.

4. The parent interrupts the child's utterance after a stutter occurs and asks the child to fix the stutter. The request for the repair may be direct, but an indirect request is usually effective and less interrupting to the conversation. The example would sound like this:

Child: C–c-c-c-can I go?
Parent: Can I?
Child: Can I go to Tim's house?
Parent: Good one! That was smooth! Yes, you can go to Tim's today.

5. The parent waits for the child to finish talking, then asks the child to correct the stuttered utterance. This form of correction is always presented as a request so that the child has the choice to refuse to repeat the utterance. A request like this is often used: "That was a bit bumpy. Can you try that again?" This form of correction is the least used of those listed here, as we find that children do not like to repeat whole utterances a second time.

For each of these forms of correction, the parent's aim is to help the child fix the stutter and avoid giving the child any impression of being punished. The clinician always models a helpful, encouraging tone of voice for parents. The parents are therefore encouraged to choose forms of correction that will be easily accepted by their child and will assist the child in increasing stutter-free speech. Over the course of treatment, several forms of correction will be used. Typically, the less direct forms of feedback listed above are used early in the Lidcombe Program. More direct feedback tends to be successful later in the Program, when the child has received frequent praise and is confident about producing stutter-free speech.

The clinician demonstrates appropriate therapy responses for the parent during clinic sessions and has the parent conduct therapy in the clinic also. Many parents are embarrassed at first and may need encouragement to begin. It is important to persist in getting even the most reluctant parent to demonstrate their therapy skills in the clinic, because it is essential for the clinician to know how the parent conducts treatment activities. Therapy conducted by the clinician and parent in the clinic is largely for the purpose of teaching the parent skills that they can apply in daily therapy at home. The therapeutic effect for the child of 20–30 minutes of within-clinic therapy once a week is likely to be negligible.

Structured therapy sessions or therapy games are carried out by the parent with the child, for 10–15 minutes, once or twice each day. The parent chooses a quiet setting away from distractions, and a time when the child is alert. Therapy materials are several books or toys that the child enjoys and a token reward. The aim is for the parent to elicit stutter-free utterances from the child, which are then praised with such comments as "good talking!" or "that was smooth!" In early therapy sessions, the child may only be consistently successful in producing stutter-free, single-syllable words. During each therapy game the parent's aim is to assist the child in being stutter-free for the entire game. When the game finishes, the child resumes natural conversational speech, and stuttering returns to its pre-therapy level. The clinician warns parents to expect this and not to be surprised that there is no immediate generalization from the game to the child's natural speech. At this early stage in the treatment process, SRs do not change.

As therapy games continue day by day, parents are taught to look for and reinforce longer stutter-free utterances that will start to occur during therapy games. They respond to the child's increasing length of stutter-free speech by increasing the length of the child's responses during the games. As children build up more and longer stutter-free utterances during therapy games, they become more confident in their new skill. Generalization begins to occur, and parents see this reflected in a change in the pattern of the child's SRs. The first change noticed with many children is a *decrease in the variability of their SRs from day to day*. The next change often is a *gradual decrease in SRs*, which indicates that generalization of stutter-free speech is taking place. The stutter-free speech that the child is practicing each day during therapy games is starting to carry over into their everyday speech *outside* therapy games.

Self-evaluation of stutter-free speech can be added to the treatment process at any stage. It is particularly useful in aiding generalization of stutter-free speech from therapy games into everyday conversation. The simplest way to introduce self-evaluation to a preschool-age child is during a structured therapy game. After praising several consecutive stutter-free responses the clinician, rather than giving praise, asks the child "Was that smooth?" The clinician asks this with a positive intonation and a smiling, expectant facial expression. The aim is to make it clear to the child that the response was smooth, and that the expected answer is "yes." The clinician then agrees with the child and adds praise for the stutter-free utterance. An example of this could be "Yes, I think it was smooth too. Good talking!"

When a child's SRs are down to 4, we expect to see many short, stutter-free utterances in everyday speech. The clinician prompts parents to be alert to this and notice the stutter-free utterances as they occur. This is also the stage of the Lidcombe Program when the clinician introduces parents to the second therapy format: online therapy. The parent is taught to praise spontaneous, stutter-free utterances as they occur—hence it is called "online" therapy. As a child increases stutter-free speech, there is a consequent increase in praise. The parent continues to also conduct daily structured therapy games, using praise for stutter-free speech and assisting the child to correct stuttered utterances.

Online correction of stutters is introduced 1 or 2 weeks later, or when the clinician and parent are confident that the child's stutter-free speech skills are robust. Online correction of stutters is introduced to the child during a clinic session, so that the child's reactions can be monitored by the clinician and parent together. If a child seems particularly sensitive to online correction of stutters, treatment can continue with online praise alone, but progress is likely to be slower.

Another change that commonly occurs around this stage of treatment is for children to self-correct stuttering. The child stutters, then pauses briefly and repeats the word fluently before continuing. Not all children will do this, but in our experience, if they do it is an indicator of a good prognosis. We do not teach preschool-age children to self-correct, as to do so would mean excessive focus on their stuttering. Rather than teaching a child deliberately to become self-conscious about stuttering, we prefer that, if anything, they become aware of how to produce effortless, stutter-free speech. The clinician monitors each child's speech for self-correction of stutters during clinic sessions and asks the parents if any instances have been noticed at home. If a child self-corrects a stutter, then the clinician and/or parent will wait until the child has finished their utterance, and then praise the child with specific feedback . Examples of praise would be "Well done, you fixed up your bumpy word!," or "Great talking, you smoothed out a bumpy word by yourself!"

As a child's SRs continue to decrease, the frequency of structured therapy games is decreased. Most commonly, parents are asked to drop one therapy game per week, so that after 7 weeks, all of the child's treatment is online therapy. This involves a mixture of praise and correction, and parents are taught to aim for a ratio of 10 praises for each correction of stuttering.

Weekly clinic visits and daily home therapy continue until the clinician and parent agree that the child's speech meets their preset criteria over 3 consecutive weeks. These criteria are based on speech measures made both within and outside the clinic. In the Stuttering Unit, the following criteria are currently used: 1. %SS less than 1.0 within the clinic, 2. SR average less than 2.0 outside the clinic, and 3. fewer than 1.5 SMST outside the clinic.

It is a complex task to learn to conduct the therapy activities of the Lidcombe Program and successfully apply them to eliminate stuttering from a preschool-age child's speech. Parents learn these skills gradually, and the clinician's role, primarily, is to assist the parent in attaining these skills.

Maintenance

Once the child's speech goals are achieved, a maintenance program is begun. The aim of the maintenance program is for parents gradually to withdraw all treatment activities, while children maintain their stutter-free speech. The maintenance program consists of a series of half-hour clinic visits which gradually decrease in frequency across the next 12 months. The clinician can vary the schedule of frequency for clinic visits, and the speech outcome criteria according to a child's individual needs; however, we routinely use the following schedule of clinic visits, which are based on a procedure developed by Ingham.[9] The first two visits are 2 weeks apart, then 4 weeks, 4 weeks, 8 weeks, 8 weeks, and 16 weeks. Of course, this is not the only schedule possible, but whatever schedule is decided on, it is set by the parent and clinician, and can be shorter or longer as they decide is necessary for the child. The child's progress through this schedule of maintenance visits is contingent on passing preset speech criteria at each clinic visit. These criteria are the same as those set for the child's entry into the maintenance program: 1. %SS less than 1 within the clinic, 2. SR average less than 2.0 outside the clinic, and 3. less than 1.5 SMST outside the clinic. The within-clinic speech sample is collected during the clinic visit during a conversation between the child and the clinician or parent. The beyond-clinic speech measures are collected by the parent during the week before the scheduled clinic visit.

In cases where a child is unable to meet the criteria, the clinician recommends that suitable treatment activities are increased or recommenced, if necessary, at home. The child stays on the same stage of the maintenance program until either speech criteria are achieved or the clinician and parent agree to return the child to weekly clinic visits and further regular treatment.

Treatment Outcomes

The expected outcomes of the Lidcombe Program are effortless stutter-free speech by the child in all situations at all times. We expect that by the time children are discharged from the maintenance program, they will have only a hazy memory of ever having stuttered. Their most enduring memory seems to be their favorite toys and games in the clinic and the stickers and stamps with which they were rewarded. A further outcome of the Lidcombe Program is one that we did not expect but has been reported by many parents. They report that their child has become a confident speaker, an enthusiastic participant in conversations at preschool, and willing to talk with older children and adults.

Our various scientific reports have presented data in support of the effectiveness of this treatment. The Onslow, Costa, and Rue[5] report incorporated objective speech data for four children, collected in everyday childhood speaking situations, and it spanned more than 12 months. In a subsequent randomized clinical trial, that preliminary report was substantiated using a larger group of subjects.[4] The preschool children in that report showed near-zero stuttering, in everyday speaking situations, during a 12-month posttreatment period. A similar result was obtained with school-age children.[6] A subsequent publication showed that preschoolers who received the Lidcombe Program were not stuttering up to 7 years after treatment,[2] and Lincoln, Onslow, and Reed[3] showed that the speech of our treated children was perceptually indistinguishable from that of matched controls. At the time of this writing, objective, scientific treatment outcome data have been reported for 61 children, all of whom have achieved zero or near-zero stuttering for clinically significant periods. Those scientific data are accompanied by hundreds of cases that we have treated successfully at the Stuttering Unit.

Final Comments

The Lidcombe Program has proved to be an effective treatment for stuttering in preschool-age children. We are confident of its effectiveness, based on results of our clinical research and our extensive experience in applying the Program to preschool-age children. This confidence is reflected also in the widespread use of the Lidcombe Program in speech pathology clinics throughout Australia. This chapter has described the way we use the Lidcombe Program at present, but we can only speculate on how we will conduct it in the future. Research and development of a "distance" version of the Lidcombe Program is now under way. This project is necessary because of the many Australian children who stutter but live in remote rural communities with limited access to health services. The project is determining methods by which such children can receive effective treatment. Another project is exploring aspects of the presentation of the treatment to groups of parents and children. Is it possible to eliminate components of the Program while maintaining its effectiveness? What are its most critical features? These are questions without answers as yet, but we are working on them in the hope of refining a procedure that has been shown to leave preschool-age children free of stuttering.

Suggested Readings

Martin RR, Kuhl P, Haroldson S: An experimental treatment with two preschool stuttering children. *J Speech Hear Res* 1972; 15:743–752.
   This extraordinarily creative laboratory experiment was the first to show that preschool children's stuttering might be controlled by verbal contingencies from adults, in a format that children would enjoy. It was our inspiration to develop the Lidcombe Program.
Onslow M: *Behavioral Management of Stuttering.* San Diego, CA, Singular Publishing Group, 1996.
   One of the things attempted in this book is to put the development of the Lidcombe Program into a historical perspective of how early stuttering has been managed during the past decades.
Onslow M, Packman A: Behavioral Treatment of Stuttering in Adults: Designing a Management Strategy, in Curlee RF, Siegel GM (eds): *Nature and Treatment of Stuttering: New Directions* (2nd ed). Boston, Allyn and Bacon, 1997.
   This chapter describes our treatment approaches for adults who stutter. It may be of interest because it highlights the contrasts between managing preschool children and managing adults.

References

1. Attanasio J, Onslow M, Packman A, Menzies R: Australian and American perspectives on early stuttering. *Australian J Human Communication Dis* 1996; 24:55–61.

2. Lincoln M, Onslow M: Long-term outcome of an early intervention for stuttering. *American J Speech–Language Pathol* 1997; 6:51–58.
3. Lincoln M, Onslow M, Reed V: Social validity of an early intervention for stuttering: The Lidcombe Program. *American J Speech–Language Pathol* 1997; 6:77–84.
4. Onslow M, Andrews C, Lincoln M: A control/experimental trial of an operant treatment for early stuttering. *J Speech Hear Res* 1994; 37:1244–1259.
5. Onslow M, Costa L, Rue S: Direct early intervention with stuttering: Some preliminary data. *J Speech Hear Dis* 1990; 55:405–416.
6. Lincoln M, Onslow M, Wilson L, Lewis C: A clinical trial of an operant treatment for school-age stuttering children. *American J Speech–Language Pathol* 1996; 5:73–85.
7. Packman A, Lincoln M: Early stuttering and the Vmodel. *Australian J Human Communication Dis* 1996; 24:45–54.
8. Onslow M, Andrews C, Costa L: Parental severity scaling of early stuttered speech: Four case studies. *Australian J Human Communication Dis* 1990; 18:47–61.
9. Ingham RJ: Modification of maintenance and generalization during stuttering treatment. *J Speech Hear Res* 1980; 23:732–745.

Stuttering and Related Disorders of Fluency, 2nd edition.
Edited by Richard F. Curlee, Ph.D.
Thieme Medical Publishers, Inc., New York © 1999.

5

Behavioral Treatment of Young Children Who Stutter: An Extended Length of Utterance Method

Janis Costello Ingham

The assessment and treatment of children who stutter have been controversial topics for decades, although behavioral approaches have become increasingly popular and accepted over the years. This may be because these are the techniques that stem most directly from known principles of human behavior and are supported most clearly by evidence obtained in laboratory and field experiments. Behavioral techniques require clinicians to rely primarily on observable phenomena in children's behavior and resist making diagnostic and treatment decisions based on speculation or intuition. What follows is a description of a method of assessment and treatment evaluated in a recent program of research[1] and used for many years in our clinic with children (aged 2–9 or so) who stutter. The treatment is referred to as Extended Length of Utterance (ELU) and is based upon behavioral principles and a combination of techniques gleaned from the experimental literature and from clinical experience.

Clinical Evaluation

In this system the purpose of clinical evaluation is threefold: 1. to make a judgment of whether the child is a stutterer, 2. to determine the need for treatment, and 3. to specify and systematically measure relevant characteristics of the child's speech to serve as a baseline against which to compare future measures.

Case History

For this kind of assessment, traditional case history information has rather limited value for the diagnosis of stuttering. Such diagnosis is based primarily on observation of the child's speech behaviors. Although information regarding the topographies of early moments of stuttering, the nature of the onset of a child's stuttering, birth history, etc., are interesting, such information does not necessarily lead to differential diagnosis of stuttering versus normal nonfluency, nor is it currently useful in predicting in which children's stuttering is likely to remit without treatment. One exception to this position is information regarding family history of stuttering. When children have immediate family members who are or have been stutterers, the possibility that those children's nonfluencies may be stutterings is enhanced.[2] However, a family history of stuttering does not appear to be particularly useful in predicting a child's ultimate response to treatment. For example, in a recent case of 3½-year-old monozygotic twin girls, stuttering resolved without treatment for one and with treatment for the other.

Other information of value sought from parents during the diagnostic interview relates to whether they consider their child to be a stutterer and, if so, how long the child's stuttering has existed. Children who have been stuttering for less that 6 months are not generally enrolled for treatment unless their stuttering is unusually severe. The parents' report of their children's reactions to their nonfluencies is also informative. Descriptions of children's expressions of frustration, anger, or bewilderment regarding why words cannot be produced at certain times, or reports of children being unwilling to attempt speech in certain circumstances, are influential in establishing the existence of stuttering and the need for treatment.

A primary function of taking a case history is that it provides an opportunity for parents to air their feelings and fears regarding their children's speech. Many parents have heard the folklore that suggests that something in their interactions with their child is responsible for stuttering.[3] Or perhaps they have their own theory of the cause of stuttering for their child, and they want to have the chance to discuss their ideas with an expert. The interview connected with obtaining case history information affords the opportunity for parents to express these notions and for clinicians to allay parents' fears with assurances that no evidence exists to support parental responsibility as a cause of stuttering,[4] to update them on recent theories and relevant research regarding potential etiologies of stuttering, and inform them of the success rates associated with treatment of stuttering in young children. During this interview, as well, the parents' role in treatment is discussed. This is a chance to ascertain whether parents are responsive to participating in their child's treatment.

Observation and Tests

STANDARD ASSESSMENT BATTERY

A child's suspected fluency disorder must not be allowed to distract the clinician from assessing whether other communication disorders exist. In fact, there is some evidence to suggest that a substantial number of stuttering children are prone to display other concomitant communication problems.[5] Therefore, standard evaluation procedures for the presence of hearing, language, phonology, and voice disorders are always employed. If such problems exist at a clinically significant level, and the child is also determined to stutter, the clinician must decide whether to design treatment that addresses those problems concurrently or concentrate on the constituent that appears most fundamental to the child's aberrant communicative status. An *articulation* problem is the most common disorder that appears with stuttering. Although much has been written about concurrent treatment of the two disorders,[6,7] no convincing evidence for the viability of such treatment exists. In terms of the ELU treatment to be described below (see Appendix A), some minimum level of *language* proficiency is needed because the treatment depends on connected speech utterances of increasing length. This does not, however, negate the possibility of using this treatment with children who have auditory processing, word-finding, or syntax problems. In fact, because the spontaneous production of conversational language is basic to this treatment, some children's language skills may be anticipated to improve along with their fluency.

As mentioned above, in the diagnostic process of discovering and describing stuttering, the most critical information is obtained from direct observation of the child's speech and the analyses that are drawn from those observations. This process extends over a substantial time period so that the chance of observing all variations in the child's speech is enhanced. Sets of audio and/or video-recorded Standard Talking Samples (STSs) are obtained from each child.[8,9,10] These are conversational speech samples recorded in multiple settings with different speaking partners representative of common speaking situations for the child. Each is generally 10–15 minutes in length. (The goal is to obtain 500 syllables of child speech from each sample.) A typical set of STSs might be 1. conversation in the clinic with the clinician, 2. conversation in the clinic with one parent, 3. oral reading in the clinic or at home (for older children), 4. conversation at home with the other parent, or a grandparent, and 5. conversation at home with a sibling or at school with a peer. It is important that at least two of these samples are obtained in natural settings outside of the clinic. The more beyond-clinic samples obtained, the better. (Such beyond-clinic recordings are one example of responsibilities parents are expected to undertake.) Our research[1,10] has indicated that making these recordings once per month for a period of at least 3 months prior to making decisions regarding treatment is useful for discovering the full range of variability inherent in a child's stuttering. An example of the kind of data obtained from such samples is contained in Figure 5-1. The data reported in this figure show the pretreatment frequency of stuttering (percent syllables stuttered, see below) in STSs obtained monthly over an 11-month period for BD, a male aged 5 years 10 months, at the time of the first measurement. Five different conversation samples were obtained on each occasion: A = in clinic with mother, B = in clinic with clinician, C = at home with mother, D = at home with father, E = with 10-year-old female cousin at her home. For purposes of illustration, consider for the moment only the data reported for the first four measurement occasions (B1–B4), the length of a typical baseline period. These data illustrate the variability for which stuttering is (in)famous. If data had been obtained on only one of these occasions or with only one of these conversation partners, which is the typical case when stuttering is assessed via one in-clinic conversation with a clinician, then an inadequate picture of the severity and inconsistency of BD's stuttering would have been obtained. Imagine that the one sample utilized to characterize BD's pretreatment level of stuttering produced data similar to Sample B at baseline 1 (11% SS) and then, following treatment, a subsequent talking sample produced data similar to Sample B at baseline 3 (3% SS). The clinician could wrongly conclude that treatment had produced a 73% decrease in stuttering because she would have no way of knowing that that range of stuttering frequency existed in BD's repertoire *prior to treatment*. In order to be considered effective, treatment for BD should produce stuttering levels considerably below 2% SS, the lowest level that occurred during this baseline period. Thus the assessment procedures that help determine whether a child is a stutterer in the first place also serve as baseline against which to measure behavior change for those children enrolled in treatment.

Another benefit of obtaining a pretreatment profile of a child's stuttering in this fashion is obvious in BD's data. This procedure allows for the occurrence and documentation of

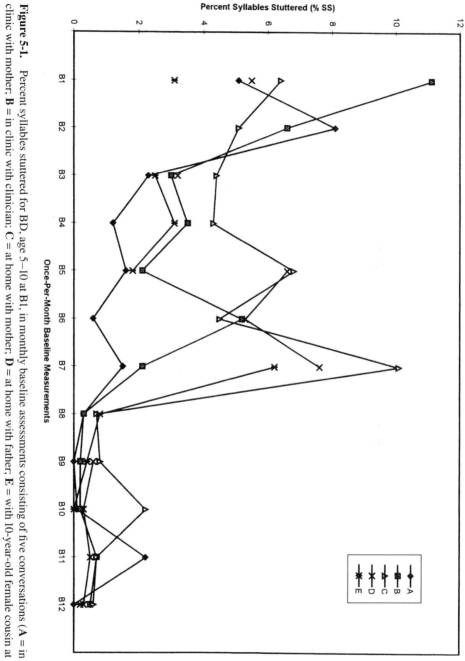

Figure 5-1. Percent syllables stuttered for BD, age 5–10 at B1, in monthly baseline assessments consisting of five conversations (**A** = in clinic with mother; **B** = in clinic with clinician; **C** = at home with mother; **D** = at home with father; **E** = with 10-year-old female cousin at her home.

untreated recovery. In fact, BD's baseline period was not considered completed at the end of 3 months because stuttering appeared to be decreasing. Therefore, treatment was withheld, and monthly measurements were maintained in order to observe whether stuttering continued to decline. Figure 5-1 illustrates that large fluctuations continued until B8 (i.e., across a 7-month period), and then stuttering frequency and variability decreased until, at the end of 11 months, BD was essentially stutter-free, *without treatment*. Had the course of pretreatment measurement been less lengthy than the predetermined 3-month period, then the opportunity to observe this untreated recovery would likely not have occurred, and BD would have been enrolled in treatment unnecessarily. Such "spontaneous recovery" is not uncommon among young children who stutter.[11] Although recent longitudinal research by Yairi and colleagues[12] is beginning to show some significant statistical relationships between certain variables and the persistence (or otherwise) of stuttering, these correlations do not yet appear strong enough to allow a clinician to predict the likelihood of untreated recovery *for a given child*. A safer bet is to make such judgments based on direct evidence produced by the particular child, as illustrated in Figure 5-1.

ANALYSES OF STANDARD TALKING SAMPLES

A number of relevant aspects of children's speech can be empirically evaluated from the STSs. Further, each can be compared across samples for a given measurement occasion as well as across time for the 3-month evaluation period. Thus, a representation of the full range of variability can be observed. The dimensions of speech that are most basic to this analysis are: frequency of stuttering, speech rate, and speech naturalness. Other measures that may be useful are the duration of typical and outlying stutterings and the duration of typical and outlying stutter-free utterances.

Frequency of Stuttering.   The occurrence of stuttering is, of course, the primary behavior of interest in determining whether a child is a stutterer and in gauging the severity of the disorder; however, measuring this phenomenon is not as straightforward as one might hope. To determine whether a child is, in fact, a stutterer, the occurrence of even only one genuine moment of stuttering ought to be sufficient. To gauge the severity of the disorder and provide objective evidence of the status of stuttering prior to treatment (and thereafter), more particular information is required. Still, both of these goals require the examiner to be able to recognize essentially every occurrence of a stutter in the speech of a child. Herein lies the rub!

Distinguishing between nonfluencies that are normal and nonfluencies that are stuttered requires perceptual judgments on the part of the listener, and currently there is no independent way to validate the correctness of those judgments. While many nonfluencies are obvious to listeners as unusual or pathological, some nonfluencies, especially those occurring in the speech of potential incipient stutterers, may be equivocal. Some researchers have attempted to differentiate nonstuttered and stuttered nonfluencies on the basis of topography (e.g., phrase repetitions and revisions versus silent and audible part-word repetitions and prolongations, respectively);[13] others have trusted the validity of the practiced listener's "perceptual threshold" for discerning which nonfluencies are stutters and which are normal disfluencies.[14] Neither method has produced satisfactory agreement among different listeners, especially when attempts are made to evaluate agreement for *each* identified moment of stuttering.[15,16]

For STS analysis purposes, the latter method is preferred. Assisted by a computerized program, the Stuttering Treatment Rating Recorder (STRR),[17] the clinician listens to the child's speech sample (e.g., the STSs) and presses the right mouse button whenever the child is judged to stutter. The button is pressed once for each new occasion of stuttering, independent of its duration. Nonstuttered syllables are indicated by left mouse button presses. The computer program converts these counts into the percentage of syllables spoken that are stuttered (%SS). No attempt is made to designate particular topographies of nonfluencies as stuttered or not stuttered; that is, clinicians do not follow *a priori* definitions of stuttering and count only those forms of speech as occurrences of stuttering. Rather, they listen to the child's speech and signal (by the button press) any event that surpasses their perceptual threshold of normalcy. They keep in mind that some nonfluencies are normal and attempt to disregard those in their counts. The computer records the number of stutters (and percentage of syllables stuttered) that are judged to occur in a particular sample.*

Reliability of Judgments of Stutterings.   Using the above-described method, it is important that clinicians assess their *self-agreement*. The value of counts of stuttering is negated if those counts are not reliable. Therefore, recounting stutter events in randomly selected speech samples and comparing second counts with the first is an important method for verifying the caliber of the data collected. (Calculation of total percent agreement is adequate for these purposes: smaller total count ÷ larger total count × 100.) Clinicians who cannot agree with themselves at a minimum level of 80% need self-training and practice until they have established consistency. Consistent identification of moments of stuttering will also be important for the clinician during treatment activities. Unfortunately, training programs that teach the skill of reliable identification of stutters are not currently available (although such a program is in the early stages of preparation in our laboratory).

At certain points in the use of a measurement system such as that described above, assessment of *interjudge* agreement is also pertinent; that is, clinicians should confirm their judgments of stuttering by asking other listeners to make the same judgments on at least some of the same samples. Certainly before the child is formally diagnosed as a stutterer, corroborating judgments of another experienced speech–language clinician should be obtained. Such confirmation is appropriate, as well, when decisions regarding termination of treatment are made.

Speech Rate.   The speed of a child's speech is important to assess for a variety of reasons. First, of course, the clinician would like to know whether the child's speech rate is within normal ranges. The presence of stuttering typically slows down overall speech rate (e.g., the number of syllables produced per minute of speaking time); therefore, increases in speech rate are to be expected as one by-product of successful treatment. Some children (and many adults) who stutter actually speak at unusually fast speaking rates. If this is recognized, then treatment directed toward speech rate modification alone may lead to reductions in stuttering. Because of the presence of stuttering, fast speaking rates are sometimes difficult to identify unless speaking rate measures are obtained exclusively from

---

*This program, in PC configuration, is available from the author. In the near future it will include additions that allow the listener to record duration of individual moments of stuttering and the occurrence or nonoccurrence of stuttering in speaking intervals of various lengths,[18] calculate reliability according to interval-by-interval agreement, and extract speech rate from stutter-free-only intervals of speech. Contact author for further information.

periods of speech that do not contain stutterings. This *articulatory rate* can be highly informative. Another reason to measure speech rate is to ascertain whether differences in stuttering frequency across different samples (i.e., in different settings or in comparisons of pre- and posttreatment speech samples) might be artifacts of abnormal reductions in speech rate rather than "real" changes in fluency.

Speech rate is measured with the STRR, as described above. At the end of the speech sample, the computer calculates overall speaking rate: the average number of syllables spoken per minute of child talking time (SPM, indicated by left [stuttered syllable] + right [nonstuttered syllable] mouse button presses).

Speech Naturalness. Stuttering frequency and speech rate have become relatively common, utilitarian measures of the speech performance of people who stutter; however, clinicians and researchers have struggled to find a method to assess empirically the rather global aspect of speech production referred to as speech quality or speech naturalness. For example, two stutterers who are similar in regard to %SS and SPM still may not be perceived as equally impaired. In spite of occurrences of stuttering, one may speak in a style that listeners judge to be relatively natural, while the other may sound highly unnatural. Likewise, at the end of treatment two stutterers may display no stuttering and speech rate within normal ranges, but sound quite different in regard to the naturalness of their speech. The speech of one may be perceived as tentative, uneven, prolonged, calculated, while the speech of the other may sound highly natural, spontaneous, and essentially indistinguishable from normal. The speech naturalness measure described by Martin, Haroldson, and Triden,[19] and now in frequent use in the literature, has been shown to be a valid and reliable indicator of this heretofore unmeasured aspect of speech production (although, interestingly, naturalness ratings for children's speech have been reported in the literature only infrequently).[20]

Using the STRR the computer keeps track of the clinician's periodic ratings of naturalness. After every 15 seconds of child speaking time has elapsed, a signal sounds. At this time the clinician rates the perceived naturalness of the child's speech for the preceding 15 seconds by touching the appropriate number between 1 and 9 on the computer keyboard. Ratings of "1" indicate the child's speech was perceived to be "highly natural"; ratings of "9" indicate the child's speech was perceived to be "highly unnatural." Research using this system with adult speakers indicates the speech of normal speakers is typically rated between "1" and "3."[19,21]*

Other Measures. For the child whose speech is judged in need of treatment, two other analyses made from the STSs are useful: durations of stutterings, and durations of stutter-free utterances (see footnote p. 85). One of the first changes apparent during treatment is typically a reduction in the duration of individual moments of stuttering, especially because the accessory feature components (ancillary facial and body movements, avoidance mechanisms, etc.) are virtually eliminated early on. This change in behavior is not necessarily reflected in %SS data, but it is revealed in measures of 1. the durations of the three longest stutters in a sample and 2. the average duration of stutters in the sample (based on a random sampling of a minimum of 10 stutters). Consideration of such stutter duration measures adds empirical information to the picture of the overall severity of a child's stuttering. Such

---

*Even when completely stutter-free, some children's speech does not achieve complete naturalness due to remaining voice, language, or phonologic disorders.

measures are also extremely potent in the evaluation of change produced by treatment (i.e., in pretreatment–posttreatment STS comparisons).*

Most of the speech sample analyses described thus far emphasize, directly or indirectly, stuttered nonfluencies; however, the aspects of the child's speech that are of primary interest during treatment are utterances that are stutter-free. For this reason, empirical information regarding the status of stutter-free utterances in a child's pretreatment speech is beneficial for treatment planning and assessment of the progress of treatment. Therefore, from representative STSs, clinicians tally the lengths of 10 stutter-free periods (i.e., the number of syllables and speaking time that occur between moments of stuttering) and then summarize the findings by reporting the average length of stutter-free speaking periods and the length of the longest stutter-free periods in the sample (see footnote p. 85).

Summary.   It is obvious from the substantial number of pages allocated to this section that diagnosis of stuttering and the treatment that ensues are predicated on thorough and detailed assessment procedures. The variability that may exist in the child's speech is examined through multiple speech samples obtained over time in a variety of settings with different pertinent speaking partners. Empirical descriptions of those speech samples are made, providing quantitative measurement of the dimensions of speech considered most relevant: frequency of stuttering, speech rate, speech naturalness, durations of stutters, and durations of stutter-free utterances. This evidence serves as the basis for the decision of whether the child is a stutterer, and this "objective" finding is bolstered by the more impressionistic judgments of parents, relatives, and teachers. Further, for the child who is diagnosed as one who stutters, these measures provide baseline data for the treatment that will follow: a base against which to compare the child's speech performance during, and at the termination of, treatment.

Case Selection Criteria

For a child whose speech characteristics cannot reliably be judged as stuttering, the continuation of monthly STSs (monitoring, or "watch and wait") will eventually establish the child's fluency status. If the child is, or becomes, one who stutters, moments of stuttering will become more consistent across settings and time and easier for the examiner to identify reliably. And, if periodic monitoring is carried out often enough, the child will be identified and enrolled in treatment soon enough to minimize negative effects on the child's social development. Further, an important finding of our recent research[1] is that *stuttering becomes more entrenched and more difficult to modify rather early in its development: past age 6 or so. This makes early identification and treatment imperative.* Therefore, any child who is reported by parents to have stuttered for at least 6 months and whose STS 3-month baseline indicates stuttering consistently above 3%SS becomes a candidate for immediate treatment.

Clinical Management

A review of the literature related to treatment of children who stutter[23] indicates that direct, behavioral treatments, even for preschool-aged children, have become acceptable and, in

---

*Although precise, reliable measurement of stutter durations is quite difficult to achieve,[22] a clinician's abilities in this realm are adequate for these general measurement purposes.

fact, popular. This may be because once tried, their effectiveness is obvious and their harm, fictional. The particular approaches to behavioral treatment advocated by this author have been described previously[23-28] and will be updated and detailed with greater specificity in the pages that follow. Through the years, the fundamental principles of this treatment have remained unchanged. The procedures rely on 1. arranging extensive talking opportunities for the child, and using these to facilitate fluent and progressively more realistic speaking experiences; 2. objectively recording relevant observable features of the child's behavior (the moments of stuttering, stutter-free utterances, speech rate, and speech naturalness, as described above), and using these records to continually evaluate the progress of treatment; 3. developing a functional feedback system, and using it to decrease the frequency of stuttering and enhance reciprocal, stutter-free speech; and 4. assessing the generalization and maintenance of fluency change in the child's speech in the natural environment, and using this information to modify treatment procedures when necessary to produce clinically significant treatment efficacy.

Treatment Goal

The goal of this treatment is to facilitate children's spontaneous and automatic use of natural-sounding, stutter-free speech under all talking conditions, in all settings, with all speaking partners and audiences. *Spontaneous and automatic* means that the speech used by the child at the termination of treatment should not require special attention or effort on the child's part. *Natural-sounding stutter-free speech* refers to speech that is indistinguishable from that of a child's nonstuttering peers. In other words, the goal of this treatment is that its beneficiaries become normal speakers.

Treatment Procedures

The specific treatment method to be described, Extended Length of Utterance (ELU),[24,28] is based on the principles listed above and elucidated further below. Its forebear is Ryan's "gradual increase in length and complexity of utterance" (GILCU).[29] This treatment method is able to be individualized so that it suits the speech characteristics and personalities of essentially all children served. It is driven by continuous evaluation of its effects, so that unsuccessful treatment components can be modified midstream.

SPEAKING TASKS

Behavioral treatments gain their label by concentrating treatment directly on child speaking behaviors considered to be "correct" and "incorrect." In the case of children who stutter, correct behaviors are periods of speech that do not contain stuttering, and incorrect behaviors are moments of stuttering. Obviously, the occurrence of these two response classes cannot be observed or modified unless the child is talking. Therefore, an important aspect of behavioral treatments is the use of activities that will generate lots of speech from the child. (For some children who may be particularly reticent or even uncooperative, treatment might begin with procedures aimed exclusively at encouraging responsiveness and talking, fluent or otherwise.)

The ELU treatment method, which is appropriate for most children from age 3½ to 6 or 7, requires speech tasks that allow the clinician to control the length and complexity of children's utterances. By first building a foundation of short, simple, stutter-free utterances, children's fluency can be expanded gradually by facilitating stutter-free utterances that are progressively longer. The length of children's utterances can be controlled by the presentation of pictures, or sentence or conversation topics, and/or written stimuli that are designed to evoke responses of the desired length. Broadly, the bulk of treatment is conducted during children's spontaneous connected speech, although treatment begins with shorter, nonconversational utterances. Monologue speaking tasks are used early in treatment because they afford children the opportunity to produce a lot of speech without having to deal with the pragmatic, interactive components of dyadic language use, such as responding to questions, taking turns, coping with interruptions, and producing utterances that are responsive to themes introduced by the conversational partner. However, the use of connected conversational speech is incorporated into later stages of the program because that is the style of speech used in the natural environment, and thus the style of speech children must practice under treatment conditions. It is also the most difficult style of speech for most children who stutter, so when they have mastered it, they are typically able to speak fluently in monologue and reading, even if they have not had direct treatment in those modalities.*

Summary.   The first step in treatment is the selection of speaking activities that meet the response length requirements of the treatment program, are within the capabilities of the child, and will sustain the child's efforts to speak so that the treatment can be applied. Speech–language pathologists are typically highly skilled at developing creative and interesting methods for getting children to talk,† so this aspect of treatment presents nothing particularly new to the practicing clinician, except, perhaps, the emphasis that is placed on it in this treatment. A general rule of treatment is that the more talking produced by the child, the more likely, and the more quickly, the treatment will be effective.

MEASUREMENT

Within-treatment Measurement.   Data collection during treatment is inherent in the ELU method and begins with the specification of target behaviors; that is, the clinician must identify observable behaviors in a given child's speech that are to be the targets of treatment: stutters (to be reduced or eliminated) and occasions of stutter-free speech (to be increased). The previous discussion of clinicians' perceptual judgments of stutters is pertinent here as well. Treatment depends upon the clinician's skill in immediately discriminating all occasions of stuttering in the child's speech. Although occasions of stutter-free speech are targeted as well, the clinician's recognition of such occasions hinges upon recognition of stutterings, because stutter-free speech is just that: speech that does not contain stuttering. The unit of stutter-free speech that is targeted at different steps of the treatment is defined by its duration in syllables or length of talking time.

ELU treatment adheres to the principles of programmed instruction,[30] in which target behavior requirements are increased slowly and in small steps. For example, early steps require stutter-free production of utterances that are 1, then 2, then 3 syllables in length, and

---

*For older children who can read and whose stuttering may be more severe in spontaneous speech than in reading, ELU treatment can be introduced via reading. Precise control over the length of utterance is made simpler by reading tasks, but generalization does not usually flow from reading to connected speech, so it is important to move to treatment spontaneous speech as early as possible. On the other hand, it is not unusual for stutter-free speech gained during spontaneous speech tasks to generalize to oral reading.

†This statement reminds me of the T-shirt designed by UC Santa Barbara NSSLHA students some years ago which read, "Speech pathologists have *ways* of making you talk!"

later the requirement becomes stutter-free utterances that are 3, 5, and 10 seconds in length, until late in the program when stutter-free responses of 3, 4, and 5 minutes are required.

Programmed instruction also stipulates mastery of each step as a prerequisite to advancement to the next step. Mastery is operationalized by specifying a minimum level of performance required at each treatment step. For example, in the ELU program, mastery of step 14 (3-min stutter-free monologue) requires that response to be produced five times, consecutively. Specification of such a "pass criterion" is made on the assumption that children's successful performance is predicated on achievement of simpler, related skills that are established as a base upon which to build the next level of behavior. Many behavioral treatments also specify "fail criteria," the level at which a child's performance on a given step of the program is deemed unsatisfactory, and change in the treatment program is sought so that the child is not forced to continue to fail. In the ELU program, for example, the fail criterion for step 14 is seven consecutive trials containing stuttering or 50 attempts to produce the specified stutter-free behavior without meeting the pass criterion.*

In order to ascertain when a child has met the pass criterion (or fallen to the level of the fail criterion) for a given treatment step, performance data must be obtained on-line during treatment. This means that the clinician scores each trial as correct or incorrect on a data sheet so that it is possible to notice when either criterion has been reached. This simple kind of event recording also allows calculation of number of trials required to meet criterion and percentage of correct trials for each step of the program. These numbers are useful reflections of the ease with which children progress through their treatment, and also highlight program steps that are too difficult (and therefore might be revised before the program is used with another child).

Beyond-treatment Measurement.   The first section of this chapter described measurement procedures used during the pretreatment assessment period, especially data collected from periodic STSs. STSs are continued throughout the duration of children's treatment (about once monthly) and follow-up (at progressively longer intervals) in a time-series fashion. Thus, information regarding the quality of the child's speech in the absence of treatment, within and beyond the confines of the treatment setting (i.e., across-settings generalization), is readily available to the clinician, which aids decisions regarding when to terminate or modify treatment to enhance its effectiveness.

Summary.   A prominent component of this treatment is continuous measurement of the child's stuttering and stutter-free behaviors. STSs continue to be obtained and analyzed as described earlier, and on-line performance data are collected for every speech attempt during treatment sessions. Thus, decisions regarding moving ahead to more advanced stages of treatment, modifying aspects of the treatment that are not productive, and

---

*While the concept of "pass criterion" is quite logical, the *particular* pass criterion specified for any treatment step within most treatment programs (including ELU) is basically an arbitrary one. That is, clinicians or program designers use their best judgment and clinical experience to suggest the level at which a response should be produced to meet the assumption of mastery. This is clearly an area in need of research. In actuality, a treatment program may be unnecessarily long if unduly high pass criteria are specified for every step; other programs may be unsuccessful in producing substantial and durable behavior change because they do not establish great enough mastery of the responses required for individual program steps. Fail criteria are equally arbitrary. Nonetheless, specification of pass and fail criteria lend consistency to the administration of the treatment program and remove possibilities for clinicians to be capricious in their judgments of how and when to move children forward or make changes in the treatment program.

terminating treatment, are all made on the basis of evidence regarding the status of a child's speech in and out of the clinic setting.

FEEDBACK

The most crucial ingredient of behavioral treatments, including ELU, is the response-contingent feedback system. This treatment relies heavily on the principles of positive reinforcement and negative feedback (sometimes referred to as punishment, although the connotations associated with that term are unduly punitive). As has been mentioned above, two response classes are of primary interest in the treatment of the speech of children who stutter: moments of stuttering, and periods of stutter-free speech. In a simplistic sense, stuttering and fluency are reciprocals, meaning that change in the frequency of occurrence of one produces covariation in the other. Therefore, procedures that reduce or eliminate moments of stuttering leave speech that is perceptually stutter-free; procedures that increase the amount of stutter-free speech necessarily reduce occurrences of stuttering. Thus, the appropriateness of the use of response-contingent feedback in treatment becomes obvious. The presentation of positive reinforcers contingent upon stutter-free speech increases the amount of stutter-free speech produced by the child; the presentation of negative feedback contingent upon occasions of stuttering reduces the frequency of stuttering produced by the child.

In theory, treatment ought to be approachable exclusively from either direction. However, the "double-barreled" approach, which combines both procedures, has certain advantages. In this process, occasions of stutter-free speech are followed immediately by presentation of functional positive reinforcers, and occasions of stuttering are followed immediately by negative feedback. Both of these contingencies play an important role in the ultimate effects of treatment. Interestingly, it appears[25,31] that reductions in stuttering are primarily dependent upon the provision of stuttering-contingent negative feedback. The tactic of reinforcing stutter-free utterances to "drive out" stutterings is not particularly powerful.* On the other hand, positive reinforcement of stutter-free utterances appears to sustain children's participation in treatment activities and give them the opportunity to discover enjoyment and self-satisfaction in talking. Further, when positive reinforcement and negative feedback are combined, milder forms of negative feedback can be used, and a positive relationship between the child and the clinician can be maintained (and even enhanced), because the clinician is associated with the presentation of positive reinforcement. The use of programmed instruction concepts in the design of treatment ensures that the balance between positive reinforcement and negative feedback always weighs heavily in favor of reinforcement.

Selection of Positive and Negative Feedback Stimuli.   Given that positive reinforcement and negative feedback are crucial components of treatment, discovery of *functional* positive and negative stimuli becomes a significant issue. It is well known that stimuli that function as positive reinforcers (or negative stimuli) for one child do not necessarily work

---

*The case for reinforcement may be different for older children whose stuttering is more severe, and for adults. That is, if their treatment is designed to teach a new or different speech pattern—for example, one that emanates from prolonged speech, the role of reinforcement in the acquisition of this response may be more important. However, for younger children, the implicit assumption is that the segments of their speech that are stutter-free are essentially normal speech. Therefore, the treatment is designed to rid that normal speech of occasions of stuttering.

in the same way for all children. While clinicians can often make good guesses based on their clinical experience with children, those guesses must be tested in order to assure that the selected stimuli actually do have the power to change behavior in the predicted direction. This basic factor is fundamental to principles of behavior change and is well known, yet too often overlooked by clinicians. (Suggestions for selecting and testing the function of positive and negative stimuli have been described previously.[28])

Feedback Schedules.   The well-known principles of schedules of reinforcement are applied throughout the course of the ELU treatment. That is, in the early stages, during the establishment of new behavior in children's repertoires, feedback (both social and tangible) is provided for every correct (nonstuttered) and incorrect (stuttered) response. However, as the treatment progresses, the reinforcement schedule is gradually "thinned" so that a reinforcer is earned after the occurrence of two fluent responses, then three, and so on. In ELU treatment, the density of reinforcement also becomes reduced as the required responses become longer. The goal is to approximate, by the end of treatment, the reinforcement schedule that exists in the natural environment (which is likely to be rather sparse).

In the spirit of altering the treatment so that it becomes progressively more similar to the contingencies that exist in the natural environment, the kinds of stimuli used as positive reinforcers also change. In the beginning, "contrived" reinforcers (such as toys, prizes, opportunities to play a game, etc.), usually paired with verbal feedback, are used as positive stimuli; however, as early as possible, these kinds of reinforcers are faded out, and greater reliance is placed on clinician praise and the child's recognition of and self-satisfaction in the production of stutter-free responses. The clinician often can recognize that this shift has occurred when children begin attending more to the plus-marks on the data sheet than to the tokens and stickers they earn, and when they begin commenting favorably about their own correct responses during treatment.

Oftentimes, this stage of treatment is one of the most difficult—for clinicians. Once clinicians observe directly the power of positive (and negative) feedback to facilitate change in children's speech, they sometimes become reluctant to reduce the density of that feedback. The use of these procedures becomes reinforcing to the clinician, and, therefore, is likely to be maintained by the clinician! However, extensive research has established that behavior that has been maintained on intermittent schedules of reinforcement is more durable and more likely to generalize than behavior maintained on continuous reinforcement schedules. Therefore, if the last steps of a treatment program still rely on frequently presented, contrived reinforcers, it should be no surprise when a child's newly acquired behavior does not generalize to the natural environment. Children's natural environments are typically not replete with tokens dropped into a cup every time a fluent utterance is produced!

In the ELU treatment program a one-to-one ratio between occurrences of stuttering and presentation of negative feedback is maintained (even while reinforcement is becoming intermittent) until quite late in the program. This is because negative feedback seems to be primarily responsible for producing reductions in the frequency of stutters. As treatment nears completion, explicit negative feedback is delayed, then removed. Ultimately, the goal of treatment is that at its termination children's stutter-free speech is completely under their own control—that is, that production of stutter-free, natural-sounding speech does not rely on positive or negative feedback controlled by external sources.

Summary. The ELU treatment described herein relies heavily on the use of functional positive and negative forms of feedback regarding the occurrence of stutter-free and stuttered utterances, respectively. Such feedback is applied frequently early in treatment and is faded in amount and form as treatment progresses.

EXAMPLE OF A BEHAVIORAL TREATMENT PROGRAM FOR USE WITH YOUNG
CHILDREN WHO STUTTER: EXTENDED LENGTH OF UTTERANCE

One example of how the above-described features come together in a behavioral treatment program is the Extended Length of Utterance (ELU) program. This strategy is a good starting place for treatment. For many children, it has been the only treatment required, with or without the addition of transfer activities. Appendix A describes the ELU treatment. (Read each step horizontally across the page.) Major characteristics of the program are discussed below, through explanations of each of the column headings.

Step. The first column simply numbers each step in the treatment sequence. Not all children are obligated to begin at step 1. Prior to treatment, probes of children's performance on the first few treatment steps are administered. In these probes, children are presented with five trials of a treatment step to determine whether the required response is already within their level of ability. No feedback regarding stutter-free speech or stuttering is provided in these probes. A total of five consecutive stutter-free trials is considered evidence of acceptable (passing) performance. If the child is able to pass, for example, step 1 (1-syllable fluent), step 2 is probed in the same way. Probes for each consecutive step of the program are continued until the child is unable to produce five consecutive stutter-free trials. Treatment then begins on the preceding step to ensure that the program begins at a level at which the child will be able to earn lots of positive feedback. Probes of succeeding steps are also administered whenever a given step is completed. Oftentimes it is possible to skip steps in the treatment sequence. In this way, treatment can take advantage of generalization across steps to accelerate progress through the program.

Discriminative Stimuli. Information contained in this column describes, for each step of the program, the stimuli (materials and clinician instructions) used to evoke responses from the child. Initially, a substantial stack of picture cards is used. It is not important that children learn to say fluently particular words (or sentences), just lots of different words (and sentences). Therefore, a minimum of 50 picture cards is used, and this number is increased and changed throughout the course of the treatment. Perusal of the items listed in this column of the treatment protocol illustrates that treatment begins by using lots of contrived visual stimuli and verbal instructions, and gradually changes so that responses are eventually evoked by more naturally occurring kinds of stimuli.

Response. The programmed nature of this treatment is evident by the specifications given in this column. The behavior that is required of the child to earn positive reinforcement at each step of the program is defined. No other form of response produces reinforcement. Responses systematically increase in length (and, thereby, in motoric and linguistic complexity) as the program progresses. The first step requires stutter-free production of one-syllable words, the last step requires 5-minute stutter-free conversations with the clinician in the clinic setting, and there are 18 "gradations" of response difficulty in between.

Consequences and Schedules.   This column contains specifications for the application of the feedback system for the child's stutter-free and stuttered responses. Correct responses are only those that meet the length requirement and are perceived as stutter-free by the clinician. As consequences for stutter-free responses, both social and token reinforcers are used in early steps of the program on continuous (1:1) schedules. Because responses judged as nonstuttered by the clinician will earn positive reinforcement and will, by definition, thereafter occur more frequently, the clinician's proper identification of stutter-free responses is crucial. If an utterance containing undesired characteristics (i.e., facial grimace or indeterminate nonfluency) is produced *and reinforced*, those undesired characteristics are likely to remain in the child's speech. Similarly counterproductive effects will occur if all stuttered syllables do not occasion negative feedback. In the ELU program, brief time-out from talking is utilized as negative feedback.* As the treatment progresses, both positive and negative feedback are faded.

It is well known that feedback that *immediately* follows the occurrence of a response is the most able to influence the probability of that response occurring in the future. Therefore, it is important to be especially careful to provide positive and negative feedback within these temporal constraints. Clinicians attempt to deliver the request to "Stop" (talking) *as soon as the beginning of a moment of stuttering* is detected. Oftentimes, then, the stuttered syllable and the stutter itself are interrupted by presentation of the negative stimulus. The procedural requirement to consequate every occasion of stuttering (1:1) and to do so essentially instantly necessitates a clinician's ability to rapidly discriminate the occurrence of a stutter in the child's speech.

With young children, typically, the contingencies are not explained—that is, the clinician does not elaborate on what is required to earn a reinforcer and what behavior produces the request to stop talking. Children respond to these contingencies rather naturally without explanations, and explanations often confound the effects of the treatment because they are confusing or misunderstood. If an occurrence of stuttering is followed by the clinician's gentle instruction "Stop," and if stutter-free utterances of the required length are followed by the presentation of a positive reinforcer, then the child will soon figure out which behaviors produce which consequences. Explanations are provided only if they are sought by the children (e.g., "Why did you say 'stop'?"). It quickly becomes clear by the way children change their behavior that, at some level, the contingencies are "understood," even though they may not be verbalized by the children or the clinicians.

In addition, children do not generally need instructions regarding *how* to be fluent; that is, clinicians do not have to teach them to use "easy" onsets or slow speech, etc., although some children appear to discover these particular solutions for themselves, if speech-pattern alterations are required for fluency. Part of the power of these procedures may result from the problem solving and hypothesis testing that children must undertake in order to discover the kind of response that will earn reinforcement and avoid negative feedback. Usually children are somehow able to generate stutter-free responses from their own behavioral reservoirs.

---

*Time-out from speaking is not an effective negative stimulus for the youngest children. It appears that their metalinguistic facility with language and communication is not well enough developed that they are able to turn their speaking on and off at will. Midsentence instructions to "Stop" are typically ignored by such children. In these cases time-out can be replaced by the presentation of a stuttering-contingent remark such as "uh oh" or "oops." If this feedback is salient enough, then it serves to highlight the occurrence of stuttering, but does not interrupt the ongoing flow of communication.

Criteria.   This column lists the Pass and Fail criteria that specify how well, or how poorly, children must perform the target behavior (stutter-free utterance) before advancing in the program, or before the program is altered due to failure.* When the Fail Criterion is met, the program is modified in some fashion by the clinician, based upon her analysis of why the step was failed. Repeating the previous step, on which the child had performed at criterion level, is not generally a solution to the problem. Sometimes the "behavioral space" between two steps is too large for the child to bridge, and an intermediate step can be inserted; sometimes the feedback system needs adjusting because the reinforcers may be weakening, or the token-backup reinforcer exchange rate is too sparse; sometimes a child may initiate a trial without obvious concentration. Whatever the nature of the "branch" step that is created when a child has failed a step, that step is taught until criterion is met, then the child is returned to the regular sequence.

Measurement.   This column describes the data that are collected, response-by-response, during each step of the program, and the calculations that are made from those data. These calculations provide evidence regarding the effectiveness of the ongoing treatment.

Comments Regarding Particular Aspects of the ELU Program.   It should be noted that imitated utterances are generally avoided in the ELU program. It would be possible to conduct the early treatment steps imitatively, but the use of imitation is reserved for children who are unable to produce stutter-free utterances even on the shortest utterances (e.g., as a branch step). An (untested) assumption of the ELU program is that learning to produce *spontaneous, self-formulated utterances* in a stutter-free fashion is fundamental to children's acquisition of requisite speech-motor skills. Experience indicates that 1. imitation does not necessarily facilitate children's production of stutter-free responses (unlike articulation responses, for example) and, 2. fluency does not necessarily generalize from imitated to nonimitated utterances.

One tricky part of the program is the transition between utterances defined by syllable length and utterances defined by time (transition from step 6 to 7). Because a fundamental principle of this treatment is control of length of utterance, children must learn to stop when they are signaled (by the click of the stopwatch or the clinician saying "OK" or "good") that the required response duration has been met, even though this may occur in the middle of a sentence or idea. A practice step is inserted to help the child learn this procedure (see Appendix A). Also at this stage, some children will have difficulty formulating phrases and sentences to describe the picture stimuli. If this occurs, it can be helpful to introduce a "story retell" task, wherein the clinician models a response of the appropriate content and duration, and the child then produces a similar response. The child does not need to use the

---

*Clinicians should not be confused between occasions when a child has earned the requisite number of tokens required to exchange for a backup reinforcer, which can occur in the middle of a treatment step, and occasions when a child's performance level has met the Pass Criterion, which signals the completion of that step. Both events are determined by the data recorded on the clinician's data sheet. When the former occurs (which is usually obvious because the last available token is delivered), treatment is momentarily halted and the child immediately receives the previously selected backup reinforcer before the next trial is administered. Also, at this time a new backup reinforcer is chosen, and the full complement of tokens is once again available for the child to earn as the treatment continues. On the other hand, when a Pass Criterion is achieved, the clinician simply changes the parameters to those appropriate for the next step of the program and continues on. No particular mention is made to the child unless the new step requires some kind of new instruction. Clinicians should *not* say something like, "Now you've passed that step, we're going to do something even harder." The prospects of "something even harder" may not be perceived by some children as the exciting, stimulating challenge we intend!

same words or even express the same ideas that the clinician modeled. The child needs only to produce stutter-free spontaneous speech of the required duration. As soon as a child catches on to this task, the clinician's model is faded out.

At step 9 (10-second stutter-free response) the program suggests that the clinician occasionally monitor children's speaking rates. This is accomplished easily by making a pencil dot on the data sheet for each syllable produced in the 10-second utterance, and then multiplying that number by 6 to extrapolate SPM. Although speaking rate is not generally a problem with very young children, older children oftentimes use speech rates that appear to be beyond their ability to manage. If this appears to be the case for a given child, reminders regarding speech rate or even contingencies for producing speech within a specified range can be added at this point in the program.

Summary.   The ELU program described herein is an example of the application of established behavioral principles within a flexible framework that fosters individualized treatment and a high level of accountability. Further, the treatment program is relatively simple to administer and enjoyable for the child and clinician alike; this is not to say, however, that learning to produce fluent speech is easy for children. Generally, focused attention and concentrated effort on the part of the children is required. This program facilitates both.

Outcomes

The outcomes expected of this treatment are the same as the previously stated treatment goals: spontaneous and automatic use of natural-sounding stutter-free speech under all talking conditions, in all settings, with all speaking partners and audiences. Evidence regarding stuttering frequency, speech rate, and speech naturalness obtained from the STSs is the primary source of information for determining when these outcomes have occurred. Because STSs are obtained periodically throughout treatment, it is possible to know well before the assumed termination point of treatment whether these goals are being met. In fact, when preschool-aged children have been treated, it has not been necessary to administer the complete treatment program in order to reach these goals.

Partial data are available from a larger research program conducted to evaluate the ELU treatment method formally and objectively.[32] At the time of this report, complete data are available for five children between the ages of 3:6 and 9:1, who ranged widely in stuttering severity and who received 20 hours of ELU treatment. Stuttering was reduced by more than 60%. In addition, the severity of remaining occasions of stuttering was also greatly reduced. Further, when children over the age of 6:0 are removed from the group, stuttering is virtually eliminated among the remaining children. For the older children, additional hours of treatment produced further reductions in stuttering. For some, the treatment was altered along the way to include slightly prolonged speech as an "additive"[24] to foster additional improvement. Such additives (speech pattern changes) are not incorporated into the early steps of treatment because 1. they may not be needed, 2. they are difficult for young children to employ, and 3. they alter the naturalness of a child's speech and must eventually be severed from the child's manner of speech production.

Overall, knowledge gained from these partial findings, from both as-yet-unpublished data on other children in this research project and clinical documentation obtained from scores of children treated in a university setting over more than 15 years, indicate consistently positive outcomes of the ELU treatment program.

ACROSS-SETTINGS GENERALIZATION

An especially important aspect of treatment outcome is whether a child's newly acquired stutter-free speech generalizes to real-life speaking conditions. Our research findings with children under age 9 demonstrate that most children spontaneously generalize their clinic-acquired, stutter-free speech to home, school, and other settings without the need of additional "transfer" steps. The younger the child, the more likely is such generalization. For older (more severe) children, generalization appears to be enhanced when one or more of the following components, aimed at transferring clinic-bound fluency to the natural environment, is included in the treatment procedures.

Self-management.   Many children are able to take greater responsibility for their own behavior change than clinicians typically allow. And if children have control over more components of the treatment, then the treatment has the potential of leaving the clinic with them. Each aspect of the treatment paradigm offers opportunities for children to take responsibility. In regard to the stimuli used to evoke speech, children can be responsible for bringing in pictures (e.g., family photograph album) and picking conversation topics. In regard to the feedback system, children can learn to monitor their responses and judge whether they contain stutters or are stutter-free. They may even be encouraged to record the data regarding their responses. (Taking this sheet home to show to parents and friends is often a powerful reinforcer for high levels of stutter-free speech.) Certainly children should play a major role in determining the reinforcers to be used in treatment, and oftentimes they can learn to award both positive and negative feedback to themselves following their judgment of the correctness of their response. Even before they are taught to do so, many children begin spontaneously to stop themselves mid-stutter, and it's certainly not unusual to observe young stutterers reminding the clinician when reinforcers are due! Teaching young children to take responsibility for more aspects of their treatment helps develop a treatment strategy that can be applied in the child's natural environment in the absence of the clinician—a goal of procedures aimed at producing transfer. The usefulness of self-management techniques depends partially on the child's age, but the best way to determine this issue is by gradually shifting control of various treatment components to the child and observing the child's ability and readiness to accept these responsibilities.

Parent Training.   Whenever possible, parents are taught to serve as adjunct clinicians. Sometimes this is done by training the parents to administer the program being used in the clinic. As soon as a child's performance has met criterion on a given step of the program in the clinic, the parent is taught how to administer that treatment step at home, and regular 10- to 15-minute sessions are held daily. In other cases, parents are informed regarding the level of stutter-free responding the child has achieved in the clinic (e.g., five consecutive syllables) and are instructed to notice and reinforce occasions of similar stutter-free speech in the child's spontaneous speech at home or elsewhere, any time it occurs. In either case, parent training is conducted systematically, by having the parent observe the clinician's sessions with the child, and by having the clinician observe the parent's sessions with the child. Direct training to recognize targeted stutter-free responses, how to reinforce them, and how to recognize and provide feedback for stuttered responses is crucial to this process. An example of behavioral treatment similar to ELU administered entirely by parents can be found in the work of Onslow and colleagues.[20,33]

Inclusion of a Peer or Sibling in Treatment.   At some point in the treatment, the earlier the better, it is useful to include someone who is in frequent contact with the child in the natural environment. The goal is for this person to become a discriminative stimulus for stutter-free speech. Such persons become salient stimuli when they are responsible for providing reinforcement for stutter-free utterances. If they have been included in the child's treatment sessions, they can learn to recognize and reinforce stutter-free speech. The assumption is that the presence of that child in the natural environment will become a "reminder" (discriminative stimulus) to the stuttering child for stutter-free speech.

Concurrent Treatment Across Settings.   Arranging for treatment to occur simultaneously in more than one setting helps produce generalization. That is, the child is less likely to learn to produce stutter-free speech only in the clinic or only in the presence of the clinician if multiple treatment settings and treatment agents are utilized. One way to accomplish this is by training both a parent and a teacher in the treatment methods used in the clinic.[34] Besides preventing narrow stimulus control, this procedure multiplies the treatment and practice opportunities available to the child.

Conclusion

Many clinicians have discovered that using behavioral treatments, such as ELU, with children who stutter can be highly reinforcing—for clinicians as well as for children who benefit by improved speech. Children are not tainted when direct attention is paid to their stuttering. In fact, they oftentimes say they are glad their speech difficulties and frustrations are being acknowledged and dealt with. On the other hand, many young children complete the treatment described herein with little awareness that they were ever in "treatment." Behavioral treatments have the advantage of being based on experimentally verified principles of behavior change and carry with them the accountability factors inherent in continuous measurement. They are relatively easy for clinicians and others to administer. They address directly the behavior of primary interest: a child's stuttering. Behavioral treatments are able to be individualized for different children and modified as needed to produce greater behavior change. And, most important, behavioral treatments, such as the ELU method described here, produce clinically beneficial treatment outcomes for children who stutter.

Suggested Readings

Costello JC, Ingham RJ: Assessment strategies for stuttering, in Curlee R, Perkins WH (eds): *Nature and Treatment of Stuttering: New Directions.* San Diego, College-Hill, 1984.
Ingham RJ, Costello JM: Stuttering treatment outcome evaluation, in Costello JM (ed): *Speech Disorders in Children. Recent Advances.* San Diego, College-Hill, 1984.
   These two chapters describe measurement procedures that facilitate judgments regarding the characteristics of a child's stuttering and how/whether those characteristics change as a function of treatment.
Costello JM: Current behavioral treatments for children, in Prins D, Ingham RJ (eds): *Treatment of Stuttering in Early Childhood: Methods and Issues.* San Diego, College-Hill, 1983.
Ingham JC: Therapy of the Stuttering Child, in Blanken G, Dittman J, Grimm H, Marshall JC, Wallesch C-W (eds): *Linguistic Disorders and Pathologies.* Berlin, Walter De Gruyter, 1993.
   These two chapters present overviews of philosophies of treatment for children who stutter, with contrasts between behavioral and other styles of treatment.
Onslow M, Andrews C, Lincoln M: A control/experimental trial of operant treatment for early

stuttering. *J Speech Hearing Res* 1994; 37:1244–1259. Also see, Erratum, *J Speech Hearing Dis* 1995; 38:386.

Onslow M, Costa L, Rue S: Direct early intervention with stuttering: Some preliminary data. *J Speech Hearing Dis* 1990; 55:405–416.

These articles describe and document experimental findings regarding a parent-administered behavioral treatment of young children who stutter. The procedures described are variants of those advocated in this chapter.

References

1. Riley G, Ingham JC: Stuttering Treatment Project Final Report. Report to National Institute of Deafness and Other Communication Disorders. Bethesda, MD, 1997.
2. Kidd KK: Stuttering as a Genetic Disorder, in Curlee RF, Perkins WH (eds): *Nature and Treatment of Stuttering: New Directions*. San Diego, College-Hill, 1984.
3. American Speech-Language-Hearing Association: Let's Talk. *ASHA* 1990; 32:63.
4. Ingham R, Ingham JC: Let's Talk about Stuttering. *ASHA* 1990; 32:42.
5. Nippold M: Concomitant speech and language disorders in stuttering children: A critique of the literature. *J Speech Hearing Dis* 1990; 55:51–60.
6. Conture EG, Louko LJ, Edwards ML: Simultaneously treating stuttering and disordered phonology in children: Experimental treatment, preliminary findings. *Am J Speech-Lang Pathol* 1993; 2(3):72–81.
7. Ratner NB: Treating the child who stutters with concomitant language or phonological impairment. *Lang Speech Hearing Serv Schools* 1995; 26:180–186.
8. Costello JM, Ingham RJ: Assessment strategies for child and adult stutterers, in Curlee RF, Perkins WH (eds): *Nature and Treatment of Stuttering: New Directions*. San Diego, College-Hill, 1984.
9. Ingham RJ, Costello, JM: Stuttering Treatment Outcome Evaluation, in Costello JM (ed): *Speech disorders in children: Recent advances*. San Diego, College-Hill, 1984.
10. Ingham JC, Riley G: Guidelines for documentation of treatment efficacy for young children who stutter. *J Speech Lang Hearing Res* (in press, 1998).
11. Ingham RJ: Spontaneous Remission of Stuttering: When Will the Emperor Realize He Has No Clothes On? in Prins D, Ingham RJ (eds): *Treatment of Stuttering in Early Childhood: Methods and Issues*. San Diego, College-Hill, 1983.
12. Yairi E, Ambrose, NG, Paden EP, Throneburg, RN: Predictive factors of persistence and recovery: Pathways of childhood stuttering. *J Commun Dis* 1996; 29:51–77.
13. Wingate ME: A standard definition of stuttering. *J Speech Hear Dis* 1964; 29:484–489.
14. MacDonald JD, Martin RR: Stuttering and disfluency as two reliable response classes. *J Speech Hear Res* 1973; 17:691–699.
15. Curlee R: Observer agreement on disfluency and stuttering. *J Speech Hear Res* 1981; 24: 595–600.
16. Young MA: Identification of Stuttering and Stutterers, in Curlee RF, Perkins WH (eds): *Nature and Treatment of Stuttering: New Directions*. San Diego, College-Hill, 1984.
17. Fowler SC, Ingham RJ: Stuttering Treatment Rating Recorder. Santa Barbara, University of California, 1986. (Available upon request from author @ $30.00.)
18. Cordes AK, Ingham RJ, Frank P, Ingham JC: Time-interval analysis of interjudge and intrajudge agreement for stuttering event judgments. *J Speech Hear Res* 1992; 35:483–494.
19. Martin RR, Haroldson SK, Triden KA: Stuttering and speech naturalness. *J Speech Hear Dis* 1984; 49:53–58.
20. Onslow M, Costa L, Rue S: Direct early intervention with stuttering: Some preliminary data. *J Speech Hear Dis* 1990; 55:405–416.
21. Ingham RJ: Speech Naturalness and Stuttering Research: A Review, in Gerber SE, Mechner GT (eds): *International Perspectives on Communication Disorders*. Washington, Gallaudet University Press, 1988.
22. Ingham RJ, Cordes AK, Ingham JC, Gow ML: Identifying the onset and offset of stuttering events. *J Speech Hear Res* 1995; 38:315–326.

23. Ingham JC: Therapy of the Stuttering Child, in Blanken G, Dittman J, Grimm H, Marshall JC, Wallesch C-W (eds): *Linguistic Disorders and Pathologies*. Berlin, De Gruyter, 1993.
24. Costello JM: Current Behavioral Treatments for Children, in Prins D, Ingham RJ (eds): *Treatment of Stuttering in Early Childhood: Methods and Issues*. San Diego, College-Hill, 1983.
25. Costello JM: Time-out procedures for the modification of stuttering: Three case studies. *J Speech Hear Dis* 1975; 40:216–231.
26. Costello JM: Operant conditioning and the treatment of stuttering. *Semin Speech Lang Hear* 1980; 1:311–325.
27. Costello JM, Ingham RJ: Stuttering as an operant disorder, in Curlee RF, Perkins WH (eds): *Nature and Treatment of Stuttering: New Directions*. San Diego, College-Hill, 1984.
28. Ingham JC: Behavioral treatment of stuttering in children, in Curlee RF (ed): *Stuttering and Related Disorders of Fluency*. New York, Thieme, 1993.
29. Ryan BP: *Programmed Therapy for Stuttering in Children and Adults*. Springfield, IL, Thomas, 1974.
30. Costello JM: Programmed instruction. *J Speech Hear Dis* 1977; 42:3–28.
31. Costello JM, Ferrer JS: The effects of three punishment procedure applied to programmed instruction with young children. *J Commun Dis* 1976; 9:43–61.
32. Riley G, Ingham JC: Vocal Response Time Changes Associated with Two Types of Treatment, in Starkweather CW, Peters HMF (eds): *Stuttering: Proceedings of the First World Congress on Fluency Disorders*. New York, Elsevier Science, 1995.
33. Onslow M, Andrews C, Lincoln M: A control/experimental trial of operant treatment for early stuttering. *J Speech Hear Res* 1994; 37:1244–1259. Also see, Erratum, *J Speech Hear Dis* 1994; 38:386.
34. Ingham JC: Measurement and facilitation of across-settings generalization. Paper presented at Annual meeting of the American Speech-Language-Hearing Association, November, 1991.

Appendix: The Extended Length of Utterance (ELU) Program

Step	Discriminative Stimuli	Response (+ & −)	± Consequences and Schedules	Criteria	Measurement
1	Minimum of 50 cards containing pictures labeled by monosyllabic words within vocabulary range of client—presented without model—one card at a time. Example: car, leaf. Instructions: "Say each word"	+: Stutter-free 1-syllable word. −: Stuttered syllable	+: *Positive social reinforcer* ("Good!" "Right!" "Excellent!" "Perfect speech!" etc.), 1:1 *Positive token reinforcer*, 1:1 (Tokens exchanged for backup reinforcers throughout the program as follows: 10:1, 20:1, 35:1. The exchange rate may be altered backward as longer responses are required or when declining levels of correct responding indicate the need for increased motivation) −: "Stop," said by clinician during or immediately following a moment of stuttering; client must stop speaking briefly; 1:1	*Pass:* 10 consecutive stutter-free responses *Fail:* 7 consecutive stuttered trials or 100 trials without meeting pass criterion	(+) Each stutter-free response (−) Each stuttered response At completion of step, calculate % correct responses and number of trials required to meet criterion.

Step	Discriminative Stimuli	Response (+ & −)	± Consequences and Schedules	Criteria	Measurement
2	Minimum of 50 cards containing a) pictures labeled by 1-syllable words presented in pairs, plus b) a minimum of 50 cards containing pictures labeled by 2-syllable words, plus c) a minimum of 50 cards containing pictures to evoke two-syllable syntactic utterances. Example, a) car-house, b) mother, c) my cat. Instructions: "Tell me what's in these pictures".	+: Stutter-free 2-syllable utterance −: Any stuttered syllable	+: Same as above −: Same as above	Same as above	Same as above
3	Same kinds of stimuli as a, b, c above except selected to evoke 3-*syllable* word strings, single words, and syntactic word combinations	+: Stutter-free 3-syllable utterance −: Any stuttered syllable	+: Same as above −: Same as above	Same as above	Same as above
4	Same kinds of stimuli as a, b, c above except selected to evoke 4-*syllable* utterances	+: Stutter-free 4-syllable utterance −: Any stuttered syllable	+: Same as above −: Same as above	Same as above	Same as above

	Stimuli	Child	Clinician	Pass/Fail	Notes
5	Same kinds of stimuli as c above except selected to evoke 5-syllable utterances (NOTE: Do not include 5-syllable words)	+: Stutter-free 5-syllable utterance −: Any stuttered syllable	+: Same as above −: Same as above	Same as above	Same as above
6	Same kinds of stimuli as c above except selected to evoke 6-syllable utterances	+: Stutter-free 6-syllable utterance −: Any stuttered syllable	+: Same as above −: Same as above	Same as above	Same as above
Practice	Minimum of 50 pictures containing lots of activity, toys and play, topic cards. Instructions: "Tell me about this" (present one stimulus) and keep talking until I say 'OK.' I want you to talk for 3 sec. I'll show you." Describe one picture in relatively slow, simple connected speech and stop at the end of 3 sec, in the middle of a sentence, if necessary, and click the stopwatch at the same time. Show the child that the stopwatch is at 3 sec. Demonstrate on two or three different stimuli.	+: Continuous talking in connected speech for a duration of 3 sec (stuttering allowed) −: Pauses, problems thinking of things to say, etc.	+: Positive social reinforcer, 1:1 −: Re-explain and/or change stimulus materials. Helpful to let child watch the clock	Be sure client learns to stop as soon as the watch stops, even if utterance is not completed. Be sure client does not increase speaking rate in an attempt to complete utterance before the time is up	Pass: 3 consecutive correct responses Fail: Continue task as practice until child meets pass criterion	Start timing with stopwatch when client begins talking. Do not initiate child's response by saying "Go!" and thereby imply that a fast speaking rate or hurried speech is appropriate. Just say "Start when you're ready" and start the clock when the child begins speaking

Step	Discriminative Stimuli	Response (+ & −)	± Consequences and Schedules	Criteria	Measurement
Practice (cont.)	Then say, "Now it's your turn. Keep talking until I stop the watch and say 'OK.'" For some clients it may be necessary to practice using "story retell" tasks wherein the clinician speaks about the picture for 3 sec and then the child repeats the task in his or her own words for 3 sec				
7	Same picture, topic cards, and toy stimuli as above, presented in random order. Instructions: "Tell me about this one and keep talking until I say 'OK,' just like you've been doing." If necessary, give "story retell" models until the child is able to generate utterances independently	+: Stutter-free 3-sec monologue connected speech utterance (monologue = uninterrupted by the clinician) −: Any moment of stuttering	+: *Positive social reinforcer*, 1:1 *Positive token reinforcer*, 1:1 −: "Stop," said by clinician during or immediately following moment of stuttering; client must briefly stop speaking; 1:1 (Be sure you *do not* say "stop" at the end of *stutter-free* utterances when the required speaking time has been reached. Say "Good," etc.)	*Pass:* Ten consecutive stutter-free monologue responses *Fail:* Seven consecutive stuttered trials or 75 trials without passing the step	(+) Each stutter-free response (−) Each stuttered response At the completion of the step, calculate percent of correct trials and number of trials required to meet criterion

8	Same stimuli and instructions as above	+: Stutter-free 5-sec monologue connected speech utterance -: Any moment of stuttering	+: Same as above -: Same as above	Same as above		
9	Same stimuli and instructions as above	+: Stutter-free 10-sec monologue connected speech utterance -: Any moment of stuttering	+: Same as above -: Same as above	Same as above	(+) Each stutter-free response (−) Each stuttered response	For every third or fourth trial, count number of syllables spoken in 10 sec and multiply × 6 for approximate SPM speaking rate. At completion of the step calculate percent of correct trials, number of trials required to meet criterion, and average SPM (based on all trials for which rate data were taken)
10	Same stimuli and instructions as above	+: Stutter-free 20-sec monologue connected speech utterance -: Any moment of stuttering -: Any utterance >160 SPM	+: Same as above -: Same as above -: Reminder to speak a bit more slowly, 1:1	Same as above		Same as above (for rate data, multiply 20-sec syllable count × 3 for approximate SPM for each trial)

Step	Discriminative Stimuli	Response (+ & −)	± Consequences and Schedules	Criteria	Measurement
11	Same stimuli and instructions as above	+: Stutter-free 30-sec monologue connected speech utterance −: Any moment of stuttering	+: Same as above: "Refreshing" the stimuli used as positive reinforcers may also be appropriate here, or at any time in the treatment when the child's attention/focus appears to wane. −: Same as above. Also, for some children it may be appropriate to increase the influence of feedback for stuttering by adding the removal of one token for each stuttered response (response cost). This can be added here, or whenever it seems apparent that additional focus/effort is required on the child's part. −: Reminder to speak a bit more slowly, 1:1	Same as above	Same as above (for rate data, multiply 30-sec syllable count × 2 for approximate SPM for each trial)
12	Same stimuli and instructions as above	+: Stutter-free 1-min monologue connected speech utterance −: Any moment of stuttering Any utterance >160 SPM	+: Same as above −: Same as above −: Same as above	Same as above	Same as above (for rate data count syllables for 15 sec of each 1-min response and multiply × 4 for approximate SPM)

Step	Stimuli and instructions	Response criteria (±)	Consequation (±)	Criterion	Rate / notes
13	Same stimuli and instructions as above	+: Stutter-free 2-min monologue connected speech utterance. −: Any moment of stuttering	+: Same as above	Pass: 10 consecutive stutter-free monologue responses Fail: 7 consecutive stuttered trials or 50 trials without passing the step	Same as above (for rate data count syllables for four different 15-sec intervals during the 2-min response and add for approximate SPM)
14	Same stimuli and instructions as above	+: Stutter-free 3-min monologue connected speech utterance. −: Any utterance >160 SPM −: Any moment of stuttering	+: Same as above −: Same as above	Pass: 5 consecutive stutter-free monologue responses Fail: Same as above	Same as above
15	Same stimuli and instructions as above	+: Stutter-free 4-min monologue connected speech utterance. −: Any moment of stuttering −: No rate requirement	+: Same as above −: Same as above −: (No feedback regarding rate unless stuttering occurs associated with high SPM)	Same as above	Same as above
16	Same stimuli and instructions as above	+: Stutter-free 5-min monologue connected speech utterance. −: Any moment of stuttering	+: Same as above −: Same as above	Pass: 4 consecutive stutter-free monologue responses Fail: 20 trials without passing the step	Same as above

Step	Discriminative Stimuli	Response (+ & −)	± Consequences and Schedules	Criteria	Measurement
17	Topics introduced by clinician and by child for conversation. Include clinician questions, interruptions, overlapping utterances, topic changes, etc.; i.e., mirroring natural conversational interactions (but keep clinician utterances short)	+: 2 min of stutter-free conversation (Note: 2 min based on cumulative child speaking time) −: Any moment of stuttering	+: Same as above −: Same as above	Pass: 10 consecutive stutter-free conversations Fail: 7 consecutive stuttered trials or 50 trials without passing the step	Same as above, plus use stop watch to cumulate child speaking time (i.e., 2 min of child talking time, rather than a 2-min conversation, including clinician talking time)
18	Same as above	+: 3 min of stutter-free conversation (Note: 3 min based on cumulative child speaking time) −: Any moment of stuttering	+: *Positive social reinforcer, 1:1* *Positive token reinforcer, 2:1* −: Report number of stutters to child at end of trial. Do not stop child at the moment of a stutter	Same as above	Same as above

19	Same as above	+: 4 min of stutter-free conversation (Note: 4 min based on cumulative child speaking time) −: Any moment of stuttering	+: Positive social reinforcer, 1:1 Positive token reinforcer, 2:1	Pass: 7 consecutive stutter-free conversations Fail: 30 trials without passing step	Same as above
20	Same as above	+: 5 min of stutter-free conversation (Note: 5 min based on cumulative child speaking time) −: Any moment of stuttering	−: Report number of stutters to child at end of trial. Do not stop child at the moment of a stutter +: Positive social reinforcer, 1:1	Pass: 6 consecutive stutter-free conversations Fail: 25 trials without passing the step	Same as above
21	If child continues to stutter, develop transfer program in natural environment		−: Report number of stutters to child at end of trial. Do not stop child at the moment of a stutter		

Stuttering and Related Disorders of Fluency, 2nd edition.
Edited by Richard F. Curlee, PH.D.
Thieme Medical Publishers, Inc., New York © 1999.

6

Therapy for School-age Stutterers: An Update on the Fluency Rules Program

CHARLES M. RUNYAN
SARA ELIZABETH RUNYAN

Choosing the most effective treatment procedure for the preschool and young school-age stutterer, given the constraints associated with the delivery of services in the public school setting, continues to challenge the speech–language pathologist. Public school speech–language pathologists are required to provide services to a significant number of students, and the resultant caseloads have been high. School-based speech–language pathologists find it difficult to fulfill their professional responsibilities for complete assessments, intervention plans, and carryover services when nationally reported caseloads average 53.[1] These large caseloads, combined with such frequent scheduling conflicts as IEP and eligibility meetings, testing, assemblies, student and therapist absences, holidays, artists-in-residence programs, state testing programs, and field trips limit the number and length of treatment sessions during a school year. One example of the effect of large caseloads and scheduling constraints occurred in Virginia where, on average, a child was enrolled for two 20- or 30-minute sessions per week but was seen for fewer than 50 sessions a year.[2] Speech–language pathologists in Virginia and in other regions of the country have continued to report that caseload size and scheduling conflicts remain unchanged. Therefore, because of these job constraints and large caseloads, public school speech–language pathologists need a stuttering treatment program that can maximize therapeutic effectiveness while creating minimal disruption in the child's normal school routine.

After the initial publication of the Fluency Rules Program (FRP),[3] numerous requests were received for additional information and clinical updates. Over the past few years public school clinicians, as well as clinicians in other treatment settings, have shared with us their clinical successes using the FRP as well as their modifications to the treatment protocol. Unfortunately, as gratifying as these interactions have been, to our knowledge, no additional data of FRP use in public school or other clinical environments have been published. Therefore, the changes in the FRP presented in this chapter reflect our experiences with young stutterers in a university clinic, a private practice setting, and through consultations to public schools. Although two of these clinical environments differ from public school environments, the suggested therapy changes and recommendations are applicable to public school treatment settings.

The Revised Fluency Rules

The FRP was developed in 1981 in an attempt to teach young grade school children to speak fluently and naturally. The individual rules were worded to instruct young children, in language they could comprehend, the physiological concepts associated with fluent speech production. Originally, 10 Fluency Rules were developed, and through clinical trial and error, the effectiveness and utility of each rule was evaluated. Subsequently, some rules remained unchanged; others were modified or deleted until the current seven rules remained. The treatment paradigm has also been tested clinically and modified. At first, the FRP treatment procedure was designed to teach a stuttering child all of the Fluency Rules. With continued use of the FRP, however, this procedure proved to be time inefficient. Teaching all of the rules consumed a significant amount of time and often required a clinician to teach skills the children already exhibited. Therefore, by 1986, when the FRP was first published, the treatment program consisted of seven rules, with therapeutic instruction provided only for those rules that were broken. Continued clinical application of the FRP has not changed the rules dramatically but has significantly altered their application.

The remainder of this chapter describes the seven Fluency Rules, presents the revised FRP, and reviews our clinical results. The seven rules are presented individually using the new treatment format which starts with two Universal Rules, followed by two Primary Rules, and finally three Secondary Rules. For each rule, background information will be provided followed by therapy suggestions regarding the application of each rule.

Universal Rules

Rule 1: Speak Slowly (Turtle Speech)

BACKGROUND

This rule for speech rate reduction allows the child additional time to develop self-monitoring skills necessary for the acquisition of the physiological skills required for fluent speech production. When this rule was first considered as a component of the FRP, minimal information was available in the literature on the speaking rates of early grade-school children. This lack of information made it difficult for clinicians to determine how much to reduce a stuttering child's speaking rate. To obtain preliminary data on the normal speaking rates of young children, Purcell and Runyan[4] conducted a study of students enrolled in grades 1 through 5. These results are presented in Table 6-1. Although this rule is labeled "speak slowly" or "turtle speech," the intent was never to have children produce speech that was abnormally slow or one word at a time. In fact, it has been our clinical experience that children acquiring linguistic competency are not concerned with their speaking rate. The message takes precedence, and attempts to manipulate rate to one sounding abnormally slow does not have the desired therapeutic effect. Furthermore, a child is unlikely to use a dramatically reduced speaking rate or produce speech one word at a time outside the clinical setting.

Table 6-1.   Means and Standard Deviations of Speaking Rate
of Children in Words and Syllables per Minute

Grade	Words per Minute	Standard Deviation	Syllables per Minute	Standard Deviation
1	124.92	12.17	147.66	13.47
2	130.44	12.05	156.72	17.14
3	133.44	10.01	158.94	14.86
4	139.32	16.33	165.66	24.58
5	141.84	16.24	170.04	23.19

A secondary benefit of this rule, supported by reports from public school speech patholo-gists, is that a slow rate of speech has an overall calming effect on the child as well as on various speaking partners. This calming effect appears to contribute to a life-style and a speaking environment that are conducive to fluent speech development. Clinically, we have noted that following a therapy session in which the goal was reduction to a slow, normal speaking rate, the child appeared more relaxed. Interestingly, during these sessions, a marked reduction in stuttering was noted; however, speaking rate remained virtually unchanged. Therefore, the reduction in the frequency of stuttering appeared to be, in part, due to the general calming effect of the therapy setting.

THERAPY SUGGESTIONS

1. *Symbolic Material*: Use symbolic therapy materials, such as turtles and snails, to characterize slow speech.

2. *More Symbolic Material*: Use modeling or choral speaking to contrast slow turtle speech, or other slow moving animals (i.e., normal speech rate), with race horse speech, using horses to portray too fast or rapid speech.

3. *Metronome*: To create a calm clinical atmosphere and encourage slow speech produc-tion use a desk-level metronome set at 60 beats per min as background during therapy.[5]

4. *Old Ears*: This technique has been applied successfully with both Universal Rules. Constructing a pair of old ears, with wrinkles and gray hair or large rubber clown ears, enhances the teaching of this rule. Tell the child your (i.e., the clinician) ears are old and tired and, if the child uses race horse speech, your old ears will become confused. An unexpected outcome of this therapy technique was having children run to the waiting room and tell their parents that it was fun coming to therapy and helping the clinician's ears by talking slowly (i.e., following this Rule). The obvious secondary value to this technique is that it places the child in the role of helper rather than a recipient of therapy.

5. *Modeling*: Clinicians and parents should adopt relaxed, slow-motion speech produc-tion. Parents are instructed to slow their speech rate, but not to prolong or use excessive pauses in their speech, because these behaviors produce speech that sounds abnormal. To prevent parents from excessive reductions in speech rate, which often occurs following this instruction, a speedometer analogy is used with the suggestion that reducing their rate by only 10 miles per hour (mph) will allow them to stay in better control without becoming a traffic hazard. In other words, slow down from 65 to 55 mph but do not slow to 25 mph, because that is too slow and could cause a traffic problem. This analogy, coupled with the clinician modeling the intended speech rate, has proven to be successful in developing the desired speech in most parents.

6. *Animal Tracks*: Clinicians can put turtle tracks (e.g., any slow moving animal footprints) and race horse tracks (i.e., horse shoes) on the floor and have the children simultaneously walk and talk symbolized by the type of animal trail that they are walking. (See Rule 6 for additional information.)

7. *Hands Down*: The clinician gives a nonverbal cue by moving his/her hand up and down in a way that traditionally means to slow down. This visual cue does not require a direct explanation, and the child's speech rate will immediately be reduced following its use. Clinically, we use this technique more than any of the previous therapy suggestions because the child's speech is not interrupted, which has proven to be extremely effective.

Rule 2: Say a Word Only Once

BACKGROUND

The dominant speech characteristics of young children who have not stuttered long are part-word and whole-word repetitions. Therefore, a fluency rule to help control this characteristic of stuttering is vital for any treatment program designed to help young stutterers. For this rule to be effectively implemented, clinicians must determine if the child has the language concepts of "once" and "word."

THERAPY SUGGESTIONS

1. *Railroad Train*: Two different trains are compared. The first train contains different cars and represents fluent speech (i.e., each car/word is different). The second train has a number of similar cars (e.g., box cars) placed in a row, which represents speech that contains repetitive speech samples. This technique can also be used by comparing different rows of coins, tokens, or zoo animals.

2. *Monitoring Clinician/Parent Speech*: The child detects instances of repetitions in the speech of the clinician. The clinician periodically produces speech repetitions and calculates the percentage of correct identifications made by the child as well as how rapidly the child accurately identifies them. As the child's ability to correctly and rapidly identify repetitions produced by the clinician increases, more therapy time is allotted to identifying repetitions in the child's speech. Therapy typically progresses from having the clinician produce part-word repetitions with several to many iterations before the child becomes aware and identifies the repetition to the child's identifying each part-word repetition immediately after the first iteration. Once a child can quickly and accurately identify part-word repetitions, his/her progress usually moves rapidly to fluent speech and dismissal from therapy. A number of our more dramatic treatment successes have occurred after a child has used this therapy technique at home and spontaneously identified instances of repeated words in the parent's speech. Apparently, once the concept of not repeating elements of speech is finally understood, a child often carries over this awareness to the home and corrects the parents' nonfluent speech. Once such spontaneous generalization occurs, progress can be quite rapid, usually going from a significant number of stutterings to zero in a very short period of time.

3. *Old Ears*: Explain to the child that a person does not have to repeat words to be understood. To illustrate this point, a humorous, exaggerated, and animated example of repeating a word 10 times or more is presented. Immediately after the child is asked if the repeated word helped to better understand the message. As a follow-up therapy technique, the clinician can feign that his/her ears are hurting when part-word repetitions are produced by the child. If the child does repeat, then the clinician can roll on the floor in mock pain.

This always gets a child's attention, and carefully produced speech without disfluencies usually follows. If fluent speech production continues for a reasonable period of time, the clinician can dance around with "happy ears" because no "repeating of words" has hurt the clinician's ears for the past few minutes. The combination of happy ears and hurting old ears provides constant reminders to the child and keeps the focus on fluent speech during therapy sessions.

4. *Different Feet*: Use the turtle or slow animal trail to facilitate this technique (see Rule 1: technique 6). Have the child say different words with each step while walking the slow animal trail. Walking is easy and smooth when different feet are used for each step, but if the same foot is used, and the child starts to hop, then walking becomes "hard and bumpy." And if the same word is said over and over, speech gets bumpy, and people may have difficulty understanding what is said.

5. *We're Number One*: Another nonverbal cue is used with this rule. When the child produces a part-word repetition, the clinician holds up a finger (i.e., similar to what people do to indicate their team is number one) to indicate that a repetition has occurred. This allows the therapist to signal, while the child is speaking, without interrupting. This signal makes the child aware of the Fluency Rule and permits his/her immediate practice of speech without repetitions. This technique has been effective for parents use outside the clinic to help their child become aware of repetitions without the perception of "badgering."

Primary Rules

These rules are always taught as a unit if a clinician determines that stuttering has advanced to a level that air flow and laryngeal control have become affected.

Rule 3: Use Speech Breathing

BACKGROUND

During the last 9 years of implementing the FRP, the Primary Rules have been applied whenever more direct physiological intervention was required. During this period, our private practice had achieved excellent clinical success using the Computer-Assisted Fluency Establishment Trainer (CAFET) with adolescent and adult stutterers.[6] A major component of the CAFET program is its measurement of chest-wall expansions and contractions which allows the clinician to make inferences regarding a client's inhalation/exhalation. The CAFET also provides both the speaker and clinician immediate visual feedback of the speech breathing curve and assists the speaker in coordinating speech breathing with the initiation of speech. Because of our success with these older clients, we wanted to simulate this clinical experience and bring speech breathing to a conscious level of young stutterers by utilizing visual and tactile procedures. Prior to beginning these therapy techniques, the difference between regular and speech breathing is explained to the child. For speech breathing, the explanation includes breath in, slowly let your air out, speak on the "out" breath, and keep the air moving (i.e., do not hold your breath). A final clinical observation on the breathing patterns of the stutterers we have treated. As was reported in the previous edition of this text, most stuttering and vocal abuse/nodule clients, except for preschool and early grade-school children are expanding or "pushing their thoracic/diaphragmatic area outward prior to the production of speech when they begin therapy with us. This is in contrast to other clients or even their own non–speech breathing, which is characterized by a steady contraction or inward movement of the thoracic/

diaphragmatic area as exhalation begins. When questioned about this unusual movement, most have reported the perception of a slight concurrent, tensing in their laryngeal area. Using the techniques described in this section has eliminated this initial irregular breathing/ laryngeal pattern.

THERAPY SUGGESTIONS

1. *The Breath Curve*: Draw a typical breath curve on a chalkboard or piece of paper, illustrating inspiration with a rising line and a gradual downward slope for exhalation. Next, place an "X" on the line shortly after exhalation starts to indicate where speech should begin. Have the child trace the breath curve with an index finger as he or she "feels" the breathing pattern. After the child understands the feeling of speech breathing, practice initiating speech at the point on the breath curve where the "X" has been placed. At first, have the child count or recite days of the week or months of the year as the breathing curve is carefully traced. The clinician must be cautious at this time to make sure that the child's tracing of the breath curve is in synchrony with the in and out motions of the child's breathing. Next, four- and five-syllable phrases (e.g., "Where is my toy?") are used for practicing speech breathing while the child still traces the breath curve.

2. *Tactile Feedback*: Just the previous activity encouraged the child to visualize speech breathing and, to a lesser degree, feel the physiological components of speech breathing, this second activity focuses on the child feeling the physiological aspects of speech breathing. To accomplish this, the clinician first positions the child's hand below his or her sternum, where the lower ribs flare, then places her hand over it. This technique focuses the child's attention on the feel of the in and out movements of the chest wall that accompany speech breathing. With the first therapy suggestion above, the child can both visualize and feel speech breathing. If needed, another clinical activity can be added. The clinician places a hand around the child's upper arm and gently squeezes it to initiate speech. As the child traces the breath cycle and feels the speech breathing movements with a hand on the chest wall, the clinician squeezes the child's arm as the tracing finger passes the "X," providing a tactile cue to begin speech. These combined therapy activities have been successful and usually require only minimal therapy time to achieve a child's awareness of speech breathing, prevoiced exhalation, and when to initiate speech.

3. *For Breath/speech Holding*: Have the child begin a typical speech breathing cycle, and, begin counting from 1 to 20 at the "X." At the count of 4, have the child vigorously pull up on the sides of the chair in which he or she is sitting until breathing and speech stop momentarily. Then instruct the child to continue to count, strongly pulling and tensing on every fourth count to contrast the feeling of a tense and relaxed neck and the corresponding changes that occur to the voice. Explain that if the neck is so tense that air flow stops, then speech will also stop. Finally, have the child repeat this procedure without pulling and feel how a relaxed neck is better for fluent speech production.

Rule 4: Start Mr. Voice Box Running Smoothly

BACKGROUND

An important modification has been made to this rule since the first publication.[3] The original wording "Keep Mr. Voice Box running smoothly" was modified to "Start Mr. Voice Box running smoothly." This subtle change was made because of the importance for young stutterers to learn the feeling of starting their vocal folds vibrating easily and smoothly. This is often referred to as a gentle onset and is a major component in a number of fluency training treatment programs for stutterers. Although this is a commonly used therapy target for stutterers, there does not appear to be a widely accepted definition of gentle onset. In our therapy program, it is defined as a gradual increase of intensity over time at the beginning of an utterance or after a pause. Therapeutic success has been achieved using this definition particularly with those children who pointed to their neck and indicated this is where they get "stuck."

THERAPY SUGGESTIONS

1. *Awareness*: A variety of caricatures have been used to represent "Mr. Voice Box" to show children that "he lives" in the neck and that when Mr. Voice Box is running you can feel the vibration. Have the child hum while touching the neck area with his or her hand to locate where Mr. Voice Box lives. The clinician can further illustrate that Mr. Voice Box lives in the neck by manipulating the larynx gently with his/her fingers while the child is vocalizing causing Mr. Voice Box to make funny noises.

2. *Contrasting*: Demonstrate two distinctly different modes of initiating phonation to illustrate the difference between a gentle and hard onset. First, have the child focus on the tension in the neck and the abrupt or hard onset of voicing as he or she pulls up on the chair. Next, ask the child to feel the absence of tension in the neck area as he or she phonates without pulling up on the chair.

3. *A Suggestion Changed*: Originally, we suggested that clinicians teach children to use a breathy voice to experience and learn to produce gentle onsets of speech. Once breathy voice production and the concept of gentle onset was learned, the clinician gradually was to return the child's voice to one that was less breathy and more natural sounding. Unfortunately, we have had considerable difficulty eliminating this newly acquired breathy component from a child's voice. The process of teaching a therapy concept, then telling the child to no longer use it, has proved to be very confusing to some children. As a result we no longer recommend teaching breathy speech production, then asking the child to eliminate its use, and we have not had substantial difficulty in teaching school-age children easy onset without using the breathy voice model.

4. *Gentle, Not Soft*: In our early attempts to teach gentle onset, some children interpreted this technique to mean a soft onset (i.e., reduced intensity) and would, therefore, begin speech at a very low intensity. To illustrate that the goal is a gentle, not a soft onset, two horizontal lines are drawn on a chalkboard or paper with a sloping line, drawn at about a 45° angle, connecting the lower to the upper line. The lower horizontal line is marked as zero intensity, which we refer to as silence; the upper horizontal line, as the child's normal speaking intensity; and the 45° connecting line, as gentle onset. Using this drawing, the child is asked to begin speech with an easy onset of phonation as he or she traces the sloping line while initiating speech with exaggerated slowness. As soon as the clinician believes the concept has been learned, the child is instructed to reduce the exaggerated slow onset to normal-sounding speech. Single-syllable, vowel-initiated words, and short phrases are used for this task.

5. *The Laryngeal Lips*: Because Mr. Voice Box "lives" in the neck and cannot be seen, there seems to a kind of mystery about the larynx for many young children. To help children visualize the vocal folds and understand "how the larynx works," clinicians can use their lips as a model. By producing what is often called a "raspberry sound" (i.e., blowing air between and vibrating lips) the clinician can demonstrate the principals of air flow and medial vocal fold compression. We also demonstrate that air flow stops if we press our lips

together too tightly, which may be similar to what some children are doing with their vocal folds when they feel tension in their neck. These demonstrations and age-appropriate explanations of these principals greatly help the child to understand the larynx and this therapeutic goal.

Secondary Rules

These rules are used as needed to eliminate secondary or concomitant behaviors presented by the stutterer and should be applied as soon as such behaviors are observed.

Rule 5: Touch the "Speech Helper" Together Lightly

BACKGROUND

The "speech helpers" (i.e., lips, tongue, and teeth) have been depicted as cartoon characters that are parts of the mouth which are important for producing "speech sounds." A number of public school speech–language pathologists have used these cartoon "speech helpers" to decorate the walls of their therapy rooms/offices, which increases the awareness of the children to these anatomical structures. Children who stutter are instructed to touch the "speech helpers" together very lightly, because if they press them together too hard, speech breathing and speech will stop.

THERAPY SUGGESTIONS

1. *The Hard Contact*: Have the child attempt to produce a bilabial plosive by pressing the lips together tightly "until a word pops out." Some older children have been encouraged by well-intentioned parents to "just try harder" and their speech will improve. Therefore, clinical explanations and demonstrations are used to show that easier not harder efforts and contacts are necessary for producing fluent speech. To illustrate, practice hard contacts in front of a mirror with a great deal of animated effort while pointing out, humorously, the futility of trying to produce speech with excessive effort. For example, clinician can press his/her lips together with a GREAT deal of effort and a contorted face while jumping up and down to demonstrate that no matter how hard he or she tries a word will just not "pop out." Then the clinician can demonstrate that by just lightly touching the lips together, fluent speech is produced with ease, not effort. Children usually enjoy practicing these contrasting methods of speech production and quickly learn the importance of easy contacts of the articulators to fluent speech.

2. *Can I Hold Your Arm?*: Another treatment technique that illustrates the goal of light contact of the "speech helpers" involves squeezing the child's arm as he or she speaks, as we described for Rule 3: suggestion 3. As the child speaks fluently, the clinician holds one arm lightly, but as soon as a hard contact occurs, the clinician squeezes the child's arm gently, but firmly. The amount of pressure applied by the squeeze should be roughly proportional to the amount of tension perceived in the hard contact.

Rule 6: Keep the Speech Helpers Moving

BACKGROUND

This rule was designed originally to eliminate prolongations but has been expanded to include easy movements from one speech sound to the next. Using this rule in conjunction with Rule 5, Touch the "speech helpers" together lightly, has also proved to be effective.

Several examples of how to combine these rules are included in the therapy suggestions that follow.

THERAPY SUGGESTIONS

1. *Turtle Tracks or Lily Pads*: With turtle or other slow-moving animal tracks, or lily pads, have the child move from one track or lily pad to the next, smoothly stepping on each one lightly. During this activity, five-syllable phrases are used as stimuli for the child to repeat. In using this phrase length, five tracks are placed close together, indicating the syllables of each phrase, then a larger space is used to represent the pause between phrases and the place for the child to start the speech breathing and gentle-onset cycle again. To demonstrate "what happens" when an instance of stuttering occurs, clinicians using exaggerated movements and animation can fall off an animal track to the floor or jump on a lily pad so hard (i.e., when a hard contact occurs) or so often (i.e., when repetitions occur) that they sink.

2. *Piano Fingers*: Moving the thumb to each finger or tapping the thumb and fingers on a table top has proved useful in teaching this speech rule. This also demonstrates that fluent speech should move easily and smoothly from sound to sound, just as we can move our thumb to our fingers or our fingers to tap the table top. With each digit representing a speech sound or syllable, the child produces short phrases, saying them while moving the thumb and fingers smoothly from sound to sound. Next, we demonstrate that if the thumb and finger stay or stick together too long, or a finger remains on the table too long, a prolonged sound will be produced. In addition, we show the child that if the thumb and finger press together with too much force, like the lips or the tongue may do, air flow and speech will slow down and stop.

3. *Keep It Short*: Another nonverbal cue can be used specifically to make the child aware of and ultimately eliminate prolongations. Ordinarily, a hand signal is used to alert the child that a prolongation occurred so that the flow of speech is not interrupted. As the child talks, the clinician holds a thumb and forefinger close together in the child's field of vision as a reminder to keep speech units short. By quickly lengthening the distance between the thumb and finger, then slowly reducing the distance, the clinician can illustrate the change from a prolongation to a correct "short" sound.

Rule 7: Use Only the "Speech Helpers" to Talk

BACKGROUND

This rule explains that fluent speech is produced by moving only the "speech helpers" and that it is not necessary or helpful to move other muscles or parts of the body when speaking. This rule is used to eliminate any secondary or concomitant behaviors that a child may have developed.

THERAPY SUGGESTIONS

1. *The Mirror*: A mirror may be all that is needed for some children to eliminate their secondary behaviors. Frequently, children are unaware of the extraneous body movements or other secondary affectations that accompany their stuttering behaviors, and once these behaviors are pointed out to them visually, they are often quickly eliminated.

2. *Too Much of a Bad Thing*: The mirror is again used with this technique. For example, if a

head turn is used as speech begins, we explain that turning the head does not help anyone produce speech. Standing with the child in front of a mirror and using exaggerated animation humor we say that "we are going to turn our heads as hard and as frequently as possible until a word comes out." Obviously nothing happens, and it is clear that turning the head to start speech is not helpful and should be eliminated. This therapy technique can be used to illustrate to a child with any inappropriate motor responses that speech does not begin until air flow begins and the "speech helpers" are moving smoothly.

Fluency Rules Program: Revised

Since the first version of the FRP was published,[3] we have become increasingly aware of the importance of their order of presentation. Originally, the steps appeared as follows:

1. Determine the Fluency Rule broken.
2. Teach language concepts necessary for complete understanding of therapy instructions.
3. Develop the child's self-monitoring skills.
4. Practice fluent speech production using the fluency rules.
5. Carry over procedures for the home and classroom.

In the current version, FRP-R, step 1 follows the order the Fluency Rules described in this chapter. Although the original FRP version was successful with many young children, with continued use, our therapeutic strategies have steadily changed. Originally, we recommended that clinicians work only on those Fluency Rules that were broken by a child. No suggestions regarding which rule to treat first or the order in which to teach other rules that are broken were given. Following review of recent clinical records, we found that therapy was always started with two rules: "Speak slowly," and "Say a word only one time." Thus, these rules are now viewed as "universal." The review of clinical records further revealed that when these two universal rules were taught simultaneously, a dramatic improvement in fluency often occurred without additional therapeutic intervention. Thus, when these two rules were used appropriately by some children, other aspects of their stuttering (e.g., struggle and/or accessory behavior) frequently disappeared, eliminating the need for teaching additional Fluency Rules.

As effective as the two Universal Rules can be, those children who struggle during their speech disruptions frequently continue to stutter. Therefore, when the two Universal Rules did not result in fluent speech production, the two Primary Rules became the focus of such children's therapy. These two rules were taught as a pair also, for example, Rule 3, Speech breathing, was explained first followed by Rule 4, Start Mr. Voice Box running smoothly. Teaching these rules simultaneously is our current procedure, which appears to be consistent with other therapy protocols that emphasize the importance of the interaction between speech breathing and gentle onset of phonation. Our rationale for designating these as Primary Rules is that a significant number of young stutterers we have seen clinically exhibit laryngeal tension and report that "words get stuck in my throat." Many of these same stutterers also do not demonstrate appropriate speech breathing patterns or consistently coordinate speech breathing with the onset of phonation. Twelve of 17 young children treated for stuttering during the past 6 years have exhibited breathing/voice onset problems, the most frequent being the tendency to "push the words out." These children appear to reverse the direction of their thoracic/abdominal wall movements, usually when about to stutter, but occasionally when fluent. Thus, as they began to exhale, their thoracic/abdominal wall would contract, but immediately prior to initiating speech production, the direction of these movements would reverse and the thoracic/abdominal area would expand, as if they were inhaling. Our clinical impression is that these stutterers are using this respiratory maneuver in an attempt to push words out. Those children who were old enough to understand our questions about such behavior verified that they were, in fact, trying to "push the words out."

The three secondary rules are used with a child only if needed. Although we now use all of these rules less frequently, Rule 5, Touch the "speech helpers" together lightly, has been used more frequently than the others. In addition, these Secondary Rules are used in FRP-R as soon as aberrant behavior first occurs. Thus, even if the current therapeutic goal is to teach the Universal Rules and a secondary behavior is observed, the clinician should immediately stop instructing the Universal Rules and teach the appropriate Secondary Fluency Rule. When satisfied that the child understands the new rule and fluency concept, the clinician should return to teaching the Universal Rules.

Carryover and Transfer

The final phase of FRP involves carryover or transfer of the Fluency Rules to the child's home and classroom. Obviously, for transfer to be effective, the child must remember the rules in new speaking environments. The most effective procedure we have found to facilitate carryover has been to place a discriminative stimulus in each environment. In school, the speech–language pathologist, the classroom teacher, subject teacher, and the student meet to select a small, unobtrusive item that will be placed in each room as a reminder of the Fluency Rules (e.g., sticker on notebooks or refrigerator magnets on the edge of chalkboards). Only the teacher and student need be aware of the item and its significance. Then, if the child forgets to use a Fluency Rule, the teacher can provide a reminder by glancing in the direction of or touching the item.

At home, the same procedure can be used. The family places similar reminders (e.g., elephants are effective symbols because elephants never forget) in conversation areas (e.g., the family room, kitchen, bedroom, and dining room) and family members call the child's attention to them as needed. The subtle nature of these stimuli and how they are used also provides a secondary benefit. They eliminate the need for direct confrontations when Fluency Rules are not used which reduces family conflicts that may arise from frequent verbal reminders, particularly during the early stages of transfer. Ideally, the transfer phase of therapy will result in the Fluency Rules being generalized away from the therapy room and ultimately lead to fluent speech in all environments.

A new and effective treatment strategy that we now use clinically as discriminative stimuli and reinforcements involves video games, toys, and other games. These materials have considerable motivational appeal for children, which is the key, and can be used to motivate children to use the Fluency Rules in therapy, at home, and at school. During scheduled therapy sessions, computer games or other play-time breaks are a regularly scheduled component of therapy which reinforces a child's correct application of the Fluency Rules. To facilitate carryover of fluency rules at home, we have a lending library arrangement which allows children to check out one video game until the next therapy session. Toys and games are used with younger children in the same way. A board game or toy can be loaned for a week with the parents' agreement to play with the child and encourage use of the Fluency Rules. In order to check out a game or toy, the child must agree to use their Fluency Rules at home or school, especially when playing the game. An additional positive effect of the lending library is that it stimulates more parental involvement in the therapeutic process. Because these games can be played competitively, parents are encouraged to set aside time to play these games with their children. This leads to enjoyable times together and allows the parents to remind the child of the Fluency Rules, when needed, and monitor how well the child is using them. The feedback received from both parents and children has been positive.

Equally impressive is the motivational value of these games in the clinic with children. When our lending library was first started, there were two difficult children on the caseload. Their renewed interest and subsequent increased cooperation in therapy after the inclusion of video games were impressive. Both successfully completed therapy, which we feel was due in part to the use of the lending library and the interest that these games brought to the therapy process.

Lastly, we also use telephone calls as discriminative stimuli to help carryover of fluency to the home environment. We begin, typically, near the end of therapy, when the child is using the Fluency Rules effectively in therapy sessions. At this point, we encourage the child to think about and use the rules at home. To assist in keeping the child's awareness high, we call him or her at home and ask about speech and if the Fluency Rules are being used. At first, with the parents' permission, we make these calls frequently, about five calls a night. This frequency of calls is continued for about a week, then calls are gradually and systematically reduced until they occur infrequently, about twice a week. Periodically, however, we call five times on randomly selected nights. The intended outcome of this procedure is that, after a short period of time, the child thinks that every time the phone rings "the crazy therapist is calling again," which serves as a reminder to use the Fluency Rules. Since the creation of the lending library, our calls are longer and more effective, because conversations can be directed toward the child's use of video games and not be limited to just checking up on speech. These calls also provide us an excellent opportunity to evaluate the child's fluency in a different setting than the clinic.

Therapy Outcome

In our first description of the FRP,[3] the therapeutic results of nine children were reported. They consisted of five males and four females with an average age of 5 years, 5 months. Based on Riley's severity scale[7] three who were treated were mild, four were moderate, and two were severe stutterers. Five of these children were followed for 2 years after therapy; four were followed for 1 year. All had been seen in a public school setting, receiving therapy two or three times a week for 30 or 40 min. The data indicated that each of these children evidenced a significant improvement in fluency while maintaining normal speaking rates and eliminating all secondary behaviors. Further data revealed that the improvements in their fluent speech production that occurred during therapy had been maintained during follow-up assessment, however, a lingering concern remained. Although each child demonstrated marked improvement in fluent speech production, each child's speech also contained slight, residual signs of stuttering. These residuals were limited to mild part-word repetitions of two or less iterations and no secondary behaviors. Unfortunately, these children could not be followed for longer periods of time and no additional data are available.

During the past few years, we have consulted with numerous public school systems regarding the implementation of the Fluency Rules Program in their schools and have supervised a number of students as they used the program. We have personally treated 17 young stutterers in a private practice, and the information that follows is based on these 17 stutterers. They consisted of three females and 14 males whose ages at the beginning of therapy averaged slightly less than 7 years. Based on the Stuttering Prediction Instrument,[8] two were severe, eight were moderate, and seven were mild stutterers. Nine of these children exhibited secondary behaviors. The seven mild stutterers and one moderate stutterer did not exhibit accessory behavior. All of the 17 children's speech were judged by us to be within the acceptable range on the 9-point naturalness scale[9] at their release from therapy. Average length of therapy was 9 months, with a range of 3–20 months.

Efficiency and adaptability were important factors in the design of the FRP because of the typical treatment format required in a public school. Results of the first group of children who were treated using this program demonstrated that it was effective in reducing stuttering when treatment was conducted in a public school setting. Of the clinical outcomes just described for our private practice, six of the 17 children received services in the public schools in addition to our private practice therapy. Therefore, it appears that the FRP can be implemented successfully in a combined effort between public school and private settings.

Finally, we hope that clinicians in all therapeutic environments who use the FRP will share their results, techniques, and experiences with us and their colleagues at professional meetings. The FRP's ultimate effectiveness and utility can only be determined when larger and more diverse groups of stuttering children are treated by different therapists in different settings and are followed over longer periods of time.

Suggested Readings

Bennett-Mancila E: *The House that Jack Built*. Staff. Garland, Texas, Aaron's Association, 1992.
Excellent analogy for helping children understand the speech process necessary for fluent speech production by using the construction of a house.

Meyers S, Woodford L: *The Fluency Development System for Young Children*. Buffalo, United Educational Service, 1992.
A commercially available treatment technique for stutterers up to age nine. The focus of this approach is on slow versus fast speech, bumpy versus smooth speech, turn-taking, and withstanding time-pressure.

Ramig PR, Bennett EM: Working with 7–12 year old children who stutter: Ideas for intervention in the Public schools. *Language, Speech Hearing Serv Schools* 1995; 26:138–150.
A very good maintenance program for children who stutter.

Conture E, Guitar B: Evaluating efficacy of treatment of stuttering: School-age children. *J Fluency Disord* 1993; 18:253–287.
A review of therapy programs and their reported effectiveness. Suggestions for future assessment and treatment efficacy is provided.

Ramig PR, Bennett EM: Clinical Management of Children: Direct Management Strategies, in Curlee RF, Siegel GM (eds): *Nature and Treatment of Stuttering: New Directions*. Boston, Allyn and Bacon, 1997.
An excellent review of therapy techniques that have been used successfully in commercially available programs/kits as well as published general/structural approaches.

Peters JT, Guitar B: *Stuttering: An Integrated Approach to Its Nature and Treatment*. Baltimore, MD, Williams and Wilkins, 1991.
Text containing information on the nature of stuttering as well as therapy and assessment techniques for beginning and intermediate stutterers.

References

1. Speech–Language-Hearing Association of Virginia: Position statement: Public school speech and language caseload reduction. *J Speech Hear Assoc Va* 1991; 32:34–35.
2. Dunlap K: A comparative study of public school speech–language pathologists in Virginia: 1982 vs 1994. Unpublished Honor's degree thesis: J Madison U 1995.
3. Runyan CM, Runyan SE: Fluency rules therapy program for young children in the public school. *Lang Speech Hear Serv Schools* 1986; 17:276–284.
4. Purcell R, Runyan CM: Normative study of speech rates of children. *J Speech Hear Assoc Va* 1980; 21:6–14.
5. Greenberg JB: The effects of a metronome on the speech of young stutterers. *J Behav Ther* 1970; 1:240–244.
6. Goebel MD: A Computer-Aided Fluency Treatment Program for Adolescents and Adults. San Francisco, Miniseminar, ASHA, November 1984.
7. Riley GD: A stuttering severity scale for children and adults. *J Speech Hear Disord* 1972; 37: 314–320.
8. Riley GD: Stuttering Prediction Instrument. Tigard, OR, CC Publications, 1981.
9. Martin RR, Haroldson SK, Triden KS: Stuttering and speech naturalness. *J Speech Hear Disord* 1984; 49:23–58.

Stuttering and Related Disorders of Fluency, 2nd edition.
Edited by Richard F. Curlee, Ph.D.
Thieme Medical Publishers, Inc., New York © 1999.

7

Treating Children Who Exhibit Co-Occurring Stuttering and Disordered Phonology

Linda J. Louko
Edward G. Conture
Mary Louise Edwards

Speech–language pathologists (SLP) who work with young children will undoubtedly encounter children on their caseloads who exhibit either stuttering or speech sound difficulties (disordered phonology); however, when a child exhibits *both* of these disorders, the SLP is presented with a potentially complex clinical situation, one that may neither be easily nor quickly resolved. As with any such speech–language problem, the SLP first must determine if the behaviors presented are of a quantity and quality to warrant a diagnosis of stuttering and/or disordered phonology. Second, the severity of each disorder must be determined before a prognosis can be made, and before the SLP can answer such questions as "Will my child recover from these problems?" and "How long will therapy last?" And finally, once a diagnosis and prognosis have been made, the SLP will need to determine the most appropriate type of treatment.

Based on our experience, decisions regarding treatment for children who exhibit *both* stuttering and disordered phonology may differ from those decisions regarding treatment for children who exhibit *only* stuttering or *only* disordered phonology. For example, the SLP may need to decide whether treatment for one of the two disorders should precede treatment for the other (i.e., serial treatment). Conversely, the specific needs of the child may lead the SLP to decide to concurrently treat the co-occurring stuttering and disordered phonology problems (i.e., parallel treatment). It is our opinion and experience that when a child exhibits *both* stuttering and disordered phonology, all of these clinical decisions are more difficult to make. We also believe that both disorders can and should be treated simultaneously in most cases. Hence, this requires a different approach to therapy for these children than the traditional serial approach of treating one problem, then the other. The purpose of this chapter is to provide an overview of how to identify children who exhibit both stuttering and disordered phonology and provide detailed information regarding one treatment program that we have found to be reasonably successful.

Prevalence Information

The frequency with which disordered phonology co-occurs with stuttering has been well documented in the literature.[1–18] It has also been documented that articulation or phonological difficulties are one of the more common concomitant speech–language problems to co-occur with stuttering.[14] However, there is a substantial range in the reported percentage of children who stutter and exhibit speech sound difficulties. This range in prevalence data is likely due to various factors, and one main factor may be the dissimilarities in methodologies (e.g., direct testing of children versus use of clinical records or parental observations) among reported studies.[19,20] Such prevalence data estimate the co-occurrence of stuttering and disordered phonology in children from as low as 16%[2] to as high as 67%–96%.[14] Results of several prevalence studies that *directly* examined the articulation/phonological disorders exhibited by children who stutter are reported in Table 7-1, with a mean percent co-occurrence of 41% (range = 19%–96%).

After reviewing the literature and records from years of clinical experience with young children who stutter, Conture[21] concluded that approximately one third of all children who stutter are likely to exhibit some articulation/phonological difficulties, compared to the 2%–6% that would be expected in the general population.[22,23] It is also interesting to note that at least one study found that more speech disfluencies are exhibited by children *with* articulation problems than by children *without* articulation problems.[24] On the other hand, some question whether there is a relatively strong relationship between stuttering and disordered phonology in children. For example, Throneburg, Yairi, and Paden[25] reported that relatively few children who stuttered (7%) also exhibited severe/profound phonological disorders; however they did not report data on the occurrence of mild to moderate speech sound difficulties. Also, Seider, Gladstein and Kidd[26] found no significant difference in the articulation abilities of a group of children who stuttered versus siblings who did not stutter. However, when considering *all* published findings, it is reasonable to conclude that young children who stutter are more likely to exhibit speech sound errors than are those who do not stutter. Or, as Bloodstein[3] suggests, "Almost without exception, studies have shown that stutterers tend to have more articulatory difficulties than nonstutterers" (p. 271).

The implications of a meaningful relationship between stuttering and disordered phonology, in terms of impairment, disability, and pathogenesis of either problem, are yet to be determined, although, some have attempted to provide theoretical explanations of the potential relationship between these two disorders.[27] For example, the results of Yaruss and Conture[27] suggest that the Covert Repair Hypothesis[28,29] has some potential for explaining the relationship of speech sound errors to stuttering in children; simply stated, this theory suggests that stutterings are the by-product of "repairs" that occur when the child tries to rectify speech sound errors.

Evaluation Needed

Information detailing the process for evaluating children who stutter is available elsewhere (e.g., see Conture,[30] for a review of this topic). Specific procedures for the identification of speech sound errors in children are available as well, whether using an articulation approach or a phonological process analysis.[31,32] Experienced clinicians will certainly want to employ their own procedures and criteria when assessing children who both stutter and exhibit disordered/delayed speech sound development; however, a brief overview of the

Table 7-1. Thirteen Studies That Directly Examine Articulation/Phonological Disorders Exhibited by Children Who Do/Do Not Stutter. The Number of Children in Each of Two Groups Is Provided: Children Who Stutter and Who Do Not Stutter

Author	Number of Stutterers	Number of Nonstutterers	% of Stutterers with Articulation Disorders	% of Nonstutterers with Articulation Disorders	Summary
McDowell (1928)	33	33	19	16	Articulation difficulties; significant differences between groups
Schindler (1955)	126	252	49	15	"Other speech disorders"
Morley (1957)	37	113	50	31	"Other speech disorders"
Williams and Silverman (1968)	115	115	24	9	Associated articulation difficulties
Riley and Riley (1979)	100	—	33	—	Associated articulation difficulties
Daly (1981)	138	—	58	—	Articulation disorders
Thompsno (1983)	48	—	35–45	—	"Suspected articulation difficulties"
Cantwell and Baker (1985)	40	—	30	—	—
St. Louis and Hinzman (1988)	48	24	67–96	—	—
Louko, Edwards, and Conture (1990)	30	30	40	7	Greater number and variety of phonological processes, more /s/—cluster reduction for children who stutter
Ryan (1992)	20	20	0	0	No significant difference on formal articulation test; but 5/20 (25%) of stutterers eventually required articulation therapy
Throneburg, Yairi, and Paden (1994)	75	—	7	—	Reported "severe phonologic deficits," no report of mild/moderate phonologic deficits
Paden and Yairi (1996)	36	36	22/36 (61%) (moderate–severe phonological deficits)	14/36 (39%) (moderate–severe phonological deficits)	Significant differences on formal test of phonology between persistent stutterers and their controls

procedures we use to diagnose both disorders and our case selection criteria provides a foundation for the management approach that follows.

Observations and Tests

In general, our goal is to determine the quantity and nature of a child's stuttering and/or phonological problems. However, as is the case with any complete speech–language assessment, some assessment of hearing sensitivity and other speech–language behaviors (e.g., expressive or receptive language, voice, etc.) should be included.

Stuttering*

The purpose of the stuttering portion of the evaluation is, of course, to determine whether the child is stuttering or is at risk for developing stuttering behavior. In order to do so, the clinician needs to identify the speech and nonspeech behaviors that are typically associated with speech disfluency: the frequency, duration, type and severity of disfluency, as well as any associated nonspeech behaviors (see Conture and Kelly[33] and LaSalle and Conture[34] for detailed descriptions of these nonspeech behaviors). The average frequency (and range) of disfluency can be determined from three to five, 100-word conversational speech samples that are recorded while the child is speaking to either his parent(s) or the clinician (and if possible, one or more other speaking situations). From the same samples, the average duration (and range) of disfluencies is measured from 10 to 15 randomly selected disfluencies. Furthermore, from this 300- to 500-word sample, the percentage of total disfluency represented by each disfluency type as well as the number and variety of associated nonspeech behaviors can be noted. The Stuttering Severity Instrument (SSI)[35], the Stuttering Prediction Instrument (SPI), as well as the Iowa Scale for Rating the Severity of Stuttering[36] are utilized to determine the chronicity and severity level of the child's disfluency. These tests may be augmented by "expert systems,"[37] a computer-based decision-support process for determining presence, severity, and chronicity of childhood stuttering, in addition to other formal/informal tests,[38,39] which are useful for assessing related aspects of stuttering, for example, the relationship between a child's stuttering and the length and complexity of his/her utterances.

Disordered Phonology

In the case of speech sound errors, an articulation or phonological approach to assessment may be taken, depending on the severity of the presenting phonological disorder. If a child has just a few speech sound errors, the clinician may choose to complete a traditional (3 position) articulation test.[40,41] On the other hand, for the child who exhibits numerous speech sound errors and/or is unintelligible, we suggest a phonological process analysis. For example, the SLP may employ Hodson's[42] Assessment of Phonological Processes— Revised, the Khan-Lewis Phonological Analysis,[43] or any of a variety of nonstandard procedures.[44,45] In this case, the clinician will want to identify the phonological processes exhibited by the child and make some determination of which processes are in need of remediation. The clinician may also want to assess the child's phonetic inventory; that is, the speech sounds that are produced (whether used correctly or incorrectly) in the child's

---

*See ref. 21 (pp. 35–84 for details).

speech sample. We have found the use of both of these procedures (i.e., phonological process analysis and phonetic inventory) to be helpful, particularly in the selection of processes and sounds to be targeted in therapy.

Case Selection Criteria

Stuttering

To be considered as "stuttering," a child typically has to meet at least two basic criteria: 1. produce three or more stutterings per 100 words in a 300-word sample of conversational speech obtained while the child interacts with his or her mother, father, or clinician at the time of the initial evaluation, and 2. have significant adult listeners who express concern over the child's speech fluency and/or believe that the child "stutters" or is at high risk for developing a stuttering problem.[21,46] Obviously, such basic criteria are augmented by other (in)formal tests (e.g., Stuttering Severity Instrument) (Yaruss, LaSalle and Conture[67]); however, all children we consider to be stuttering must meet at least the two aforementioned criteria.

Disordered Phonology

As noted previously, some clinicians may choose to use a traditional articulation approach when assessing the speech of children with speech sound difficulties, using the categories of substitutions, omissions, and distortions. On the other hand, especially if the child exhibits numerous speech sound errors, the clinician may want to assess the child's phonological system by identifying the phonological processes exhibited. For reasons that we will explain below, we have chosen to use a phonological approach in most cases.

To be identified as phonologically disordered, in our research and clinical work, children must fulfill *either* of the following criteria: (a) exhibit at least two age-inappropriate phonological processes, each of which has at least four opportunities to apply and affects at least 25% of all relevant items (see also Grunwell[47] and McReynolds and Elbert[48]) or (b) exhibit one or more "atypical" phonological processes (i.e., processes not typical of normal development at any age[49,50]), each of which has at least four opportunities to apply and affects at least 25% of all relevant items.

Management Approach

The management/treatment approach we use has been described previously.[51] It involves the simultaneous treatment of stuttering and disordered phonology using "indirect"* methods. We hasten to point out that there is of a gap between the research (theoretical and empirical) and the applied knowledge base needed to conduct therapy in this area. Simply put, the basic and applied information needed to support our clinical procedures is not well developed at present. Therefore, what we do presently is based, in large part, on what works and on what makes sense in terms of our clinical experience. Thus, our discussion of therapy procedures provides few literature citations and must rely heavily on our own clinical work. Although we would like to cite a variety of published articles in refereed

---

*An indirect approach to therapy is "an approach that does not explicitly, overtly or directly try to modify or change the child's speech fluency [or speech sound production] in specific, and oral communication skills in general.[21]

journals to support our clinical work in this area, such information is simply not available. This is not to suggest that we are overly egocentric in terms of our clinical approach in this area; rather it suggests that there is not a great deal of information available regarding therapy for children who exhibit both stuttering and disordered phonology.

Treatment Objectives

In general, the goal of treatment is for the children to acquire a normal level of disfluency and normal (age-appropriate) phonology. We believe that these goals are best achieved through the concurrent or simultaneous treatment of both disorders, rather than choosing to treat one disorder before or after the other in serial fashion.[51] While our distinct preference is to carry out this approach in group therapy, many of our procedures can be adapted and applied to individual sessions. In our opinion, groups clearly provide the opportunity for a large variety and number of adult and peer communicative interactions, which can be used to the advantage of the client and clinician. For example, group therapy often provides the "natural" conditions under which other speech, language, and pragmatic skills can be developed, which may facilitate improvement in the child's speech fluency.

Treatment Procedures

In general, our approach to simultaneous treatment of stuttering and disordered phonology is modeled after the Parent–Child Stuttering Group that has been described elsewhere.[52,68] The parents meet together (Parent Group) during the same period of time (approximately 45–60 min) that their children are receiving therapy for fluency and phonological difficulties (hereafter we will refer to this particular parent–child group as the Stuttering–Phonology Group or SP Group). The parent aspect of the SP Group allows parents to obtain information about their child's speech/language difficulties and related issues, ask questions about their concerns, interact with parents having similar concerns, receive guided observations of the children's group, and participate with their children in an activity at the end of the group therapy session. We believe that the education and active participation of parents is essential to the success of this type of therapy. This belief is based on the assumption that changes in the home environment may be needed to facilitate the child's speech and language development. Thus, at least one parent is required to attend each Parent–Child Group session.[52]

Session Organization

Both the Parent and Child's sections of the SP Group meet at the same time but in separate rooms. Therefore, two SLPs usually administer the program. Sessions are weekly and last for approximately 45–60 min.

STUTTERING–PHONOLOGY GROUP (SP GROUP)

The main goal of the children's therapy in the SP Group is to "develop age-appropriate phonology within the context of increasing speech fluency."[51]

General Treatment Guidelines.   The following guidelines apply to the SP Group as a whole.

1. An *indirect* therapeutic approach is used; that is, there are *no* overt references made to identifying and/or modifying stuttering, and no specific directions are given to alter speech disfluencies. Likewise, we avoid traditional direct sound training for the children's articulation errors. Instead, children are rewarded for success on tasks within an activity,

rather than on the "correctness" of their phoneme production. Therefore, when a child makes speech sound errors, clinicians do not identify, highlight, or point out the error. Neither do they correct, reprimand, or "punish" the child for an error or ask the child to repeat the word correctly. The rationale for this indirect approach is that *direct* intervention for phonological errors may lead to increased fluency concerns, at least for some children, particularly those who appear to have sensitive temperaments and/or be more behaviorally inhibited (see Oyler[53] and Guitar[69] for a discussion of temperamental variables relative to childhood stuttering). In fact, a few published case studies have reported that during or shortly following treatment for speech sound disorders, some children do begin to stutter.[54,55]

2. The most "natural" strategies possible are used to facilitate fluency and correct speech sound production. For example, a child learns to wait for his or her speaking turn during conversation in order to minimize any undue tendency to begin talking too soon and/or interrupt a conversational partner.

3. Emphasis is placed on group dynamics and peer interaction. Therefore, the emphasis is *not* on an individual child's speech disfluencies or speech sound difficulties. As a result, other language skills, specifically pragmatic skills are emphasized, which may subsequently facilitate speech fluency.

4. Some attempt is made to address the two disorders therapeutically during all of the activities within each session.

5. *Both* problems are consistently monitored throughout treatment, although the behavioral changes in the two disorders may have to be measured differently. However, because treatments for both disorders are interactive, the clinician will need to continually monitor how change in one problem may influence the other.

6. Overtraining of skills. All children are given frequent opportunities to learn desired skills in the hope that "overlearning" or very frequent production of skills will generalize to the children's regular environment in the form of acceptable rates of performance.

Specific Treatment Procedures for Stuttering.   The specific treatment procedures for stuttering comprise attempting to change 1. inappropriate temporal aspects of, and 2. physical tension levels associated with, speech production.[21,52] This is based on our assumption that most instances of stuttering involve a physical tensing during articulatory contact, at one or more places in the vocal tract, then a pushing with air pressure "behind" the point of contact, as if the child is attempting to push through or blast out a "frozen" or "stuck" articulatory contact. In essence, changes in such behaviors are encouraged by the clinician modeling slow, physically relaxed speech and other natural communicative strategies which are thought to facilitate fluency.[56] A variety of activities are used that incorporate or easily demonstrate these strategies at a variety of cognitive/linguistic levels. Whenever possible linguistic demands are kept at a level that maximizes the chances that the children will be fluent. Our strategies include clinician modeling and use of the following:

1. Slower speaking rate (slow normal 130–160 words per minute).
2. Longer turn-switching pauses (approximately 1 sec in length).
3. More comments (especially about topics of interest to the child) and fewer questions asked of the child.
4. Shorter, simpler sentences (three to six words in length).
5. Less interrupting, speaking for and/or "over" the children.

In addition to the above, the clinician reiterates and/or creates activities or games that teach specific interaction rules that support/facilitate the child's speech fluency in every session. These rules are 1. do not talk for others; 2. wait for your conversational turn; 3. do not talk while others are talking; 4. use appropriate turn-taking. Our rationale for these rules is that by controlling the amount of interrupting, speaking out of turn, correcting the speech of others in the group, and so forth, the children should begin to experience less time urgency and less communicative pressure, all of which, we believe, should facilitate a child's fluency. It should also help a child to become more accepting and tolerant of his or her speaking mistakes. Such acceptance and tolerance should make speech a less onerous, simpler, more enjoyable experience for the child, which, in turn, should help the child to become more fluent. If a child *continues* (after several weeks of modeling) to correct other children, speak for other children, finish their sentences, etc., the child is gently reprimanded, in private if possible. We have found, however, that most children respond well and appear to appreciate these interaction rules because of their understanding that *they too* can finish what they have to say without undue interruption or criticism, that their thoughts are valued and will be listened to.

Specific Treatment Procedures for Disordered Phonology.   The specific treatment procedures for disordered phonology focus on the discrimination and production of speech sounds, sound sequences, and/or sound classes. Like the treatment procedures for stuttering, an indirect approach is used. Consequently, there is an emphasis on clinician modeling and clinician acceptance of both accurate, as well as inaccurate productions of target sounds.

As we noted in the evaluation section, we prefer to use a phonological process approach, instead of a traditional articulation approach. Thus, entire processes are targeted in treatment, instead of focusing on the precise and/or "perfect" production of individual speech sounds. A "modified cycles" framework is used, in which several phonological processes are targeted sequentially over a period of several months.[57,58] Generally, one process is targeted from 1 to 4 consecutive weeks, and within each session, one sound or consonant cluster is generally the focus of activities and games. As with most therapies, changes in phonology begin at the isolated sound level and progress to increasingly greater levels of linguistic complexity (e.g., sentences, conversation). The following list of intervention strategies have been successful for us in this type of therapy. (For a description of specific activities and games that are appropriate, see Kelman and Edwards.[59])

1. *No Direct Phonetic Placement.* One of the key features of this type of therapy is that there is *no* direct phonetic placement work or traditional drill-like therapy. We believe that direct therapy with these children can result in an inappropriately tense speech mechanism and physical struggle as children hold their speech articulators in a specific position to achieve articulatory perfection, precision, or "correctness."

2. *Modeling.* Clinician modeling is an integral part of this treatment procedure. For example, a type of "auditory bombardment"[57] is used in which children in the group are exposed to repeated/multiple models of a target sound in isolation, words, sentences, etc., within various naturalistic activities. Naturalistic therapy has been defined as a type of phonological remediation in which "target sounds and words are presented and produced as a natural part or consequence of the activity in which the children are involved" (Kelman and Edwards, p. 17[59]). In turn, these activities facilitate/encourage repeated *productions* of the specific targets as well.

3. *Auditory Discrimination.* Early in the treatment of any phonological process, several activities focus on auditory identification of target sounds affected by the process, versus the specific error sounds produced by the children. Again, these activities or tasks are carried out within naturalistic activities. For example, the clinician produces "sssss" instead of "shhhh" to quiet a "baby" and waits for children in the group to notice the production of "sssss" and then correct it).

4. *Minimal Pairs.* Different pairs of words are contrasted in which one member of the pair contains the children's error sound and the other contains the target (correct) sound.[60]

5. *Facilitating Contexts.* Target sounds are purposely placed in phonetic contexts that should make them easier to produce; for example, if the palatal fricative "sh" is the target sound, it can be placed next to the high front vowel /i/.

6. *Modified Paired Stimuli.* Several pairs of words are presented in which the first member of the pair is a word in which the target sound is produced correctly, and that word is systematically followed by other words in which the target sound *is not* produced correctly.[60] For example, in the case of the phonological process of Velar Fronting, if the child is able to produce the target /k/ correctly in the word "key," the word pairs might be *key*-car, *key*-cake, *key*-kite.

Each session has a different phonological goal, which is specifically chosen to vary the communicative demand on the children in the group. The linguistic/cognitive demands must, of course, be balanced with communicative demands which the children can handle (i.e., their capacity) relative to their stuttering. Adams[61] and Starkweather and Gottwald[62] provide overviews of the demands and capacities model relative to stuttering.

PARENT GROUP

The first goal of the SP Parent Group is to educate and inform parents about normal speech and language development, particularly with regard to both stuttering and disordered phonology. For example, parents receive current information on how and when children acquire speech sounds and how "normal disfluency" may differ from the types of disfluencies that put children at risk for stuttering. Throughout this process, they are encouraged to ask questions of the clinician and interact freely with the other parents, many of whom will share their same concerns.

Indeed, a second goal of the group is to provide parents an opportunity to ask any questions they may have about their own child's specific speech, fluency, language, or other developmental behaviors and share their concerns about their child's development. Whenever possible, the clinician facilitates these discussions and provides an atmosphere in which parents feel free to express concerns about their children's speech difficulties with the clinician and each other. As a result of this experience, most parents realize that other parents are having similar experiences, which typically helps remove some of the burden and stress they feel about having a "different child." Not infrequently, parents provide advice, insights, and support for one another, advice which is generally accepted because, within a group setting of this kind, parents come to realize that they are "all in the same boat."

A third goal of the parent group is to instruct parents how to make a number of simple, natural changes in their own speech and in their home environment to facilitate improvements in their child's speech. Such changes in parental communication behavior are depicted in a 30-min videotape produced by Conture and Guitar.[63] Many of these changes are related to a child's fluency disorder; however, others are more general in nature or are related to a child's phonological disorder. Specifically, clinicians model and instruct parents to do the following:

1. *Reduce speaking rates.* Parents are encouraged to speak at a slower rate of speech (slow normal: 130–160 wpm) when talking to or even in the presence of their child.

2. *Increase conversational turn-taking pause times.* Parents are taught to increase the pause time to approximately 1 sec, between the termination of their child's speech and initiation of their own speech. By increasing their own pause time before initiating speech, parents can attempt to decrease their child's overall time urgency to speak, that is, the child's feeling of being "rushed" to begin or continue communicating.

Initially, parents are taught to carry out 1. and 2. for only 5–10 min per day, *every* day, and when their child is particularly disfluent. After a period of time, however, many parents find that changing these speech behaviors becomes more "natural" and, therefore, much easier to do. Thus, with practice and experience, all such changes can be employed more naturalistically by parents *primarily* during those periods when their child is particularly disfluent.

3. *Minimize interruptions and talking for their child.* By decreasing the number and duration of their interruptions of their child's speech, parents have another way of trying to decrease their child's overall time urgency and increase the feeling that he or she has all the time needed to finish what he or she has to say. Interruptions may include finishing the child's utterances, supplying words for him or her, or starting a new topic which ignores what the child was saying. Kelly and Conture[52] provide objective data pertinent to these variables.

4. *Stop all implicit or explicit correction of stuttering.* This involves decreasing any direct corrections, criticisms, or instructions parents may have for changing, or attempts to modify their child's speech disfluency. For example, such comments as "Slow down," "Take a deep breath," "Think about you're saying," or "Relax" should be discontinued.

5. *Stop all implicit or explicit correction of speech sound production.* This involves decreasing any direct corrections, criticisms, or instructions for changing or attempts to improve their child's speech sound production. For example, parents should discontinue/ minimize comments such as "Watch me," "Say it this way," "Try it again this way," "Pronounce it like this." Such comments will probably not improve the child's speech sound production, and may, in fact, result in the child physically tensing his/her speech mechanism when speaking, in an attempt to "get it right" and may even encourage the child to rush to "get it out."

6. *Model correct speech sounds following their child's error.* Parents learn how to provide good speech models for their child simply by repeating a misarticulated word in a sentence slightly altered from the one the child said. The point of this procedure is to prevent a child from feeling that a word needs to be repeated "the right way," thus avoiding his/her use of undue physical tension in their speech mechanism. For example, if the child says "Look at my wing," the mother or father might repeat back "Yes, that is a nice *ring.*"

7. *Increase comments about the content of the child's message.* By commenting on what the child has said, parents can emphasize the importance of the *content* of speech, rather than the *manner* it is said. For example, parents are instructed to paraphrase what their child has said, as a way of reaffirming that they are, in fact, listening to the child's content.

8. *Listen to and talk about what the child is interested in.* Parents can help their child find speaking more enjoyable and less stressful if they listen to and talk about what their child wants to talk about. For example, when the child comes home from school, rather than asking "How did school go today," parents can simply say "Hi, nice to have you home" and wait for the child to bring up what he or she wants to discuss.

The clinician needs to do more than just instruct parents on what and how to change their speech; she needs to *model* these behaviors frequently for the parents as well. She also needs to listen constructively and empathetically when parents talk about the difficulties they are having learning to do this. The parent group setting provides an opportunity for the clinician to model these behaviors and for parents to practice them in a comfortable, supportive setting.

During the last half or third of the parent group, parents receive guided observations, usually via a one-way mirror, of their child's group therapy. Therefore, parents directly observe how the clinician carries out many of the same *natural* strategies that they will be asked to carry out in their homes (e.g., changing their rate of speech, using longer conversational pause times).

Although it is ideal to conduct an SP group with two clinicians, one assigned to the parent group and one to work with the children, a single clinician can manage an SP Group effectively on her own. In such cases, the clinical situation is altered to accommodate the parent portion at another time. Some school clinicians, for example, conduct their parent group in the evening on a weekly, biweekly, or monthly basis. Obviously, separate meetings of this type do not allow parents to observe or participate with their children in the SP Group on a regular basis. In this case, school SLPs can supplement group meetings with written suggestions sent home with the child, telephone contacts, or, if parents are properly trained in advance, audio/videotapes for the parents to review. It is our opinion, however, that some form of parent involvement/parent group is important to the success of this therapy approach.

It should also be noted that school SLPs can also have a positive influence on the child's speaking environment by working with his/her classroom teacher. In this situation, a group meeting of teachers, all of whom have children who stutter in their classrooms, can be used to disseminate information about stuttering and discuss what they can do to facilitate fluency in that environment.

9. *Expected outcomes.* A successful outcome of this therapy approach is for a child to achieve typical disfluency, and reasonably articulate speech. In essence, the child should be able to exhibit "… the ability to communicate readily and/or easily whenever, wherever and to whomever, whatever he or she wants" (Conture and Guitar, p. 254[64]). In addition, such talking abilities should occur not only with the clinician, but also with parents and siblings, while talking at the dinner table, asking/answering routine questions, or sharing information about their daily activities. We also expect this level of speech production to occur with the children's peers on the playground or in the classroom. In order to achieve this outcome, the clinician needs to monitor each child's carryover and maintenance over time. We frequently suggest maintenance sessions every few months which serve to "renew" both parents and children behavioral changes. Indeed, we have learned the importance of "phasing-out" therapy slowly, over time, from one session/week to one every other week, then one/month, then one every other month, etc. This "phase-out" procedure, we have found, significantly aids with carryover and helps transfer in-clinic change to the child's outside-clinic life.

Conclusions

There is a growing body of literature suggesting that young children who stutter exhibit disordered phonology much more frequently than do young children who do not stutter. There is also some evidence that more speech disfluencies are exhibited by children with articulation problems. Although we do not precisely understand the relationship between these two disorders, prevalence data suggest that most SLPs will undoubtedly encounter children on their caseloads who exhibit *both* disorders.

This chapter describes our approach to evaluation, and the simultaneous treatment of both stuttering and disordered phonology in children. Our treatment involves a Parent–Child SP Group, whose purpose is to improve the children's phonology to age-appropriate levels, while improving, or at least maintaining, their speech fluency. Rather than treating these disorders in a serial fashion, we employ a treatment that involves an interaction between techniques applied in parallel that are hoped to bring about positive changes in stuttering as well as speech sound errors.

We believe that therapy of this kind also allows SLPs to monitor both disorders continually and observe how changes in one may result in changes in the other. This approach takes into account the balance that we believe is necessary between the communicative demands that children can handle relative to their stuttering and the increasing demand that comes from efforts to improve their phonological systems. Although a group approach is preferable, adaptations can be made for individual sessions and to other settings (e.g., schools) as well. Above all, this approach aims to minimize the chances of winning the battle with the child's phonology, but losing the war by exacerbating and/or worsening the child's stuttering.

Acknowledgments.   Preparation of this paper was supported in part, by NIH/NIDCD research grant (DC00523) to Syracuse University. Requests for reprints should be directed to Linda J. Louko, Department of Speech Pathology and Audiology, State University of New York at Cortland, Cortland, NY 13045, USA.

Suggested Readings

Conture E, Louko LJ, Edwards ML: Simultaneously treating stuttering and disordered phonology in children: Experimental treatment, preliminary findings. *American J Speech–Language Pathol* 1993; 72–81.
    This article describes a treatment program designed to treat co-occurring stuttering and disordered phonology in young children. It also reports results of an experimental therapy study (based on eight children) which compared changes in stuttering behavior that resulted from an SP treatment group to changes in stuttering behavior observed in treatment designed for children who stutter only.

Kelly E, Conture E: Intervention with school-age stutterers: A parent–child fluency group approach. *Seminars Speech Language* 1991; 12(4):309–322.
    Kelly and Conture describe a parent–child treatment group they use with school-age children.

Kelman M, Edwards ML: *Phonogroup: A Practical Guide for Enhancing Phonological Remediation.* Eau Claire, WI: Thinking Publications, 1994.
    This treatment manual contains over 200 activities designed to target specific phonological processes in groups of children. The approach is indirect and naturalistic, utilizing extensive clinician modeling, auditory bombardment, and such other techniques as choices and foils.

Louko LJ: Phonological characteristics of young children who stutter. *Topics in Language Disorders* 1995; 15(3):48–59.
    The author provides a review of the literature concerning the prevalence of co-occurring stuttering

and disordered phonology, the specific types of speech sound errors produced by young children who stutter, and approaches to treating children who exhibit both stuttering and disordered phonology.

Yaruss S, Conture E: Stuttering and phonological disorders in children: Examination of the covert repair hypothesis. *J Speech Hearing Res* 1996; 39:349–364.

This article describes the covert-repair hypothesis[29] in relationship to systematic (phonological processes) and nonsystematic ("slips-of-the-tongue") speech errors and stuttering in children. Results suggest that self-repairs of nonsystematic speech errors may be related to children's speech disfluencies.

References

1. Andrews G, Harris M: *The Syndrome of Stuttering*. London, England, Williams Heineman Medical Books, 1964.
2. Blood G, Seider R: The concomitant problems of young stutterers. *J Speech Hearing Dis* 1981, 46:31–33.
3. Bloodstein O: *A Handbook on Stuttering*. Chicago, IL, National Easter Seal Society, 1995.
4. Cantwell D, Baker L: Psychiatric and learning disorders in children with speech and language disorders: A descriptive analysis. *Advances Learning Behav Disabil* 1985; 2:29–47.
5. Daly D: Differentiation of stuttering subgroups with Van Riper's developmental tracks: A preliminary study. *J National Student Speech Lang Hear Assoc* 1981; 9:89–101.
6. Darley F: The Relationship of Parental Attitudes and Adjustments to the Development of Stuttering, in Johnson W, Leutenegger R (eds): *Stuttering in Children and Adults*. Minneapolis, MN, University of Minnesota Press, 1955.
7. Louko L, Edwards M, Conture E: Phonological characteristics of young stutterers and their normally fluent peers: Preliminary observations. *J Fluency Dis* 1990; 15:191–210.
8. McDowell ED: *The Educational and Emotional Adjustments of Stuttering Children*. New York, Columbia University Teachers College, 1928.
9. Morley M: *The Development and Disorders of Speech in Childhood*. Edinburgh, Livingstone, 1957.
10. Preus A: *Attempts at Identifying Subgroups of Stutterers*. Oslo, Norway, University of Oslo Press, 1981.
11. Riley G, Riley J: A component model for diagnosing and treating children who stutter. *J Fluency Dis* 1979; 4:279–293.
12. Ryan B: Articulation, language, rate, and fluency characteristics of stuttering and nonstuttering preschool children. *J Speech Hearing Res* 1992; 35:333–342.
13. Schindler M: A Study of Educational Adjustments of Stuttering and Nonstuttering Children, in Johnson W, Leutenegger R (eds): *Stuttering in Children and Adults*. Minneapolis, University of Minnesota Press, 1955.
14. St. Louis K, Hinzman A: A descriptive study of speech, language and hearing characteristics of school-aged stutterers. *J Fluency Dis* 1988; 13:331–335.
15. Thompson J: *Assessment of Fluency in School-age Children: Resource Guide*. Danville, Illinois, Interstate Printers and Publishers, 1983.
16. Van Riper C: *The Nature of Stuttering* (2nd ed). Englewood Cliffs, New Jersey, Prentice-Hall, Inc., 1982.
17. Williams D, Silverman F: Note concerning articulation of school-age stutterers. *Percept Motor Skills* 1968; 27:713–714.
18. Wolk L, Edwards M, Conture E: Co-existence of stuttering and disordered phonology in young children. *J Speech Hearing Res* 1993; 36:906–917.
19. Louko LJ: Phonological characteristics of young children who stutter. *Topics Lang Dis* 1995; 15(3):48–59.
20. Nippold MA: Concomitant speech and language disorders in stuttering children: A critique of the literature. *J Speech Hearing Dis* 1990; 55(1):51–60.
21. Conture EG: *Stuttering* (2nd ed). Englewood Cliffs, New Jersey, Prentice-Hall, Inc., 1990.
22. Beitchman J, Nair R, Clegg M, Patel P: Prevalence of speech and language disorders in 5-year-old kindergarten children in the Ottawa-Carleton Region. *J Speech Hearing Dis* 1986; 51:98–110.

23. Hull F, Mielke P, Timmons R, Willeford J: The national speech and hearing survey: Preliminary results. *ASHA* 1971; 13:501–509.
24. Ragsdale JD, Sisterhen DH: Hesitation phenomena in the spontaneous speech of normal and articulatory-defective children. *Language Speech* 1984; 27:235–244.
25. Throneburg R, Yairi E, Paden E: Relation between phonologic difficulty and the occurrence of disfluencies in the early stage of stuttering. *J Speech Hearing Res* 1994; 37:504–509.
26. Seider RA, Gladstein KL, Kidd KK: Language onset and concomitant speech and language problems in subgroups of stutterers and their siblings. *J Speech Hearing Res* 1982; 25:482–486.
27. Yaruss J, Conture E: Stuttering and phonological disorders in children: Examination of the covert repair hypotheses. *J Speech Hearing Res* 1996; 39:349–364.
28. Postma A, Kolk H: The covert repair hypothesis: Prearticulatory repair processes in normal and stuttered disfluencies. *J Speech Hearing Res* 1993; 36:472–487.
29. Kolk H, Postma A: Stuttering as a covert repair phenomenon. In Curlee R, Siegel G (eds). *Nature and Treatment of Stuttering: New Directions.* Boston, Allyn and Bacon, 1997.
30. Conture E: Evaluating childhood stuttering, in Curlee R, Siegel G (eds). *Nature and Treatment of Stuttering: New Directions.* Boston, Allyn and Bacon, 1997.
31. Bernthal J, Bankson N: *Articulation and Phonological Disorders* (3rd ed). Englewood Cliffs, NJ, Prentice Hall, 1993.
32. Bleile K: *Manual of Articulation and Phonological Disorders: Infancy Through Adulthood.* San Diego, CA, Singular Publishing Group, Inc., 1995.
33. Conture E, Kelly E: Young stutterers' nonspeech behavior during stuttering. *J Speech Hearing Res* 1991; 34:1041–1056.
34. LaSalle L, Conture E: Eye contact between young stutterers and their mothers. *J Fluency Dis* 1991; 16:173–199.
35. Riley G: *Stuttering Severity Instrument for Young Children.* Tigard, OR, C.C. Publications, 1980.
36. Johnson W, Darley F, Spriestersbach D: *Diagnostic Methods in Speech Pathology.* New York, Harper & Row, Pub., 1963.
37. Curlee R, Bahill T: *Childhood Stuttering: A Second Opinion.* Tucson, AZ, Bahill Intelligent Computer Systems, 1993.
38. Stocker B: *Stocker Probe Technique for Diagnosis and Treatment of Stuttering in Young Children.* Tulsa, OK, Modern Education Corporation, 1976.
39. Riley G: *Stuttering Prediction Instrument for Young Children.* Tigard, OR, C.C. Publications, 1981.
40. Goldman R, Fristoe M: *The Goldman-Fristoe Test of Articulation.* Circle Pines, MN, American Guidance Service, 1972.
41. Weiss CE: *Weiss Comprehensive Articulation Test.* Boston, Teaching Resources Corp., 1979.
42. Hodson B: *Assessment of Phonological Processes—Revised.* Danville, IL, Interstate Publishers and Printers, 1986.
43. Khan L, Lewis N: *Khan-Lewis Phonological Analysis.* Circle Pines, MN, American Guidance Service, 1986.
44. Edwards ML: In support of phonological processes. *Language, Speech, Hear Serv Schools* 1992; 23:233–240.
45. Edwards ML: Phonological process analysis, in Williams EJ, Langsam J (eds). *Children's Phonology Disorders: Pathways and Patterns.* Rockville, MD, American Speech-Language-Hearing Association, 1994.
46. Zebrowski P, Conture E: Judgments of disfluency by mothers of stuttering and normally fluent children, *J Speech Hearing Res* 1989; 32:307–317.
47. Grunwell P: *Clinical Phonology.* Rockville, MD, Aspen Systems Corporation, 1982.
48. McReynolds L, Elbert M: Criteria for phonological process analysis. *J Speech Hearing Dis* 1981; 46:197–204.
49. Edwards ML, Shriberg L: *Phonology: Application in Communicative Disorders.* San Diego, College-Hill Press, 1983.
50. Stoel-Gammon C, Dunn C: *Normal and Disordered Phonology in Children.* Austin, Texas, PRO-ED, Inc., 1985.
51. Conture EG, Louko LJ, Edwards ML: Simultaneously treating stuttering and disordered phonology in children: experimental treatment, preliminary findings. *Am J Speech-Lang Pathol* 1993; 2(3):72–81.

52. Kelly E, Conture E: Intervention with school-age stutterers. *Sem Speech Lang* 1991; 12:309–322.
53. Oyler ME: Vulnerability in stuttering children (no. 9602431). Ann Arbor, MI, Dissertation Services, 1996.
54. Comas RC: Tartamudez o espasmofemia funcional. Relato y aportes conceptuales. *Rev Cubana Pediat* 1974; 46:595–605.
55. Hall P: The occurrence of disfluencies in language-disordered school-age children. *J Speech Hear Dis* 1977; 42:364–369.
56. Starkweather W: Learning and its role in stuttering development, in Curlee R, Siegel G (eds). *Nature and Treatment of Stuttering: New Directions.* Boston, Allyn and Bacon, 1997.
57. Hodson B, Paden E: *Targeting Intelligible Speech: A Phonological Approach to Remediation.* San Diego, College Hill Press, 1991.
58. Tyler AA, Edwards ML, Saxman J: Clinical application of two phonologically based treatment procedures. *J Speech Hear Dis* 1987; 52:393–409.
59. Kelman M, Edwards ML: *Phonogroup: A Practical Guide for Enhancing Phonological Remediation.* Eau Claire, WI, Thinking Publications, 1994.
60. Weiner F: Treatment of phonological disability using the method of meaningful minimal contrast: Two case studies. *J Speech Hear Dis* 1981; 46(97):1–3.
61. Adams MR: The demands and capacities model I: Theoretical elaborations. *J Fluency Dis* 1990; 15:135–141.
62. Starkweather W, Gottwald SR: The demands and capacities model II: Clinical applications. *J Fluency Dis* 1990; 15:143–157.
63. Conture E, Guitar B: Stuttering and your child: A videotape for parents [30 minute videotape]. Memphis, TN, Stuttering Foundation of America, 1994.
64. Conture E, Guitar B: Evaluating efficacy of treatment of stuttering: School-age children. *J Fluency Dis* 1993; 18:253–288.
65. Paden E, Yairi E: Phonological characteristics of children whose stuttering persisted or recovered. *J Speech Hear Res* 1996; 39:981–990.
66. Riley G: Stuttering prediction instrument (SPI) for young children. Austin, Tx: Pro-Ed, 1981.
67. Yaruss S, LaSalle L, Conture EG: Evaluating stuttering in young children: Diagnostic data. *Am J Speech-Lang Pathol* (in press).
68. Conture EG, Melnick K: Parent-child group approach to stuttering in preschool and school-age children. In: M. Onslow, A. Packman, eds. *Early Stuttering: A Handbook of Intervention Strategies.* San Diego, CA: Singuler Publishing Group. (in press)
69. Guitar B: *Stuttering: An Integrated Approach to Its Nature and Treatment.* Baltimore, MD: Williams and Wilkins, 1998.

Stuttering and Related Disorders of Fluency, 2nd edition.
Edited by Richard F. Curlee, PH.D.
Thieme Medical Publishers, Inc., New York © 1999.

8

Intensive Treatment for Stuttering Adolescents

Deborah Kully
Marilyn Langevin

Introduction

Adolescence is a transitional period between the worlds of childhood and adulthood. It is often seen as a stormy time when the search for identity becomes central.[1] However, some investigators argue that more stability exists during adolescence than is recognized;[2] and although the peer group becomes increasingly influential, studies suggest that the family continues to maintain considerable influence.[3] Adolescence also marks the beginning of formal operational thought.[4] Adolescents become more capable of thinking about thinking, considering multiple possibilities, and reasoning hypothetically. Similarly, they can take the thoughts of others into account; however, development of these skills is gradual and varies across individuals. Adolescents are a distinctive population and warrant their own approach to treatment. We believe that treatment programs should be sensitive to the unique developmental changes and adjustments that occur during this period.

Our treatment approach addresses both overt and covert aspects of stuttering. We believe that neurophysiological, genetic, and environmental factors[5] as well as internal reactions to self and listeners[6] contribute to the development of stuttering. Like Smith and Kelly,[7] who propose a dynamic, multifactorial model of stuttering, we believe that the interaction among variables is complex and dynamic, changes over time, and has differential weighting from one individual to another. We also believe that secondary features of stuttering are acquired through a complex process of escape and avoidance learning.[5] Treatment procedures include fluency-enhancing techniques ("fluency skills"), which deal with core stuttering and learned struggle behaviors, and cognitive–behavioral strategies, which deal with the emotional and attitudinal aspects of stuttering. In addition, stuttering modification and anxiety and avoidance reduction strategies[8,9] are integrated with fluency shaping and cognitive–behavioral methodologies to achieve both speech and emotional–attitudinal goals. We also encourage family participation in treatment. Their degree of participation is determined by the developmental level of the client and the nature of the client–family relationship. Inherent in the process of treatment is the on-going collection of behavioral and self-report data to evaluate a client's progress and make needed adjustments.

139

Evaluations Needed

Our evaluation procedure involves advance completion of a case history form and self-report questionnaires, a brief parent interview (younger adolescents only), a client interview, a speech assessment, and a concluding meeting with the adolescent and parents. In addition to evaluating overt and covert stuttering characteristics, we determine the adolescent's needs and strengths and any special needs for transfer. This information is used to formulate prognoses for short- and long-term change and determine whether treatment is appropriate for the teen. Of course, evaluation does not end with the first meeting, but continues throughout all subsequent stages of treatment.

Observations and Tests

SPEECH

Speech samples include 5 min of conversation and 2 min of reading which are audiotaped and analyzed on-line using an electronic button press event counter.[5] Stuttered and fluent syllables are rated using counting guidelines developed at our center. In view of the variability of stuttering, teens also judge how representative these samples are of their usual speech. If speech is judged as unusually fluent, a sample of the client talking on the phone is obtained or the client is asked to make a recording in a difficult situation and forward it to the clinic.

Measures of stuttering include percent syllables stuttered (% SS) and syllables spoken per minute (SPM). Global ratings of stuttering severity based on both overt and covert features are also made using a 5-point severity scale. Reliability of such global ratings appears to be equivalent to that of formal tools like Riley's[10] Stuttering Severity Instrument.[11] All clinicians receive training in the measurement and evaluation of stuttering and complete periodic reliability checks to evaluate both intra- and interclinician agreement.

In addition to the above measures, a detailed description of the teen's core stuttering behaviors and accessory characteristics is completed using Wingate's[12] definition of stuttering. Other remarkable features of the client's speech pattern, including voice quality, prosody, naturalness, articulation, and intelligibility are also described.

Other tasks include brief probes to assess the teen's likely responsiveness to therapy and determine particular needs. A self-recording probe, based on the work of La Croix,[13] provides information about clients' sensitivity or awareness of stuttering and the effects of self-recording on stuttering frequency. Stimulability probes are administered for fluency skills and prolongation of speech pattern. Results provide a basis for tentative prognoses about clients' possible responsiveness to fluency-enhancing techniques and for planning initial treatment steps.

FEELINGS AND ATTITUDES

A major problem in assessing attitudes and feelings is that the information sought is not directly observable and must, therefore, be obtained primarily through self-report or inferred from parent observations. The limitations inherent in gathering and interpreting self-report data are well recognized.[14,15] These concerns notwithstanding, we believe that clients' perceptions and beliefs are important to evaluate, because they provide an indication of the nature and scope of the stuttering problem. Furthermore, self-report data provide the clinician with insights into the climate of ideas, beliefs, and misperceptions which may affect clients in treatment.

In our clinic, information about attitudes and feelings is obtained from client interviews and self-report questionnaires. Questions asked during the interview help in formulating impressions about clients' 1. conception of their stuttering—their beliefs about its cause, factors that contribute to situational variations, and their sense of control over the problem; 2. perceptions of the effects of stuttering on home, school, and social situations (using the SRES questionnaire referred to below); 3. avoidances and beliefs about the consequences of avoidance; 4. feelings and thoughts associated with the experience of stuttering; 5. experiences and beliefs about past therapy; and 6. expectations for change and motivation for therapy. In addition to providing insight into clients' belief systems and negative adaptations, interview responses may give an indication of their capacities for introspection and reflection about thoughts and feelings. These preliminary impressions help in planning the cognitive–behavioral component of treatment.

In addition to the interview, teens complete three questionnaires: the S24 scale,[16] the Perceptions of Stuttering Inventory (PSI),[17] and the Self Rating of Effects of Stuttering (SRES),[18] an instrument we are developing. Older adolescents also complete the Locus of Control of Behavior (LCB)[19] and the Self-Efficacy Scale for Adults who Stutter (SESAS).[20] These scales are intended to evaluate clients' attitudes about communication, perceptions of stuttering, and sense of personal efficacy. It should be recognized, however, that most were designed for adults, and their appropriateness for adolescents has not been determined. The use of adult questionnaires with adolescents is a common practice among clinicians in other disciplines, such as psychology.[21] Nonetheless, there is clearly a need to develop scales that are specific to adolescents.

We use questionnaire measures to supplement the objective measures of speech just described. Although questionnaire scores have limited prescriptive value, they do provide additional measures of treatment outcome. Furthermore, an analysis of specific questionnaire items may provide information that is useful in treatment planning.

Case Selection Criteria

There are three major factors we consider in determining whether the intensive program is suitable for an adolescent.

Desire for Change

This is a key factor in determining suitability or readiness for treatment, but it is often difficult to assess. Many adolescents appear ambivalent about undertaking treatment. In some cases, their reluctance to obtain help may reflect a true lack of concern about stuttering. In others it may reflect such reasons as apprehension about what treatment might involve, doubts about the efficacy of therapy, or reluctance to acknowledge that a problem exists. Thus, one of our aims is to facilitate their ability to identify and express concerns about stuttering and therapy. It is important that they have the opportunity to express concerns or reservations about therapy openly and candidly, without fear of negative evaluation. Rustin and colleagues[22] provide a thoughtful discussion of this issue as it pertains to adolescents.

Understanding or Expectations of Treatment

For treatment to have lasting benefits, clients must not only have the desire to improve but also be willing to take responsibility for using new skills and making life-style changes that support new communication patterns. Many adolescents express the desire to "get rid of stuttering" but expect it to be removed by treatment, much as a tonsillectomy removes the problem of sore tonsils. It is crucial, therefore, that clients and families are fully informed about the treatment process before making decisions about therapy. In a meeting with the adolescent and family at the end of the evaluation, we provide an overview of treatment, discuss possible outcomes, and demonstrate the target-controlled speech pattern. We want to ensure that the client and family understand that there is no cure for stuttering but that it is possible to control or manage the problem; that significant energy will be required during the 3-week intensive clinic and afterward to maintain treatment gains; that controlled speech can be the expected result; and that the intensive clinic is only the beginning of a long-term process of change.

Ability to Handle Treatment Requirements

To participate successfully, the adolescent must be able to sustain attention for long periods, possess adequate social skills to interact within a group, and have at least average cognitive abilities. The intensive program may not be the best placement for teens with delayed cognitive or social–emotional skills, though we sometimes include them when no other treatment is accessible. In these cases, we make extensive modifications to the treatment program and arrange to work individually with the client.

In a few cases, the decision about suitability is very clear: the client is eager, aware, and able to meet program requirements. In such cases, we enroll the teen in the clinic and encourage parents to make arrangements immediately for follow-up therapy. When readiness for treatment is not as apparent, however, we encourage the teen and family to discuss issues further before making a decision or consider individual therapy on a trial basis. When teens decline treatment entirely, we strive to gain the parents' understanding and acceptance of this decision and encourage them to maintain open communication about the teens' speech.

If intensive treatment is recommended, we determine the most suitable age group for the client. Our center offers intensive programs for three age groups: 1. children (7–12); 2. young teens (12–14); and 3. older teens and adults (15+). Several factors are considered in a placement, including chronological age, social–emotional maturity, and cognitive skills. For instance, a 12-year-old child with attention, language, or social–emotional difficulties may be placed in the children's clinic which has more structure, greater parental involvement, and shorter therapy sessions (3 hours a day). A 14-year-old with good linguistic, academic, and social skills may be placed with older teens and adults who are able to work more independently. These skills are evaluated informally on the basis of information obtained from the client and parent interviews and reports of school performance. If information is inadequate to make a confident judgment about age grouping, we rely heavily on parents' judgments in making final decisions.

Sometimes results of an evaluation suggest that treatment is appropriate but that timing is not. If intensive treatment is to be maximally beneficial, clients must be able to devote most of their energy and attention to therapy activities. Furthermore, they will need to integrate new skills into their everyday life when they return home, a process that also requires time and special effort. If a teen is engaged in activities that will compete with therapy or is experiencing high emotional or environmental stress, such as the loss of a loved one, then we may recommend that therapy be deferred.

Management Approach

The program has been developed over 25 years. It is an updated version of the Comprehensive Stuttering Program (CSP)[5] which drew from the work of many clinicians and researchers.[8,23–28] The CSP has been and continues to be modified as we learn more from basic, applied, and clinical research and from our own experience with teens and adults who stutter.

Treatment for adolescents is offered in two formats: 3-week intensive programs held every summer and nonintensive programs that span several months. The treatment goals and procedures we describe provide the foundation for both formats; however, the majority of adolescents are treated in the intensive program which provides approximately 85 hours of therapy. They attend the clinic each weekday for 5.5 hours per day and complete about 1 hour of home practice each evening. Approximately 15 additional hours are devoted to parent meetings. Therapy consists of individual, small-group, and large-group activities. The clinician–client ratio varies from 1:1 to 1:2, depending on the needs of the client and the demands of the activity. In most cases clinician–client and client–client pairings are rotated daily to facilitate generalization.

Treatment Goals

Speech, emotional–attitudinal, self-management, and environmental goals are outlined as follows:

SPEECH-RELATED GOALS

- Ability to sustain controlled fluency in all speaking environments with prosody and rate approximating normal
- Ability to manage residual stuttering
- Improved communication, social skills, and confidence

EMOTIONAL–ATTITUDINAL GOALS

- Positive attitudes toward communication
- Openness about stuttering and fluency enhancing techniques
- Reduced avoidance behavior
- Ability to manage fear and anxiety
- Ability to handle regression and recognize when relapse is occurring
- Ability to deal with teasing and negative listener reactions

SELF-MANAGEMENT GOALS

- Increased understanding of the etiology and development of stuttering and the long-term process of change
- Problem solving skills
- Self-monitoring and self-evaluation skills
- Ability to manipulate the environment to support needs
- Ability to sequence practice activities

ENVIRONMENTAL GOALS

• Increased parental understanding of the etiology and development of stuttering and the long-term process of change
• Parental ability to support the client during and after therapy

Treatment Procedures

CLINICAL STRATEGIES

There are several clinical strategies that we believe facilitate client success.

Maintaining client individuality. Because treatment programs may sometimes be viewed as unalterable,[29] it is important to emphasize that we focus on each adolescent with whom we work. In all respects, treatment is alterable and responsive to the needs of each client. Client individuality is maintained through constant tailoring of every phase, step, and activity to meet individual needs. Fluency skill emphasis, target speech rates, task demands and feedback, hierarchies, transfer exercises, maintenance plans, and family education and counseling are all adjusted according to each client's particular responses and needs.

Modeling. The tenet of vicarious observation[30,31] suggests that modeling can facilitate the acquisition of concepts and new behavior patterns. Accordingly, clinicians continuously model cognitive–behavioral skills and prolonged speech (within and outside the clinic). Former clients also act as role models. They are incorporated into discussions of emotional–attitudinal issues and act as transfer agents. In sessions that do not include clinicians, they share with teens their experiences with regard to anxiety management, avoidance reduction, and challenges in maintaining speech and attitudinal gains.

Integration of self-management strategies into all therapy activities. Self-management refers to a set of cognitive–behavioral processes that promote generalization and help clients extend new behaviors into their home and daily lives, under their own direction and control.[32] Self-management strategies are incorporated in both speech and emotional–attitudinal components of therapy. Clinicians are facilitators who strive to help clients become their own clinicians.

Speech practice in non-English languages. For bilingual or English-as-a-second-language clients, speech practice in their primary language is incorporated as soon as they achieve proficiency with fluency skills in English. It has been our experience that it is not necessary for clinicians to understand the other language. To ensure that the integrity of stress patterns and word meanings are preserved, however, we involve clients and families in evaluating these aspects when fluency skills are practiced in other languages. Homework exercises and transfers are also completed in the other languages.

TREATMENT PHASES

The first half of the clinic is primarily devoted to acquisition of fluency and cognitive–behavioral skills. The remaining time is devoted to transferring these skills outside the clinic. Preparation for maintenance begins in the acquisition stage but is more concentrated during transfer. Post-clinic maintenance activities occur in the months and years following the intensive clinic. Although fluency skills and cognitive–behavioral strategies used to achieve speech, emotional–attitudinal, and environmental goals are discussed separately, they are integrated in the acquisition, transfer, and maintenance phases of therapy.

PRE- AND POSTTREATMENT SPEECH MEASURES

Video- and audio-taped speech samples are routinely obtained immediately pre- and postclinic. Video samples consist of 3 min of conversation with an interviewer and 2 min of reading; audiotaped samples comprise 2 min of telephone calls made to businesses. In addition, a preclinic sample is obtained in a group setting as an additional measure of stuttering against which subsequent change can be compared.

FLUENCY-ENHANCING TECHNIQUES IN ACQUISITION

This phase consists of three general stages.

1. *Identification.* Teens learn that overt stuttering is a result of what they do physically to interfere with the smooth flow of speech. Following a brief description of the speech production process, they discuss how stuttering interrupts the speech flow at various levels in the vocal tract and identify where and how this occurs in their own speech.

2. *Introduction to Fluency Skills.* Fluency skill introduction and practice generally proceed in the order listed in Table 8-1. Although this order is used with most teens, it may be varied to fit the needs of differing stuttering patterns and abilities to acquire fluency skills. A brief description of these skills is provided in Table 8-2. Fluency skill practice begins with single syllables and progresses to longer utterances.[24,33,34] Throughout acquisition, clients are encouraged to focus on the kinesthetic feeling of each skill.

After teens achieve 80% accuracy in producing skills with clinician feedback, they learn to monitor and evaluate their own productions on-line. At the end of each breath group, clients use a gesture or a $+/-$ tally system to indicate whether or not a target skill was accurately produced. Clinicians give feedback on the accuracy of this evaluation and, if necessary, provide corrective feedback. When appropriate, peer monitoring is also incorporated in which one client monitors the skill accuracy of another client and gives feedback. Peer monitoring facilitates acquisition of self-evaluation skills; however, it needs to be implemented judiciously. Each client's sensitivity, skill proficiency, and tact and diplomacy are considered. For example, if a teen is overly critical of peers, peer monitoring by that client may be more harmful than beneficial. If a teen is highly sensitive to feedback, then peer monitoring will not begin until that client appears better able to handle the feedback.

Table 8-1.   Progression of Sessions in Acquisition

Identification	
Introduction to fluency skills	• Prolongation • Easy breathing (EB) • Gentle starts (GS) • Smooth blending (SB) • Light touches (LT) • Refining prosody/naturalness • Preparation for sustained prolongation
Rate increase and fluency skill refinement	• Slow stretch: EB, GS, SB, LT, all skills, Self-correction (SC), Self-assessment (SA) • Medium stretch: EB, GS, SB, LT, all skills, SC, Rate change session, SA • Slight stretch: as for medium • Control rate: as for medium

Table 8-2. Fluency Skills

Skill	Brief Description
Prolongation	Vowels are prolonged; transitions through consonants are slowed but not prolonged; stressed syllables receive more prolongation than unstressed syllables; natural prosody is maintained
Easy breathing	Full unrushed diaphragmatic inspiration; smooth movement into expiration; appropriate breath grouping
Gentle starts	Slow, smooth initiation of speech with a slight prevoice expiration and a gradual increase in loudness; full loudness achieved on the first syllable
*Smooth blending**	Continuous air flow and smooth continuous movement of articulators within breath groups; manner and voicing characteristics of phonemes are preserved
*Light touches**	Lightened but distinct articulatory contacts; manner and voicing characteristics of phonemes are preserved

*It is important to note that in producing smooth blending and light touches, manner and voicing characteristics of phonemes are preserved. Stops are not fricated, voiceless phonemes are not voiced, and consonants are not slurred.

Before progressing to the next skill, teens complete a self-evaluation task. The criterion is 80%–90% accuracy in self-evaluating at least 10 productions of short phrases, usually four syllables long. Teens rate their skill proficiency immediately after each production, using a +/− tally system while the clinician covertly makes her own tally. After five utterances, they compare their ratings. In most cases the self-evaluation criterion is easily achieved; however, a few clients experience great difficulty with self-monitoring, a behavioral observation that is consistent with the brain-imaging research by Fox et al.[35] which shows deactivation of centers involved in self-monitoring in a sample of adults who stutter.[10] For these clients, extra self-monitoring training is provided.

A session devoted to refining speech naturalness concludes the introduction to fluency skills. Teens review the features of natural prosody and practice various stress patterns in words and sentences. Voice and resonance characteristics are evaluated to ensure that clients are using their natural pitch and resonance. Naturalness is an ongoing goal in all speech practice throughout the program.

3. *Rate Increase with Fluency Skill Refinement.* Fluency skills are practiced within the context of systematically increasing rates of speech. Prolongation is now called "stretch." Speech rates increase from "slow" (40–60 SPM), to "medium" (60–100 SPM), to "slight" stretch (100–140 SPM) and, finally, to a "controlled rate" (140–210 SPM). Terminal rates are usually between 150 and 190 SPM. At each stage, teens find an optimal rate that allows them to use the fluency skills well and maintain a feeling of control and stability.

In each stretch rate, fluency skills are practiced in 5-min rating sessions. Each skill is practiced individually at first, then all skills are practiced together. The progression of rating sessions is outlined in the lower portion of Table 8-1, and sessions are carried out within the context of drill, games, and physical activities. Practice is carefully sequenced, moving from easier to more challenging tasks by manipulating the variables listed in Table 8-3, although sequences are individualized for each teen. The last minute of each rating session is devoted to client self-monitoring and self-evaluation using the gestures or written tallies described earlier. To meet criteria for completing each rating session, teens must 1. be within the SPM range for the target rate, 2. have less than 1% stuttering, and 3. have no more

Table 8-3. Variables Manipulated in Sequencing Tasks

Variable	*Hierarchy*
Length	From single syllables to connected speech
Complexity	From linguistically and conceptually simple to complex and abstract (clients generally progress from reading to answering and asking questions to monologue and then conversation)
Cuing	From strong to minimal cuing
Feedback	From continuous to intermittent feedback
Emotionality	From low to high emotion
Interest level	From low to high interest
Spontaneity	From structured to natural exchanges
Time pressure	From low to high time pressures
*Environmental variables such as physical setting, audience, and distracters**	From easier to more challenging

*One distracter that is incorporated into later rating sessions—which senior clinicians find challenging and adolescents thoroughly enjoy—is the inclusion of popular background music.

than five fluency skill errors, except in the "all skills" sessions, in which errors must not exceed 10. Clients typically have 0% stuttering; however, a few may exhibit mild stuttering during prolongation. In such cases, self-corrections are practiced extensively and stutters that are self-corrected are not counted.

After completing the "all skills" sessions, clients practice self-correction (SC) which incorporate aspects of Van Riper's[8] cancellations and pullouts. The first level of SC is called a "re-breathe" in which clients stop when they begin to stutter, slowly release tension and remaining air, re-breathe, and begin the word again using exaggerated fluency skills. Once proficiency with the "re-breathe" strategy has been achieved, clients progress to using a pullout. This involves releasing tension during the moment of stuttering and easing through the remainder of the word using exaggerated fluency skills. In both strategies, rate of speech is reduced after the stutter until control is regained. Practice begins with simulated stutters and progresses to real stutters.

Rate change sessions are introduced at the medium stretch rate. Teens learn to reduce their rate of speech on-line, as both a preventative and recovery strategy. As a preventative strategy, rate changes incorporate aspects of Van Riper's[8] preparatory sets by having clients reduce their rate slightly and exaggerate fluency skills when approaching a feared or avoided word or are feeling a loss of control or increased anxiety. As a recovery strategy, clients reduce their rate and exaggerate fluency skills to regain control after a stutter. In both cases, the reduced speaking rate is maintained until a feeling of stability has been reestablished.

To progress from one rate to the next, teens complete a formal self-assessment (SA) task. The purposes of SA are, first, to ensure that clients can produce fluency skills accurately before moving to a faster rate, and second, to ensure that self-evaluation skills are accurate. Clients evaluate their fluency skill proficiency, rate of speech, number of stutters identified and self-corrected, naturalness, sense of control felt, and loudness. To meet criteria they must 1. achieve 80% accuracy in fluency skill production and evaluation; 2. have an SPM that is within the target rate range; 3. identify and self-correct 80% of any stutters;

4. achieve good naturalness; 5. have adequate levels of loudness; and 6. feel a strong degree of control.

Beginning on the third day of therapy, rating sessions are preceded by a fluency skill "warm-up." To foster self-management, responsibility for designing and conducting the morning warm-up is shifted to the teens at the beginning of the second week. They design and lead warm-up practice, first in the clinic room, then in large groups within and outside the clinic. During the transfer phase, they are responsible for completing a warm-up practice before coming to the clinic.

FLUENCY-ENHANCING TECHNIQUES IN TRANSFER

Although transfer is a distinct treatment phase, the following self-management strategies are introduced early in acquisition to promote generalization:

1. As soon as teens are able to use fluency skills in sustained prolongation in question and answer activities during rating sessions, they are required to use prolongation in off-task comments within the therapy room, then in all talking within the clinic with clinical and support staff. This generally occurs when teens are nearing the end of their slow stretch rating sessions.

2. During lunch and other breaks outside the clinic, teens monitor each other and provide cues and feedback. They record the percentage of time they used stretch during breaks and the number of times they used self-corrections.

3. Each evening, beginning on the 3rd day of the program, teens complete structured home practice in pairs and groups. Tasks are always at a level at which they can be expected to achieve 70%–80% accuracy. They self-evaluate their tape-recorded practice and bring their recording and evaluation for checking by the clinician the following day.

4. Parents and family members are involved in completing home practice activities with teens and may also support or facilitate group evening practice.

In transfer, morning rating sessions in controlled rates continue to help teens refine fluency skills. Transfer activities are preceded by pretransfer activities which act as a bridge between the controlled clinic environment and real-life situations. Within each category there are recorded and unrecorded transfers that progress from contrived to natural situations; simple to complex; easier to harder; shorter to longer; low to high interest; strong to minimal cuing; and in-clinic to out-of-clinic activities. Pretransfers are completed first in slight stretch, then in controlled rate. Transfers are completed ordinarily in a controlled rate and are repeated several times at each level of difficulty to ensure that clients develop stability. To further develop self-management abilities, clients learn how to sequence transfer tasks.

As previously indicated, skill and rate goals, hierarchies, and types of transfers are individualized. Teens having special needs receive extra practice. For instance, if a client has to make many class presentations, extra opportunities for such presentations will be arranged.

Prior to beginning each transfer task, teens specify their skill and rate goals. They also examine and, if necessary, change their self-talk which we will describe in a later section. To meet criteria for completing a transfer task, they must achieve 80% accuracy in 1. fluency skill production; 2. maintaining the target rate; 3. self-evaluation; and 4. identifying and self-correcting stutters. Clients must also identify areas of strength and areas for improvement. Unrecorded transfers are evaluated using the same parameters; however, clients estimate their percentages of accuracy in achieving fluency skill and target rate goals. If criteria are not met, then clients redo the transfer.

Pretransfer activities include the following: 1. conversations with staff and volunteers within and outside the clinic. 2. "walk-n-talk" tasks which are tape-recorded conversations while walking outside in pairs or groups. 3. telephone calls made to and received from clinical staff and volunteers. 4. a simulated classroom activity within the clinic in which clinicians act as teachers and conduct tasks involving such subjects as language arts, math, or science and such activities as reading aloud, group work, presentations, and discussions in which teens brainstorm solutions to problems presented. 5. scavenger hunts that require teens to make as many contacts as possible with staff and volunteers within and outside the clinic. The scavenger hunts also have timed components that can require teens to run from point to point. These activities expose teens to time pressures that simulate those experienced in the real world and to the feeling of "being out of breath." Humorous situations are also included so that teens can practice using fluency skills while laughing and having fun.

Transfer activities comprise the following: 1. conversations with strangers on campus and in a variety of other locations. 2. telephone calls to businesses and from volunteers the teens have not met; messages are also left on answering machines and long-distance calls are made to family and friends. 3. opinion surveys that involve approaching people on campus and asking a series of questions about stuttering. 4. shopping activities in which shopkeepers are asked for items and items of interest are discussed. 5. presentations on various aspects of stuttering and subjects of special interest to each client are made; a "classroom education presentation" is practiced which also promotes openness about stuttering and fluency skills. 6. a simulated job interview conducted with older adolescents by personnel at a career and placement center on campus; and 7. at the end of the program, a speech in a lecture theater on campus to an audience of family, friends, and other guests.

Unrecorded transfers involve a variety of short natural exchanges (e.g., asking for directions) as well as a simulated classroom situation. The classroom simulation mirrors a usual school day with a real teacher from a local school following a schedule that includes core subjects such as math, language arts, science, and physical education activities.

Within each of these recorded and unrecorded situations, certain transfers are devoted to practicing self-corrections with simulated stutters, making rate changes, or practicing voluntary stuttering.

FLUENCY-ENHANCING TECHNIQUES IN MAINTENANCE

Preparation for maintenance is a focus throughout the program. Discussions regarding the need for, requirements of, and challenges of maintenance begin during assessment and are included in client and family discussions throughout the program. In addition, the self-management strategies incorporated in acquisition and transfer prepare the clients to plan and carry out maintenance activities.

In-clinic Preparation for Maintenance.   In their final week of therapy, teens attend special maintenance seminars and learn about the speech-related and attitudinal components of a maintenance plan. The speech-related components are as follows:
1. *Warm-up*: Warm-up consists of fluency skill practice in the morning and for short periods throughout the day. In the morning, clients focus on specific skills while prolonging

at various rates and end with a conversation in slight stretch with a family member. They are encouraged to vary the speech stimuli and place of practice daily to counteract boredom. Practice can include reading from books or magazines, reviewing school work, and discussing daily activities, news items or anything else of interest to the adolescent. Parents are urged to be involved in warm-up practice as much as possible and when appropriate so that warm-up becomes part of the family's routine.

2. *Ongoing practice*: Ongoing practice can be completed using any daily talking activity and is both preplanned and spontaneous. In preplanned exercises, teens use fluency skills in such routine activities as talking during dinner and nonroutine activities as asking for a special book at the library. In spontaneous activities, they take advantage of unexpected situations that occur and are encouraged to keep a record of their performance in these ongoing activities.

3. *Transfers*: Any daily or special talking activity can be used, but a transfer differs from ongoing practice in that it is formally evaluated and specifically related to the long- and short-term goals. Transfers should include both easy and more difficult situations as well as those that have been avoided in the past. Teens are encouraged to tape-record at least one transfer per week and to keep a record of their transfers. They are also encouraged to be creative, seek out talking situations, and take risks.

Teens then identify short- and long-term goals, learn how to sequence practice activities, and plan specific practice activities for the first 3 days posttreatment. Long-term goals are those that clients want to achieve within 1 year. Most often they are related to increasing their comfort in talking in avoided or feared situations, like class presentations or asking questions in class. They may also be attitude based. For instance, some clients want to be more open about stuttering and more comfortable using fluency skills with friends. Short-term goals are those that clients want to achieve by the end of the first month after treatment. They often are substeps in achieving long-term goals. An example might be giving a class presentation to a group of three friends in the classroom after school as a substep toward giving a presentation to the whole class.

Daily and weekly transfers are designed around short- and long-term goals. Teens plan and write a hierarchy of transfers for each month. This gives the transfers purpose and promotes goal-directed transfer practice. In planning practice activities for the first 3 days posttreatment, clients identify what they will be doing in the course of the day, decide where and when they will do their warm-up, and write out a warm-up plan. They think about the usual or special talking events that will occur in the day and decide which ones can be used for ongoing practice or transfers. They also think about how to create talking situations that are substeps in achieving short-term goals for the month. As a final step in preparing for maintenance, they identify barriers to carrying out speech practice and brainstorm solutions for dealing with these challenges.

Post-treatment Maintenance.   Maintenance activities in the posttreatment period consist of daily home practice with fluency skills, transfers, and attention to attitudinal issues, and one or more maintenance therapy options: 1. follow up sessions with a local speech–language pathologist;[5,36] 2. participation in regularly scheduled refresher clinics as needed; and/or 3. participation in a long-distance maintenance program in which taped and evaluated transfers are sent to a clinician for evaluation and feedback regarding skill proficiency, sequencing of speech practice, attitudinal issues, and self-talk. Teens are also encouraged to maintain contact with fellow clients for speech practice and support and participate in self-help groups.

COGNITIVE BEHAVIORAL SKILLS

We believe that positive attitudes toward communication and the ability to manage feelings associated with stuttering facilitate maintenance of improved fluency. The use of cognitive–behavioral strategies to help clients achieve these goals is grounded in theoretical tenets and research on the efficacy of cognitive–behavioral therapies.

According to Ivey, Ivey, and Simek-Downing,[37] cognitive–behavioral theory integrates thought and action. The task of therapy is twofold: "1. To examine how one thinks and if necessary, to change thinking and cognition; and 2. ensure that clients act on those cognitions through behavior in their daily life" (p. 302). A third dimension is the process of decision-making in which "one must *decide* how one will act" (p. 303). In a metaanalytic study,[38] cognitive–behavioral therapies were found to be effective in treating a variety of disorders. Although not superior to other forms of treatment, it was postulated that these therapies may be the best mode of therapy for some disorders. The only study of stuttering therapy included in this metaanalysis was that of Moleski and Tosi[39] in which rational–emotive therapy was more efficacious than systematic desensitization in reducing anxiety and negative attitudes about stuttering as well as overt stuttering behavior. Although cognitive–behavioral methods are often used in stuttering treatment, we believe that much additional research is needed to investigate the effectiveness of specific cognitive–behavioral strategies.

In our program, applications of cognitive–behavioral strategies are highly individualized. Although adolescents have many emotional–attitudinal issues in common, each individual has a unique constellation of concerns. Each adolescent's stage of cognitive and emotional development, state of readiness to discuss emotional issues, and desire to make changes is considered in designing group and individual discussions and exercises.

We introduce cognitive–behavioral concepts and strategies in a series of seminars that are supported by readings. Readings are drawn from *Do You Stutter: A Guide for Teens*[40] and strategies are incorporated from *Facilitating Fluency*[36]; however, the presentation and depth to which concepts are discussed are adjusted to meet the developmental level of clients. These discussions are supported by behavioral exercises which follow hierarchies of difficulty progressing from contrived to natural situations, simple to more complex, and easier to harder tasks.

The following discussion of emotional–attitudinal concepts addressed in therapy is not exhaustive. Only the main concepts are presented. Always, there is a myriad of other social and emotional issues which are interrelated, client specific and of great concern to adolescents. Dating issues and making good impressions are two such issues for older adolescents. Vast differences in interests and social–emotional maturity within adolescent groups and their move toward independence often make for most interesting therapy sessions.

Etiology and Development of Stuttering.   Teens acquire an understanding of the neurophysiological, genetic, environmental factors, and internal reactions that are presumed to contribute to the development of stuttering. This tends to 1. relieve guilt (that they did not try hard enough to stop stuttering) and shame (about being different) and 2. facilitate acceptance and openness.

Process of Change.   Knowing that change takes time, that there are ups and downs, that it is important to be pleased with small successes, and that therapy initiates a long-term process helps clients develop realistic expectations. It also prepares them to deal with and keep difficulties in perspective.

Positive Attitudes.   The tripartite definition of attitude[41] proposes that attitudes have affective, cognitive, and behavioral components. Common to each of these components are verbal evaluative statements. Examining and changing verbal evaluative thoughts, or "self-talk," about one's cognitions, emotions, or behavioral responses is one way to change attitudes. We believe that attitude change is facilitated and maintained through a combination of effective self-talk which we call "helpful thoughts," and success in using fluency skills, confronting avoidances, dealing with listeners, and managing feelings.

Teens learn that thoughts affect how feelings and reactions are handled. They identify helpful and unhelpful thoughts. Drawing from Webster and Poulos[36] and our own clinical experience, we describe helpful self-talk as that which 1. reminds clients of the fluency skills they have acquired to manage stuttering; 2. tells clients exactly what they can do to manage speech (e.g., "slow my rate" or "use a gentle start"); 3. puts feelings into perspective (e.g., "it's okay to feel anxious. This will be a chance for me to practice" or "I know I'm still afraid to stutter and it's important that I do this whether or not I stutter"); 4. is encouraging and positive; 5. is realistic (allows mistakes from time to time); and 6. is reality based. Unhelpful thoughts 1. make it harder to use skills; 2. are negative and show helplessness; 3. demand perfect fluency; 4. make it harder to enter feared situations; 5. make it harder to talk in social and other speaking situations; 6. focus on what listeners might think, do, and say; and 7. are maladaptive.

In a series of preparatory written exercises, teens identify unhelpful self-talk they have had before and after difficult situations in the past, and brainstorm effective self-talk which they could use in place of the unhelpful thoughts. They then practice identifying and changing self-talk before and after each transfer. They are also encouraged to keep a record of their self talk in maintenance. This process of examining self-talk is integral to all our discussions of emotional–attitudinal issues, including those described below.

Acceptance and Openness.   Openness facilitates self-acceptance and supports the use of fluency skills. It is imperative that clients do not use fluency skills as a way to hide stuttering. We focus discussions on acceptance of stuttering; acceptance of the sound and feel of fluency skills; being open about stuttering and using fluency skills—how, when, and who to be open with; and perceptions of listener reactions to stuttering and fluency skills. Teens prepare a presentation which can be given to their class when they return home. In it they discuss, in their own words, why people stutter, how they have learned to manage stuttering, and how listeners can help people who stutter. The presentation they have prepared is also delivered to an audience during the treatment program. Although many teens do not deliver their presentations to classes when they return home, they often proudly report being open with listeners and family in individual or small-group situations. Teens are also encouraged to take the lead in arranging and carrying out meetings with teachers to discuss what they learned in treatment and how teachers can help in the classroom. During the transfer phase, openness exercises are carried out with family members who have accompanied them to the clinic and with family members at home, by telephone. These exercises are taped and analyzed. Clients are also encouraged to use voluntary stuttering as a way of being open and desensitizing themselves to the fear of stuttering. In our experience this is one of the more challenging concepts for adolescents to understand and one of the most anxiety-provoking strategies to apply. Consequently, some transfers specifically incorporate voluntary stuttering.

Listener Reactions.   Clients need to develop an awareness of the potential difference between what is perceived and listener's true reactions. So we have them discuss why listeners' seemingly negative reactions may relate to uncertainties in knowing how to react. They also discuss reactions that have been unmistakenly negative and brainstorm and role-play different ways of responding to such reactions and educating listeners.

Confronting Avoidances. Clients learn how avoidances develop, how they are reinforced and perpetuated, and why it is important to confront them. They also learn how to sequence antiavoidance activities, beginning with easier and moving to more challenging situations to increase the likelihood of success. Transfer exercises always include avoided situations.

Feelings. Discussions of feelings are conducted in both group and individual sessions throughout the program, and we try to foster an environment in which clients feel free to express and discuss their feelings. Most adolescents talk readily about the fear and anxiety felt before, during, and after communicating in different situations; however, many are reluctant to talk about such feelings as shame, guilt, or humiliation. Indeed, it is often difficult for some adolescents to separate and identify different feelings. We respect a client's stage of readiness to acknowledge and discuss feelings, and ensure that contributions in group discussions are always voluntary. These discussions focus on identifying and acknowledging feelings rather than denying them; understanding the role that fear and anxiety play in perpetuating avoidances and interfere with the use of fluency skills; understanding normal levels of speech-related anxiety; managing feelings through effective self-talk; scanning for tension and using relaxation techniques; and systematically confronting feared situations. Like Luterman,[42] we believe that "feelings are neither good nor bad; they just are. They need to be acknowledged, and accepted but not judged." (p. 50). We try to help clients move toward a stage of being comfortable with normal levels of speech-related anxiety. Too often, clients want and expect to have no anxiety or apprehension after improved fluency has been achieved.

Expectations for Fluency. Clients need to understand that a realistic, long-term goal is maintaining the ability to manage stuttering rather than expecting to have 100% fluency.

Residual Stuttering, Handling Regression, and Recognizing Relapse. We distinguish between regression and relapse. *Regression* is defined as some slippage in fluency which includes variations in stuttering across time and situations, variations in the ability to monitor and use fluency skills, and temporary setbacks. In contrast, *relapse* is defined as a pronounced and persistent return to pretreatment levels of stuttering. Our discussions include the antecedents and cues for stuttering; adaptive ways of dealing with stuttering, which include use of effective self-talk and self-correction techniques; adopting a problem solving approach; dealing with related feelings of fear, anxiety, and disappointment; identifying internal and external factors that contribute to relapse; and getting back on track after a setback.

Confidence. Improved self-confidence is built by experiencing success in managing stuttering in a variety of situations and through discussing how one builds self-confidence. Beginning in the first week of therapy, clients record their successes in a Success Diary and are encouraged to continue this practice during maintenance.

Communication and Social Skills. Clients vary in the degree to which stuttering has affected their development of communication and social skills. For those with limited skills, intervention is both direct and indirect. Indirect interventions occur when clients practice fluency skills in various speaking situations within the clinic and in transfer. Direct instruction includes learning how to 1. initiate, sustain, and end conversations; 2. present ideas; 3. include the listener by asking questions; 4. interrupt or get one's turn when necessary; and 5. take turns. Role plays and scripts are incorporated in their fluency skill practice.

Teasing and Bullying.   Generally, bullying occurs less often in adolescence than in elementary school. Olweus[43] found that the frequency of bullying in grades 7–9 was approximately half as high as that in grades 2–6. Also, there was a clear trend toward less physical behaviors in grades 7–9. A Canadian study by Ziegler and Rosenstein-Manner[44] found that 23% of the children who were victims of bullying indicated that teasing was the only form of bullying they had experienced. In our teasing and bullying discussions and workshops, which sometimes included nonstuttering teens, adolescents have reported that the primary forms of bullying experienced were 1. social alienation, for example, being excluded, ignored, or avoided—with peers sometimes walking away while they were trying to talk— and not being taken seriously and 2. verbal aggression, such as being teased about their speech, looks, strength, cognitive abilities and so forth, and being the brunt of jokes. Stuttering teens also report being sensitive to peers, whom they believe feel uncomfortable around them. In our discussions, teens explore helpful and unhelpful ways of dealing with teasing and bullying. Helpful strategies include conflict resolutions strategies[45] and rules for fighting fair.[46]

FAMILY INVOLVEMENT IN THERAPY

The extent of family participation in speech practice sessions depends on the needs of the teen and the dynamics of the relationship; however, all accompanying parents and families participate in a series of regularly scheduled group meetings. When necessary, individual parent/family sessions are scheduled to deal with specific needs. In addition, families participate in the adolescent's homework and transfer exercises.

Generally, the topics covered in family meetings parallel those in client seminars. In discussing the etiology and development of stuttering, parents often express relief in learning the presumed neurophysiological basis of stuttering. Many still harbor guilt that they may have caused their child's stuttering. Parents are also introduced to the cognitive– behavioral strategies we use, particularly self-talk, and learn about common teen responses to our discussion topics. Of course, the confidentiality of an individual teen's response is always preserved. When needed, clinicians facilitate individual client–family discussions to help families and clients come to an understanding and resolution of issues. By the time children have become adolescents, many have learned that sharing the least information with those who have control over them is one way to keep out of trouble.[47] Therefore, we encourage adolescents and parents to engage in discussions in which the teens are free to share information, beliefs, and feelings without judgment or penalty. Likewise, parents are encouraged to share their feelings and experiences with the teen.

Parents and families learn how to support an adolescent during therapy and maintenance. They learn about 1. fluency skills and the rationale for each skill and how to monitor and evaluate skill production; 2. fluency disruptors and strategies for facilitating the use of fluency skills and cognitive–behavioral skills; 3. components of the maintenance plan; 4. when and how to remind adolescents and avoid constant reminding; 5. reinforcing the use of techniques and cognitive–behavioral strategies; and 6. facilitating and supporting their teen's meetings with teachers. In addition, parental expectations for fluency and maintenance are discussed. It is important that they understand that continual monitoring is challenging, that variations in fluency and the ability to use fluency skills will occur, that there likely will be residual stuttering, and that some regression can be expected. We also discuss how they can help their child get back on track after a relapse.

Treatment Outcomes and Conclusions

Since 1986, approximately 120 adolescents have completed an intensive clinic at our center. They came from all parts of North America, ranged in age from 10 to 17, and in severity from mild to profound. Several clients had coexisting problems such as Tourette's syndrome, dysarthria, dysphonia, misarticulations, attention deficit disorder, cluttering, or a learning disability. These teens were included in our intensive program because they were unable to obtain other treatment. Treatment programming for many of these clients was highly modified and individualized, and referrals were made to other specialists, such as neurologists and psychologists, in some cases.

As indicated earlier, we routinely obtain several measures of clients' speech, self-perceptions, and attitudes before and after therapy. With few exceptions, clients have shown marked improvements on all objective and self-report measures immediately after treatment. Of far greater interest, however, is the extent to which treatment gains are sustained across time and we have conducted several investigations of the effects of therapy on the longer term.[5,48,49] In one recently reported study,[49] which assessed the outcomes of an earlier version of the program described here, 25 adolescents and 17 adults were monitored up to 2 years posttherapy. Follow-up measures included surprise phone calls to clients at home or work, the S24 scale,[16] and a modified version of the Speech Performance Questionnaire (SPQ),[50] a scale designed to assess clients' perceptions of their postclinic performance. Mean speech and S24 measures obtained by the adolescent group are summarized in Table 8-4. The first column presents the adolescents' mean frequency of stuttering, expressed in percentage of syllables stuttered, before therapy, at the end of therapy, and 4 and 12 months later. Column two presents mean raw scores obtained on the S24 scale for the entire group pre- and postclinic and for the 11 adolescents who returned questionnaires at the 12-month follow-up.* As these data reveal, %SS scores for the adolescent group decreased sharply immediately posttreatment and then rose somewhat at the 4- and 12-month follow-up. The authors noted, however, that the increase in posttreatment scores was due largely to six of the 25 adolescents. When they deleted the scores from this subgroup of six adolescents, mean scores for the remaining 19 were 2% and 1% at 4 and 12 months, respectively. Results of the S24 scale showed a similar pattern (Table 8-4). The mean raw score for the group decreased from preclinic to a normal level immediately after the clinic. The 12-month mean score was somewhat higher, but still within ½ standard deviation of the mean for normally fluent adults (9.14; SD 5.38).

Results of the SPQ sent to clients 12 or 24 months posttherapy substantiated the findings from speech and attitude measures. Seventy-nine percent of the 14 adolescents who returned questionnaires rated their speech fluency at the time as "good" or "fair." Ninety-three percent indicated that they had the ability to control their speech, and 86%, the skills to sound fluent. All 14 reported that they "sometimes" or "almost always" were able to speak normally without thinking about controlling their speech. Ninety-two percent of these teens rated the stuttering program as "very" or "moderately" helpful; the remaining 8% (one client) judged it as "slightly helpful."

The foregoing results suggest that this group of adolescents experienced substantial

---

*Data from the S24 Scale were not reported in the Boberg and Kully study.[49]

Table 8-4. Treatment Outcomes for 25 Adolescent Clients.
Means of Speech and Attitude Measures Before Treatment,
on the Last Day of Treatment, and 4 and 12 Months After Treatment

Evaluation Occasion	% Syllables Stuttered (%SS)*	S24 Scale Score
Pretreatment	14.32	16.81
Posttreatment		
Immediate post	1.75	8.76
4 months post	3.65	
12 months post	3.89	11.57

*Data for "% syllables stuttered" are from Boberg and Kully.[48]

gains in their fluency and speech-related attitudes as a result of treatment. Although follow-up measures showed a small increase in the group's mean %SS, the majority of teens retained much of their improvement over a 12-month period. Taken together with findings from similar studies conducted recently on clients of similar age,[51,52] results indicate that treatment can be effective in reducing both stuttering and the negative reactions and adjustments to it in this age group.

The teen years are a critical time, when individuals are establishing a sense of personal identity[1] and actively formulating plans for the future. It is likely that persistent stuttering may exacerbate the already high social and developmental pressures on teens and influence their behaviors, beliefs, and decisions in ways that could have enduring adverse effects. It is unfortunate that there is a widespread belief that adolescents are extraordinarily difficult to treat[53,54] and do not respond as well to treatment as do adults. Indeed, some clinicians have suggested intensive treatment be postponed until adulthood.[55] Findings of the Boberg and Kully[49] study revealed, in fact, that both adults and adolescents show similar patterns of response to treatment. Although our experience suggests that many adolescents can indeed be challenging to work with, it is equally true that many teenagers are no more difficult to treat than an adult or child. In fact, adolescents have given us some of our most fascinating and rewarding clinical experiences. For us, challenges are part of the reward.

In sum, our experience, along with that of other clinical researchers seems to suggest that effective treatments are available and should be offered to adolescents who are willing and able to undertake them. Of course, further study is needed to evaluate the extent to which treatment gains are sustained over longer periods of 5 or 10 years, and we are now collecting such data. Although the clinical outcomes we have obtained are encouraging, there is an urgent need for systematic testing of the functional value of the various components and strategies that comprise current treatments. Furthermore, as Schwartz[56] observed, considerably more research is needed to enable us to better understand the unique needs and characteristics of adolescents who stutter.

Suggested Readings

Boberg E, Kully DA: Long-term results of an intensive treatment program for adults and adolescents who stutter. *J Speech Hear Res* 1994; 37:1050–1059.
This article describes a careful analysis of the long-term effects of treatment on a large group of clients.

Rustin L, Cook F, Spence R: *The Management of Stuttering in Adolescence: A Communication Skills Approach.* San Diego, CA, Singular Publishing Group, Inc., 1995.
The authors present a good overview of the developmental, social, and family issues relating to adolescents.

Webster W, Poulos M: *Facilitating Fluency: Transfer Strategies for Adult Stuttering Treatment Programs.* Edmonton, AB, Institute for Stuttering Treatment and Research, 1989.
This manual is appropriate for older teens and adults. A series of readings and exercises focus on changing attitudes, attacking avoidances, managing tension, and enhancing social skills.

Fraser J, Perkins WH (eds): *Do You Stutter: A Guide for Teens.* Memphis, TN, Speech Foundation of America, 1988.
This very readable booklet helps develop adolescents' understanding of stuttering, avoidances, and the process of managing speech.

References

1. Kail RV, Wicks-Nelson R: *Developmental Psychology.* New Jersey, Prentice Hall, 1993.
2. Bandura A: The stormy decade: Fact or fiction? *Psychol Schools* 1964; 1:224–231.
3. Bowerman CE, Kinch JW: Changes in Family and Peer Orientation of Children Between the Fourth and Tenth Grades, in Gold M, Douvan E (eds): *Adolescent Development.* Boston, Allyn & Bacon, 1969.
4. Piaget J: Intellectual evolution from adolescence to adulthood. *Hum Dev* 1972; 15:1–12.
5. Boberg E, Kully D: *Comprehensive Stuttering Program.* College-Hill Press, San Diego, CA, 1985.
6. Bloodstein, O: *A Handbook on Stuttering*, ed 5. San Diego, CA, Singular Publishing Group, Inc., 1995.
7. Smith A, Kelly E: Stuttering: A Dynamic, Multifactorial Model, in Curlee RF, Siegel GM (eds): *Nature and Treatment of Stuttering.* Boston, Allyn & Bacon, 1997.
8. Van Riper C: *The Treatment of Stuttering.* Englewood Cliffs, NJ, Prentice-Hall, 1973.
9. Sheehan J: Conflict Theory and Avoidance-Reduction Therapy, in Eisenson J (ed): *Stuttering: A Second Symposium.* New York, NY, Harper & Row, 1975.
10. Riley G: *Stuttering Severity Instrument for Children and Adults*, ed 3. Austin, TX, PRO-ED, 1994.
11. Lewis K: Do SSI-3 scores adequately reflect observations of stuttering behaviors? *Am J Speech Lang Pathol* 1995; 4:46–55.
12. Wingate ME: A standard definition of stuttering. *J Speech Hear Disord* 1964; 29:484–489.
13. La Croix ZE: Management of disfluent speech through self-recording procedures. *J Speech Hear Disord* 1973; 38:272–274.
14. Watson JB: Exploring the attitudes of adults who stutter. *J Fluency Disord* 1995; 28:143–164.
15. Patterson DR, Sechrest L: Nonreactive measures in psychotherapy outcome research. *Clin Psychol Rev* 1983; 3:391–416.
16. Andrews G, Cutler J: Stuttering therapy: The relationship between changes in symptom level and attitudes. *J Speech Hear Res* 1974; 39:312–319.
17. Woolf G: The assessment of stuttering as struggle, avoidance and expectancy. *Br J Disord Commun* 1967; 2:158–171.
18. Langevin MJ, Kully DA: *Self-rating of the Effects of Stuttering.* Unpublished questionnaire. Edmonton, AB, Institute for Stuttering Treatment and Research, 1997.
19. Craig AR, Franklin JA, Andrews G: A scale to measure locus of control of behavior. *Br J Disord Commun* 1967; 2:158–171.
20. Ornstein A, Manning W: Self-efficacy scaling by adult stutterers. *J Commun Disord* 1985; 18:313–320.
21. Craig RJ, Horowitz M: Current utilization of psychological tests at diagnostic practicum sites. *Clin Psychol* 1990; 43:29–36.
22. Rustin L, Cook, F, Spence R: *The Management of Stuttering in Adolescence: A Communication Skills Approach.* London, England, Whurr Publishers, 1995.
23. Perkins WH: Replacement of stuttering with normal speech: II. Clinical procedures. *J Speech Hear Disord* 1973; 38:295–303.

24. Ryan BP: *Programmed Therapy for Stuttering in Childhood and Adults.* Springfield, IL, Charles C. Thomas, 1974.
25. Martin RR: The Experimental Manipulation of Stuttering Behaviors, in Sloane, Jr. HN, Macaulay BD (eds): *Operant Procedures in Remedial Speech and Language Training.* Boston, Houghton Mifflin Co., 1968.
26. Ingham RJ, Andrews G: Details of a token economy stuttering therapy programme for adults. *Aust J Human Commun Disord* 1973; 1:13–20.
27. Gregory H (ed): *Controversies About Stuttering Therapy.* Baltimore, University Park Press, 1979.
28. Owen N: Facilitating Maintenance of Behavior Change, in Boberg E (ed): *Maintenance of Fluency.* New York, Elsevier North-Holland, 1981.
29. Shames GH, Rubin H: Concluding Remarks, in Shames GH, Rubin H (eds): *Stuttering Then and Now.* Columbus, OH, Charles E. Merrill Publishing Co., 1986.
30. Bandura A: Self-efficacy: Toward a unifying theory of behavioral change. *Psychol Rev* 1977; 84:191–215.
31. Rosenthal TL: Modeling Therapies, in Hersen M, Eisler RM, Miller PM (eds): *Progress in Behavior Modification.* New York, NY, Academic Press, Inc., 1976.
32. Rehm LP, Rokke P: Self-Management Therapies, in Dobson KS (ed): *Handbook of Cognitive–Behavioral Therapies.* New York, NY, The Guilford Press, 1988.
33. Costello JM: Current Behavioral Treatments for Children, in Prins D, Ingham RJ (eds): *Treatment of Stuttering in Early Childhood: Methods and Issues.* San Diego, CA, College-Hill Press, 1983.
34. Costello JM: Behavioral Treatment of Stuttering Children, in Curlee R (ed): *Stuttering and Related Disorders of Fluency.* New York, Thieme Medical Publishers, Inc., 1993.
35. Fox PT, Ingham RJ, Ingham JC et al: A PET study of the neural systems of stuttering. *Nature* 1996; 382:158–162.
36. Webster WG, Poulos MG: *Facilitating Fluency: Transfer Strategies for Adult Stuttering Treatment Programs.* Edmonton, AB, Institute for Stuttering Treatment and Research, 1989.
37. Ivey AE, Ivey MB, Simek-Downing L: *Counseling and Psychotherapy*, ed 2. Englewood Cliffs, NJ, Prentice-Hall, Inc., 1987.
38. Berman JS, Miller RC: The efficacy of cognitive behavior therapies: A quantitative review of the research evidence. *Psychol Bull* 1983; 94(1):39–53.
39. Moleski R, Tosi DJ: Comparative psychotherapy: Rational-emotive therapy versus systematic desensitization in the treatment of stuttering. *J Consult Clin Psychol* 1976; 44(2):309–311.
40. Fraser J: *Do You Stutter: A Guide for Teens.* Memphis, TN, Speech Foundation of America, 1988.
41. Rosenberg MJ, Hovland CI: Cognitive, Affective and Behavioral Components of Attitudes, in Rosenberg MJ, Hovland CI, McGuire WJ, Abelson RP, Brehm JW (eds.): *Attitude Organization and Change: An Analysis of Consistency Among Attitude Components.* New Haven, CT, Yale University Press, 1960.
42. Luterman D: *Counselling the Communicatively Disordered and Their Families.* Boston/Toronto, Little, Brown and Company, 1984.
43. Olweus D: *Bullying at School: What We Know and What We Can Do.* Cambridge, Blackwell Publishers, 1993.
44. Ziegler S, Rosenstein-Manner M: *Bullying at School: Toronto in an International Context*, No. 196R, revised ed. Toronto, Toronto Board of Education, 1991.
45. Schmidt F, Friedman A: *Creative Conflict Solving for Kids.* Miami Beach, FL, Grace Contrino Abrams Education Foundation Inc., 1985.
46. Schmidt F: *Mediation: Getting to Win Win.* Miami, FL, Grace Contrino Abrams Peace Education Foundation, Inc., 1994.
47. Butterfield WH, Cobb NH: Cognitive–Behavioral Treatment of Children and Adolescents, in Granvold DK (ed): *Cognitive and Behavioral Treatment.* Pacific Grove, CA, Brooks/Cole Publishing Company, 1994.
48. Langevin MJ, Boberg E: Results of an intensive stuttering therapy program. *J Speech Lang-Pathol Audiol* 1993; 17:158–166.
49. Boberg E, Kully D: Long-term results of an intensive treatment program for adults and adolescents who stutter. *J Speech Hear Res* 1994; 37:1050–1059.
50. Perkins W: Measurement and Maintenance of Fluency, in Boberg E (ed): *Maintenance of Fluency.* New York, Elsevier, 1981.

51. Craig A, Hancock K, Chang E, et al: A controlled clinical trial for stuttering in persons aged 9 to 14 years. *J Speech Hear Res* 1996; 39:808–826.
52. Ryan BP, Ryan BVK: Programmed stuttering treatment for children: Comparison of two establishment programs through transfer, maintenance, and follow-up. *J Speech Hear Res* 1995; 38: 61–75.
53. Daly DA, Simon CA, Burnett-Stolnack M: Helping adolescents who stutter focus on fluency. *Lang Speech Hear Serv Schools* 1995; 26:162–168.
54. Van Riper C: *The Nature of Stuttering*. Englewood Cliffs, NJ, Prentice-Hall, 1971.
55. Neilson, M: Intensive Training of Chronic Stutterers, in Curlee RF (ed): *Stuttering and Related Disorders of Fluency*. New York, Thieme Medical Publishers, 1993.
56. Schwartz HD: Adolescents who stutter. *J Fluency Disord* 1993; 18:289–302.

Stuttering and Related Disorders of Fluency, 2nd edition.
Edited by Richard F. Curlee, PH.D.
Thieme Medical Publishers, Inc., New York © 1999.

9

Management of Adult Stuttering

WALTER H. MANNING

Clinicians working in the area of fluency disorders, especially those who have accumulated several years of clinical successes along with some failures, appreciate that decreasing the handicap of stuttering is going to be a rigorous process for an adult. It is rigorous because, by this stage of development, the problem requires a multivariate solution. Adults who have stuttered for several decades are likely to have become sophisticated travelers within the culture of stuttering. There is a lengthy history of thinking about their speech and about themselves as a person who stutters. They have made many choices, sometimes important life decisions, based on the fact that they are a person who stutters. Much learning has taken place, and, often, because of the shame and stigma associated with stuttering earlier in life,[1] they have learned subtle ways to hide and avoid exposing themselves. It is not unusual for the original fluency breaks to be so well disguised that their stuttering behavior is not apparent. Instead of disclosing themselves as someone who stutters, they may look as if they are nervous, shy, unintelligent, or a little strange.

As a young man in college, on those occasions when someone would ask me where my hometown was, I would do nearly anything to avoid saying the name "Williamsport." Instead, I would often say "It's a small town in Pennsylvania." If they inquired further as, of course, they often did, I would say "Well, it's in central Pennsylvania" or "It's a city about 85 miles north of Harrisburg" or "It's a little east of Lock Haven." "Bloomsburg?" they would query. And I would respond, "No, it's actually west of Bloomsburg." Sometimes we would go on for awhile, gradually narrowing down the possibilities, until they correctly guessed the name of the city. I would do whatever it took, including acting as though I had no idea where I lived, in order to hide my stuttering. During such moments I certainly must have appeared to be, at the very least, a little strange or, at most, not very bright. I frequently did the same thing when asked about the schools I attended, the names of my teachers or classes, or my street address. The problems presented by stuttering went far beyond my speech. Stuttering was a way of living.[2]

Because adults who stutter have lived many years with the threat as well as the reality of stuttering, the problem has evolved far beyond the issue of fluently communicating a message. Often the adult who stutters arranges his or her life by narrowing options. Certainly, more fluent adults do this also. Few of us take as many risks or push the envelopes of our lives to the degree possible. Every so often we realize how much we live, as Maslow[3] suggests, in the "psychopathology of the average." But people who stutter are usually more likely to step back from the edge of the speaking situations that life has to offer. There are important exceptions to this, of course, and many people who stutter successfully forge ahead despite all types of challenges. However, we don't often see such people in our clinics and research centers. Most don't seek help, and the professional community seldom has the opportunity to study their response to the problem. The people whom we see are those who have become stuck with their stuttering. For them, the problem has become a major obstacle to professional and personal growth.

Changing the features of stuttering that are readily observable is usually not difficult. At least this is the case as long as the client attends to basic techniques of fluency and stuttering-modification practices with some responsibility. But changing surface behaviors, as important as that may be for an adult, is only a portion of the process. The features of the problem that lie under the surface must also shift and move off center. These intrinsic features have been referred to as cognitive and affective aspects of the problem, and, often, these are the features that create the biggest part of the stuttering handicap. Obviously, such behaviors as repetitions and prolongations, facial and body movement, contribute to the severity and handicap of the problem. But it is the roads not taken socially, educationally, and vocationally, that can have the greatest handicapping impact on the lives of people who happen to stutter. These are aspects of the problem that are often at the source of the client's complaints when they come for help.

The large majority of research on stuttering has focused on surface behavior, especially the frequency of stuttering events. Relatively little effort has been devoted to the nature of the intrinsic features of stuttering. They may not be assessed during diagnosis, they often go unattended during treatment, and they may not be used as indicators of progress during or following treatment. One of the reasons for this, undoubtedly, is the lack of measurement procedures and techniques that allow identification and quantification of the cognitive and attitudinal features of stuttering. In addition, dealing with these features may be scary for some clinicians, for it requires an understanding of the nature of stuttering, in general, and of the person who stutters, in particular. This form of treatment requires using some counseling techniques and that can be threatening to clinicians who have not had such training.

The intrinsic characteristics of a person who is stuttering are not always difficult to identify or alter. For a few people, it may not be necessary to spend a great deal of time desensitizing and altering their way of thinking about themselves and their speech. In these cases, it is possible to inform them about the basic nature of the speech mechanism, instruct them in techniques for modifying the features of their speech, and alter their communication style in ways that will facilitate communication. As a result they can begin to use more efficient ways of communicating both within and outside the treatment setting. Of course, this is not the case typically, but it does occur.

Even with more difficult cases of stuttering in adults it is rarely necessary for clinicians to become involved with in-depth counseling. This is, of course, more likely to be the case when stuttering coexists with psychiatric disorders. However, for the large majority of adults with developmental stuttering, it will be necessary to devote some time to helping clients restructure what they think and say about themselves, their stuttering experience, and their speech successes and failures.

Evaluations Needed

The process of growth and change is circular rather than linear. In that regard, the process is similar to the course of loss and grief; we make progress for awhile and then, for a time, find ourselves falling back to additional mourning. This circular process is also apparent during fluency treatment when one appreciates that more than behavior is changing during successful treatment. Attitudes and ways of interpreting one's self and others must also change, particularly if long-term success is to result. Thus, the change process is best seen as being spiral or circular both during and following treatment.[4,5]

Changing complex human problems such as stuttering should hardly be expected to be linear. Change is not linear even for relatively less complicated forms of growth. It takes months of consistent effort to modify patterns of weight loss, smoking, and exercise. For an assortment of reasons, there are peaks and valleys along the way. Motivation for change increases and decreases. It takes adjustments of schedules and priorities (one's own and often others) in setting aside the time to spend on the task. So, it should not be surprising if changing something as complex as stuttering will be a circular and rigorous process. It is necessary for the client, as well as the clinician, to understand this at the outset of treatment so that no one gets frustrated and quits whenever there is a dip in energy or achievement. It is essential for all involved to appreciate the larger pattern of change. Both the clinician and the client must keep their eyes on the prize and not become discouraged by temporary cycles and setbacks that are the norm.

Key Case History Information

Each client has a story. At its most basic level, that is what a case history is about. Obviously, I want to learn about significant physical, psychological, and educational events of each person's history. I want to find out about any previous treatment and the person's response to those experiences. I want to determine if there are any concomitant learning or communication problems that may affect future intervention. I want to find out all of these things, but more than anything else, we want to find out why the person is here with me at this moment.

As with many things in life, timing is the key. Having been more or less successful in dealing with the problems presented by stuttering for many years, what has made the person ask for help now? What has caused this speaker to reach out to a professional after dealing with the problem for decades? One possibility is that one may feel "stuck" and, despite years of trying, finally realizes that he or she cannot change this situation without some form of outside assistance.[6]

The reason clients come for help should be bigger than a temporary obstacle that they must face. I have had clients come to me because they faced a crisis and the pressure for change was on. One man who had avoided any form of treatment for more than 50 years was faced with giving the toast at the rehearsal dinner for his son's wedding. Another man in his 40s, also having postponed a commitment to treatment for years, was unable to avoid giving a speech to a large regional gathering of fellow business people. Both of these men were extremely motivated for the short term. Using strategies of both stuttering modification and fluency shaping, along with large doses of desensitization and basic public speaking techniques, I was able to assist them through these temporary crises. Both men were able to experience and appreciate their success in spite of a few minor stuttering moments. They didn't avoid the challenge, and they were genuinely proud of their accomplishments, but, of course, once the events had passed and the pressure was off, they quickly tired of the long term and rigorous process of making enduring changes and terminated treatment.

Of course, I wanted to provide more than temporary relief and would have preferred to have helped both of them become even better communicators, but, they got what they wanted. As Peck[7] points out, choosing treatment is often the more difficult path, and many clients drop out of treatment long before they have reached the goals the clinician has in mind. Long-term motivation was lacking once the threats had passed and this is undoubtedly why so few older speakers are seen in stuttering treatment programs.[8,9] The two men I saw had adapted to their speech and were, by nearly any standard, highly successful individuals.

Long-term change requires long-term commitment and is more likely to occur during significant nodes in the life cycle of most people. Such moments occur throughout life but seem to occur with greater frequency while a person is in their 20s. During this decade, people are likely to complete formal schooling, change their living status and location, enter and leave military service, initiate careers, get married, have children, and sometimes, go through a divorce. It is at such "nodes" in a person's life when self-awareness and introspection may be heightened, and consequently, when decision-making and restructuring take place.[10–12] During these periods, people are more likely to assume responsibility for their lives and begin the journeys that are required. This was reflected in the comments of adult stutterers who had made significant changes in the quality of their speech at a recent meeting of the American Speech–Language–Hearing Association.[13] Each of the eight people who spoke at this session described major changes, occurring as a function of treatment during their early to mid-twenties. I know of no research to support the notion, but I suspect that individuals who decide to enter treatment following the reflection and restructuring that occurs during significant nodes in their life cycle are much more likely to achieve long-term success than are those individuals who are responding to a temporary speech crisis.

Thus, during the evaluation process, it's important to determine a person's readiness for change. I ask them why didn't they seek help a year ago. Why are they coming now and not 6 months from now? What is it about this period in their lives that makes changing their speech important? The answer to that question may tell me much about the likely direction and slope of long-term change.

Finally, the timing of the relationship between a client and clinician may also be crucial to the success of treatment. At the time when a client makes the choice to seek help it is probably critical that the clinician selected is a person with whom he or she can be compatible. The matching of client and clinician is not a simple one and undoubtedly is an area in need of considerably more study than it has received. It involves more than locating some one with experience and a good reputation or finding a clinician who has specialized in working with people who stutter. To be sure, all of these characteristics help to insure a minimal level of competency. But more than this, the clinician should be congruent with the treatment and the techniques that will be employed.[14] As Luterman points out, the strategy and associated techniques of treatment must be "congruent" with the personality of the clinician. Techniques must blend into the treatment process. If not, then such techniques may be discontinuous with the process and even have the possibility of undermining the authenticity of the clinical relationship. This would be unfortunate for often, it is this relationship that is at the core of the change process for adults who stutter.[15,16]

Observations and Tests Used

One of the characteristics of developmental stuttering is that the behaviors we are able to observe are highly variable. As Bloodstein[17] states "The great variability of stuttering from time to time under different conditions is liable to result in assessments that are unrepresentative" (p. 386). While this is more obviously the case with younger children, which can make accurate assessment particularly problematic,[18] it may also be true for adults. Because so much of stuttering is under the surface and the behaviors that are readily apparent are so inconsistent, assessment must be an ongoing process. Even the most experienced clinician may need two or three individual sessions to become calibrated to a client and his or her behavioral patterns.

There is a wealth of information for the clinician to acquire and process during the initial treatment sessions. Not only is it important to appraise the nature of the verbal and nonverbal behaviors accompanying stuttering, but it is also important to learn about the person in a more general sense. What does this person sound and look like when not stuttering? What are the linguistic and acoustic qualities of his or her nonstuttered speech; is it truly flowing and easy or does it sound unstable, irregular, rapid, or unnatural? Does it seem as though many moments of stuttering are about to break through to the surface. Does body language provide clues that stuttering almost occurred or is about to take place? In what ways are an avoidance or word substitution signaled? Many of these clues are likely contained in a speaker's body language, choice of vocabulary, and syntax. Obviously, with all this information to process, it often takes more than a single meeting for the clinician to begin to know and understand a client.

Many formal assessment procedures and techniques may be used to assign severity ratings and measure change in stuttering as a function of intervention.[16,19] Although many of these procedures measure the surface features of stuttering, some attempts have been made to quantify the under-the-surface or intrinsic features of stuttering. These include the Locus of Control Behavior Scale[20] and the self-efficacy scaling techniques for adults (Self Efficacy Scale for Adults who Stutter)[21] and adolescents (Self-Efficacy for Adolescents Scale).[22] The most recent scale developed to quantify and track some of the internal dynamics of clients is the Subjective Stuttering Scale (SSS) by Riley.[23]

The *Locus of Control of Behavior* (*LCB*) is a 17-item, Likert-type scale designed to indicate a person's ability to assume responsibility for performing new or desired behaviors. Clients record their agreement or disagreement to the 17 statements using a 6-point scale. Items 1, 5, 7, 8, 13, and 16 are reverse scored before item scores are summed to obtain a total score. Intended for use with adults, the scale has good reliability. Lower scores indicate greater internal control (which is desirable) and higher scores indicate greater perceived external control over the person's actions. LCB scores do not seem to be related to a person's fluency[24] and may be influenced by whether or not increased assertiveness and responsibility are a focus of the treatment program.[25]

The *Self Efficacy for Adults who Stutter Scale* (*SESAS*) follows the work of Bandura[26] on perceptual self-efficacy scaling and is intended to measure the confidence with which an adult who stutters can approach and maintain fluent speech in a wide variety of extra treatment speaking situations. Ornstein and Manning[21] found that adults who stutter scored significantly lower on both the Approach (66.2) and Performance (55.8) portions of the SESAS than did nonstuttering speakers. The latter speakers scored 94.2 and 98.0 for the approach and performance portions, respectively. Several investigators have reported increases in SESAS scores as a result of treatment,[27–29] and, in some cases, adults who consider themselves recovered from stuttering have recorded SESAS scores that exceed those of nonstuttering adults.[30] A new version of this scale provides for self-efficacy scaling of participation and fluency for 20 typical speaking categories and 5 communication dimensions.[31]

The *Self-Efficacy for Adolescents Scale* (*SEA-Scale*) consists of 100 items referring to extra-treatment speaking situations in 13 categories of situations[32] and is designed to enable clinicians to map clients' predicted performance in a variety of extra treatment speaking activities. Clients score each item using an interval scale of 1 through 10. Overall reliability for the 100 items in the scale was 0.98. Manning[22] found that the scale discriminated between adolescents who stutter (mean of 7.21) and those who do not (mean of 8.65) ($p < .001$).

The *Stuttering Severity Scale* (*SSS*) is the newest scale for quantifying intrinsic aspects of stuttering and is designed to determine which individuals could benefit from changing their internal belief systems. The scale was created to provide information about a person's internal, as well as external changes as a result of treatment. The scale is composed of 17 statements (e.g., Item 13: "Does your level of self-confidence have an effect on your fluency?") to which the client responds by using a 9-point semantic differential format. The scale is composed of three subtests (I. Self-Perception—6 items; II. Locus of Control—7 items; and III. Avoidance—4 items). At present, data are being gathered on behavioral changes and SSS scores in a double-blind, placebo-controlled study of 36 adults who stutter.

One informal procedure for obtaining a client's self-assessment of his stuttering and relating it to that of the clinician is described by Manning (pp. 95-96).[16] This procedure also provides an opportunity for trial therapy. The client is first asked to indicate the severity of his stuttering on an equal interval scale ranging from 0 (no stuttering) through 1 (mild), 4–5 (moderate) to 8 (severe). The scale, easily drawn on a piece of paper, is placed in front of the client who is asked to indicate the typical, everyday level of stuttering severity. The act of providing a pen to this scale can be the first step in assigning a client the responsibility for change. The client is then asked to indicate on the scale the point that corresponds to the severity of stuttering during the assessment. Although these two points on the scale may be the same, often they are not. This gives the clinician an opportunity to discuss the variability of (developmental) stuttering. Of course, it is important to consider how closely the clinician's rating agrees with that of the client. The clinician can also ask the client to indicate how far up and down the scale his or her stuttering ranges? If the client is like most people who are assessed for fluency disorders, then the range of severity reported will be wide. This, along with case history information, provides the clinician with an opportunity to inform the client that this is typical and normal behavior for an adult who stutters. Depending on what the client may have heard or read about theories of stuttering onset and development or seen portrayed in the movies, these comments may provide a large measure of relief. Once the range of stuttering behavior has been established, usually with the clinician leading the way, the client can experiment a bit with some trial therapy. I usually have the client follow my lead and stutter along with me. This begins some preliminary desensitization activities and helps me to determine the client's motivation and willingness to experiment a bit with behavior that, until now, seemed to be completely adversative and uncontrollable.

As noted earlier, it is important at the outset to determine a client's motivation and provide him or her with a realistic idea of the demands of treatment. On the other hand, the assessment period is also a time when clinicians can "hook" prospective clients and help them move from contemplating their problem to taking action. The initial interview provides me with an opportunity to show the clients that I have both empathy and insight about the process of change for someone who stutterers. Regardless of the quality of fluency they may eventually achieve, I can show them what success can look, sound, and feel like. I can show them that I am willing to accompany them in this quest.

Case Selection Criteria

The adult clients usually seen in speech–language clinics are probably determined by a variety of nontherapeutic factors such as cost, distance, and how well the openings in clinic schedules coincide with clients' work schedules. The key element in who should be seen, in my opinion, is the client's willingness and readiness for change. Inclusion and exclusion criteria can be highly selective, a factor that is important to consider when evaluating the outcomes of treatment programs. Everything being equal, intensive treatment programs generally require higher levels of motivation and commitment in the form of their immediate cost and the time spent away from work and family.

Clients come to therapy when they feel that they need help. They enter or reenter a program when they feel no longer able to deal with the problem by themselves. They are likely to stay in treatment until they make the changes desired or until their motivation falls below that required for continued change.

A Management Approach

Whatever overall treatment strategy and associated techniques are used, the clinician as well as the client should be in agreement concerning the nature and direction of treatment. There is no single overall treatment strategy that is best for all clients, and this is certainly true for adults who stutter. There has been increased interest recently in considering the efficacy of various treatment approaches for fluency disorders.[33–35] But plugging clients into different forms of treatment, then asking which program might, by some criteria, be best is the wrong question. Such a question is analogous to questions about which car, religion, or political party is the best. Prochaska and DiClemente[5] argue that most research in behavioral therapy has concentrated on trying to determine which treatment is best for a particular problem. They refer to this as "horse race research" and point out that its results have been "a disappointing abundance of ties" (p. 204). In addition, they propose that one of the major research issues in the 1990s is how those interested in modifying human behavior can match more effectively treatment strategies and techniques to people. Thus, a better question to ask is what behavioral processes are best for whom and when?

Client motivation typically is high at the outset of treatment. The person has accepted the fact that a problem exists, at least at some level, and has initiated the process of change by contacting a professional who can provide helpful information and begin to demystify the problem. Thus, begins the process of clients becoming more objective about their predicament. Some clients appear to be highly motivated, saying all the right things. But since it is never what one says, but rather what one does that determines one's true level of motivation, how can a client's true motivation be assessed? One way is to clearly describe the nature of the treatment process. The clinician can explain that it often is an arduous and lengthy process. She can provide examples of the tasks that will have to be done, making it clear that, while the clinician is the coach, it is the client who runs the laps. To be sure, at times clinicians demonstrate or model desired behavior changes and perform some of the tasks asked of clients, but it is the client's problem, and it is their responsibility to take action. Clinicians can provide specific examples and give concrete assignments to be completed by the following treatment session. Clinicians can be supporting and encouraging but clinicians also need to be candid in explaining the long and often difficult road of change that is the case for most people who suffer from the handicap of stuttering.

Stages of Change

Prochaska, DiClemente, and Norcross[36] suggest five stages that individuals go through during the process of change. Although much of their work is in the area of changing addictive behavior, their ideas have many applications to the treatment of other complex human behavioral problems, including stuttering. Their stage model of change can be summarized as follows:

1. Change is cyclical through specific stages.
2. There is a common set of processes that facilitate change.
3. Ideally, there can be a systematic integration of the stages and processes of change.

The experienced clinician needs to determine clients' readiness for change, then adjust treatment techniques accordingly. The success of these techniques will depend not on the inherent utility of the techniques themselves but on applying the right techniques at the right time. The five stages of change described by Prochaska and colleagues[36] are as follows:

1. **Precontemplation**: During this initial stage persons are generally unaware of their problem. Even if there is some awareness and a wish to change, they have no intention of doing something about their problem in the near future (i.e., the next 6 months). Some may have enough awareness of their problem to be defensive, but they generally feel that it is under control. Because significant others often see the problem, when people in this stage come for treatment, they do so typically as a result of pressure from others. In such cases, they may be capable of change as long as the pressure is on, but are likely to cease treatment once the threat is past. A hallmark of people in this stage is their *resistance to recognizing or modifying a problem.*

2. **Contemplation**: During contemplation persons have become aware of their problem and are actively beginning to consider the possibility of change (i.e., within the next 6 months). They may begin seeking information about the problem but still have no formal plan to take action. Even with this increased awareness and concern about their problem, some may stay in the contemplation stage for years. After they begin to weigh the pros and cons of their behavior and the time, effort, and money it will take to change, serious consideration of the possible ways to resolve the problem is the key element in contemplation.

3. **Preparation**: People in this stage are ready to change and intend to take action during the next month. They may demonstrate some small behavioral changes but have not yet reached a level of effective action. They are, however, now making decisions in terms of goals and priorities.

4. **Action**: Individuals in this stage are now beginning to modify specific behaviors and/ or their environment. They use newly acquired skills to make overt changes. Because

behavioral changes are now noticeable, they are apt to receive recognition by others. Altered behavior is defined by their achieving a specific criterion.

5. **Maintenance**: People in this stage are stabilizing both behavioral and cognitive changes. Because it takes a long time to reduce the occurrences of old behaviors, attitudes, and cognitions and replace them with new ones, this period lasts from 6 months to an undetermined period of time. A marker of this stage is the appearance of new and incompatible behavior in real-life situations.

Change throughout the stages of this model is not viewed as linear. A spiral or cyclical pattern of change is more likely to occur with relapse being the rule rather than the exception. Individuals may move through these stages with professional assistance or the changes may be self-initiated. Furthermore, as Prochaska et al.[36] indicate, people often move into the action stage and into maintenance and then back to precontemplation. As clients learn from their mistakes, they again advance to the next stage of change.

Relatively few people from a population having a chronic or long-standing problem are actually ready to make changes. Summary data obtained on smoking cessation by Prochaska et al.[36] illustrate this point. They noted that 50%–60% of smokers are in the precontemplation stage and 30%–40%, in the contemplation stage. Only 10%–14% of this population can be categorized as being in the action stage. A key implication of this stage model is that people in different stages of change need to be matched with different treatment processes, or change will be less likely to occur. This way of considering the process of treatment coincides with the client-centered approach that is advocated by many clinicians.

The second part of this trans-theoretical model is how the processes of change are linked to clients' stages of change. DiClemente (1993)[4] described 10 categories of processes that facilitate change. Gathered from various clinical approaches to psychotherapeutic intervention, these processes are grouped together regardless of the theoretical construct in which they are typically used.

1. *Consciousness Raising*: These processes involve helping clients to increase information about themselves and the problem. This is accomplished using such techniques as observation, confrontation, interpretation, and bibilotherapy.

2. *Self-reevaluation*: These are processes that help clients to assess how they feel and think about themselves with respect to their problem behaviors. This is accomplished by techniques of value clarification, imagery, corrective emotional experience, and challenging beliefs and expectations.

3. *Self-liberation*: Such processes involve helping clients to choose and commit to taking action. This also relates to increasing their belief in the ability to change. This can be accomplished by decision-making therapy, developing resolutions, logotherapy, and commitment-enhancing techniques.

4. *Counterconditioning*: These processes enable clients to substitute alternatives for the anxiety related to problem behaviors. This may be accomplished by techniques of relaxation, desensitization, assertion, and positive self-statements.

5. *Stimulus Control*: These processes help persons to avoid or counter stimuli that elicit problem behaviors. Such techniques include restructuring the environment, avoiding high-risk cues, and fading techniques.

6. *Reinforcement Management*: These processes involve showing clients how to reward themselves or create rewards from others for the changes they make. This can be

accomplished by contingency contracts and overt and covert reinforcement for self-reward.

7. *Helping Relationships*: These processes help clients to be open and trusting about problems with people who care. This may be accomplished by the development of therapeutic alliances, increased social support, and association with support groups.

8. *Emotional Arousal and Dramatic Relief*: These processes have to do with helping clients to experience and express feelings about their problems and possible solutions. This can be accomplished by techniques such as psychodrama, grieving losses, and role playing.

9. *Environmental Reevaluation*: These processes enable clients to evaluate how a problem affects their personal and physical environment. This can be accomplished by using techniques of empathy training and documentaries.

10. *Social Liberation*: These are processes that help clients to increase alternatives for non-problem behaviors that are present in society. This can be accomplished by advocating for rights of the repressed and empowering policy changes and interventions.

Prochaska et al.[36] suggest that stage/process mismatches by clinicians may prevent or impede successful change by clients. This commonly occurs, for example, when clinicians select processes associated with the contemplation stage (e.g., consciousness raising, self-evaluation) at a time when a client is moving into the action stage. Becoming more aware and gaining insight, alone, do not bring about behavioral change, so these are not efficient processes at this stage of change. Such mismatches may explain some of the criticisms directed at counseling and nondirective approaches for changing behaviors. Another common mismatch is using action-orientated processes (e.g., reinforcement, stimulus control, counterconditioning) with clients in the contemplation or preparation stages of change. Accordingly, attempts to modify behaviors without clients' awareness have been a frequent criticism of radical behaviorism. In addition, behavioral changes achieved in the absence of insight are likely to be temporary, according to Prochaska et al.[36]

Treatment Goals

The most basic goal of fluency treatment for an adult who stutters is to decrease the *handicap*, the disadvantages experienced because of the stuttering impairment, disabilities, or reactions to them, that are related to the *impairment*, the disruption of speech–language function or other psychosocial or communicative processes. To the degree possible, I would also like to significantly modify the *disability*, the limitations in ability to perform tasks because of the stuttering impairment or reactions to it. During the assessment or treatment process, I am not especially concerned about issues of presumed *etiology*, the possibility of abnormality of motoric, psycholinguistic, or neural processes underlying normal speech production.[37]

Changes in these surface behaviors, which are most easily observed as the frequency and form of the stuttering, are obvious indicators of change, but changes under the surface are also essential, particularly for long-term success. Each client's handicap is a little different, for not only does the person come to treatment with a different story, but each person has different goals for his or her life and speech following intervention.

Transfer and maintenance of communication skills and attitudes to outside treatment situations can begin at the outset of treatment. For example, it's probably a good idea to have treatment in different places, certainly not in the same treatment room. It is good also to have clients practice in as many real-life settings as possible if the clinician expects them to perform in those settings. Shooting foul shots in the nonthreatening environment of a home driveway is far from performing the same act under the pressure of real game conditions. To perform under game conditions, one must practice under those conditions.

Other desirable treatment outcomes include widening clients' choices, increasing their risk taking in both speech and nonspeech activities, and improving the naturalness of their speech and their communication abilities. On occasion, it is necessary to work on communication disabilities including pragmatic, word finding, language, and voice problems. Finally, I want adult clients to be able to evaluate their negative and positive self-talk as well as their speech quality and prescribe appropriate responses for themselves. Sometimes, following successful treatment, clients may need to make the wise choice of seeking additional assistance as they experience a shallow or deep relapse.

Throughout formal treatment it is important for both the clinician and client to recognize progress and appreciate the small victories that are taking place. Such successes can be overlooked if everyone involved holds to the single-minded and unrealistic goal of perfect fluency. Even a temporary return to severe stuttering includes victories to be identified and appreciated. For example, it is an important victory for speakers to choose not to avoid or substitute a feared word and take a risk and enter a feared speaking situation. Even if obvious stuttering occurs and they are unable to modify their speech as they hoped, they may be able to step back from the emotional experience and accurately self-monitor their behavior as well as the reactions of listeners. They can also give themselves positive feedback, in contrast to their old, negative and reflexive, self-punitive statements about the experience.

Treatment Procedures

The most important statement that I can make about treatment procedures is that procedures are not the treatment. Treatment by technique results in a micromanagement of a complex, dynamic, multilayered problem. Clinicians who think that the techniques selected for use during treatment *are* the treatment are likely to miss the bigger picture. More importantly, they may be less likely to focus on the client and the client's needs.

Many therapeutic procedures have been shown to be effective in the treatment of stuttering. There are, for example, a variety of techniques that will yield, often rapidly, a decreased frequency of fluency breaks. The techniques associated with rate control, fluency shaping, and stuttering modification strategies have an important place in the repertoire of an experienced clinician. For some clients, the easier ones, changing surface features of the problem will yield long-term change and that, of course, is grand. Sometimes techniques "work" well, and sometimes they don't. As Culatta and Goldberg[38] insightfully suggest, failures of a client to make effective use of a technique are more often due to an inappropriate selection of the technique by the clinician rather than the characteristics of the technique. I suspect this is more likely to happen when a clinician is focusing on techniques, rather than the client, and the larger process of change across both surface and intrinsic features of stuttering.

A better way to consider treatment procedures and techniques is to think of them as part of the fabric of the clinical interaction and the dialogue of change and growth. Clinicians should be aware of the many different techniques that are available and constantly look for new ideas. But more important, they need to select those that are most appropriate for the person they are attempting to help. As DiClemente[4] argues, in the context of counseling, successful treatment is not the result of using techniques, but of using the right techniques at the right time. This has also been pointed out in the area of fluency disorders.[16,38,39] Egan[6] notes in discussing the techniques of counseling, that people come for help because they are stuck and that it takes more than knowledge and techniques to get them unstuck; it requires wisdom. I believe that the same view should be taken of the clinical decisions that are made when treating adults who stutter.

Techniques are more likely to be the primary focus of less experienced clinicians, teachers, and coaches. People who are beginning to learn a profession are under pressure to have something to say and do in a treatment session, in class, or on the practice field. New coaches tend to focus on techniques, as if the techniques, in and of themselves, were the athletic event. I did this at the outset of my lecturing and coaching careers. At that level of experience, I was more likely to stick to my notes and my clipboard. My decisions were based on the techniques I was selecting. I believed in them and was determined to make them work. As I gathered more experience, however, I gradually found that I was much better off when I began focusing on the needs of my clients, my students, and my young soccer players rather than techniques, and so were they. A mantra for new clinicians or coaches might be "It's not the techniques, stupid!"

On many occasions in recent years, clinicians have asked me to suggest techniques for them to use with clients. During my initial years as a university professor I did my best to respond with a series of suggestions, only to have some of them later inform me that "the techniques didn't work!" Now when asked what I could suggest for a client, I often answer by saying "I have absolutely no idea." Of course, that is not a very impressive answer for an "expert" from the university, but it is a much more honest response. It is more honest, because I have no idea what would be the best clinical decision. I have not had an opportunity to become calibrated to the person. I don't know how they stutter or how they are fluent. I don't know the nature of their stuttering or their patterns of avoidance. I have not observed their struggle behavior or their body language and if they react with shame and embarrassment during and following stuttering. When I have not had the opportunity to observe and tune into the client, I don't know whether or not some of their speech, although not stuttered, is shaky and unstable; if they are "talking on thin ice" with the loss of control and overt stuttering lurking just under the surface. And finally, I have absolutely no idea how motivated or resilient they are, so I don't know how they will respond when I push them into the process of change. Clinicians can make plans to use all types of therapy techniques, but good clinical decisions can be made only in response to a specific person in a specific stage of the change process.

Refinement of Some Common Treatment Procedures

Having argued that treatment is not equivalent to employing specific techniques, I will proceed now to discuss aspects of some of the techniques I use. Stuttering modification techniques I use are also referred to as traditional, Van Riparian, nonavoidance, or stutter-more-fluently approaches, and the goal of these techniques is to change the form of a person's stuttering to an open, flowing, and easy, but not necessarily normally fluent form of speaking. The goals of stuttering modification have been described in detail in a number of sources.[40–42] I will, however, point out a few key elements that are sometimes overlooked when using these techniques.

Because the primary emphasis of this approach to treatment is on decreasing avoidance behavior, desensitizing a speaker to his own fluency breaks, and seeking out and modifying stuttering moments, it is easy to presume that fluency is not a primary or long-term goal. With this approach, stuttering has to be out in the open and exposed in order to be identified and altered. As a result, especially early in treatment, there can be an *increase* in the client's frequency of stuttering. If the client is beginning to make telephone calls, ask questions in meetings, and participate socially, more frequent fluency breaks will often be the result. The client, of course, is making better decisions and using less avoidance behavior. But more stuttering events as well as possible increases in struggle and escape behaviors may also occur. Despite this temporary increase in stuttering, a realistic long-term goal of the stuttering-modification approach is certainly spontaneous fluency.

A primary principle of stuttering-modification techniques is to monitor and change old automatic, reflexive, and struggled fluency breaks into easier and smoother forms of stuttering. Clients initially learn to do this following (cancellation or post-event), then during (pullout or para-event), and finally, prior to (preparatory set or pre-event) moments of stuttering. Modification proceeds in this order (from after to before) to give clients time to overcome their anxiety of this experience and make it easier for them to catch and change their fluency breaks.

A goal throughout each stage of stuttering modification is not to become fluent but rather to "take charge" or "control" of the stuttering event and selectively modify the speech pattern. A common mistake of clients when performing the cancellation technique is to simply say the stuttered word again, but fluently. Instead, they should repeat the word again using a form of smooth or "easy stuttering." Although not spoken in a normally fluent manner, their speech is open, flowing, and smooth. The fluency-enhancing techniques of full breath, light articulatory contact, continuous voicing, and blending of sounds and syllables as articulatory transitions are made from one position to another, are also helpful. Once the cancellation technique is mastered in a variety of speaking situations, most clients quite naturally begins using para- or even pre-event modifications. Again, however, the key aspect of this technique is to take charge of the moment, rather than helplessly fighting through stuttering while feeling out of control.

As these modification techniques become (over)learned, a client achieves more success in progressively more difficult extratreatment speaking situations. Prestuttering modifications are, of course, preferred. If this is not possible, then the client has a second opportunity to modify stuttering by using the pullout technique. Finally, if unsuccessful in taking charge of the stuttering moment using these techniques, the client's final opportunity is the cancellation technique. Although this may take several attempts, clients should not move forward with the sentence until they have taken charge of the word. This is often difficult for clients to do, especially at the outset of treatment. They may even feel that it is an impossible task, particularly during more difficult speaking situations. If someone is having little success in modifying stuttering events, it is often because he or she has not yet become desensitized to the stuttering experience. But once a person begins to think of stuttering moments as an opportunity for victory, he or she can begin to score some runs. Of course, the score at this point is roughly Stuttering: one million, client 0. So, naturally most clients are going to feel a little behind. Even though old habits are always the strongest, they can begin by starting to win a few innings!

If the client is in hot pursuit of fluency rather than control when using any of the stuttering modification techniques, they will not be as effective. Thus, many clients have to become more comfortable with stuttering, to be able to "stay in the stuttering moment" rather than trying so hard to escape from the experience. They have to stay with the moment of stuttering, to vary it, to allow themselves to experience it fully. Although it will seem contradictory to clients, only by getting to know stuttering by experiencing it is it possible to achieve some distance from the fear and helplessness of that experience.

It is also beneficial not to try too hard to "overcontrol" speech during modifications of stuttering. Improved ease of fluency will follow as a client stops fighting stuttering, speaks with a more open vocal tract, and goes with the flow of his speech and thought process. If the client or the clinician are in a rush toward fluency and fail to appreciate more basic successes, the risk of overcontrol is greater. In the videotapes produced by the Stuttering Foundation of America,[43] Van Riper takes an adult who stutters (Jeff) through the stages of treatment. In the follow-up tape, made some 20 years later, Jeff describes what a valuable lesson he learned when Dr. Van encouraged and allowed him to play with his stuttering, to have fun (in place of fear) with the experience. It has been suggested[16,44] that humorous interpretations of the stuttering experience provide a window for observing the cognitive changes that take place during successful treatment. The appreciation of humor requires some distance and objectivity about a situation. As the client, with the leadership of the clinician, achieves both a distance from the fear of stuttering and a mastery of modification techniques, the paradoxical aspects of the stuttering experience become apparent. Only then does much of the humor of the situation become obvious. Nothing is funny when one feels overwhelmed, but as distance from a problem as well as the feeling of mastery takes place, humor can be one indicator of progress.

The client's decision to substitute or avoid sounds, words, people, or situations is one of the more insidious features of stuttering and one of the most difficult to alter. This decision can be so subtle that the client may not even be aware of it. It is a form of stuttering that may never reach the surface. The decision not to speak will not be identified as stuttering but is, in fact, a profound stuttering event. Along with the changes in surface behaviors of the problem, the choices that a client makes because of the *possibility* of stuttering must also change. The stuttering-modification strategy requires a good deal of introspection, self-awareness, self-monitoring, motivation, and courage on the part of the client, as well as good leadership and support on the part of the clinician.

Fluency-modification strategies (also called fluency-shaping or speak-more-fluently approaches) are closely related to the rate control and rate reduction therapies that became popular in the 1960s and 1970s. These approaches focused on reducing the frequency of stuttering behavior, often using behavioral modification techniques to decrease stuttering. Speech rate was slowed using delayed auditory feedback as well as clinician modeling and instructions. Rate control, in some form, remains a popular approach for modifying stuttering[45] and has been shown to significantly reduce the frequency of stuttering, particularly in the clinical setting. As Max and Caruso[39] point out, reductions of speaking rate can be viewed as a treatment goal in and of itself, a temporary goal to promote fluency before the client's rate is gradually increased, or a technique for smoothing an anticipated stuttering event. In any case, the emphasis of treatment is not on modifying a specific moment of stuttering but rather on changing the client's overall speech pattern. Rate reduction often emphasizes the use of prolonged speech in which the duration of articulatory movements is increased and smooth articulatory transitions between sounds and syllables are accentuated. Such slowing and smoothing of speech promotes the coordination and integration of respiratory, phonatory, and articulatory movements. Once such movements are well learned and integrated, the client is able to gradually increase speed of performance, often without fluency breaks. In addition, a reduction in the length of phrases, even as short as two to five syllables,[46] with pauses at natural syntactic junctures,[47] promotes an open vocal tract and provides clients the opportunity to achieve a full breath. Continuous phonation,[48] or constant vocalization,[39] of both voiced and unvoiced sounds is recommended to promote continuous air flow and articulatory movement. Boberg and Kully[49] suggest blending the sounds, syllables, and words of an utterance together as if saying one continuous word. Although earlier fluency-modification approaches focused almost exclusively on surface features of stuttering, recent versions[49] are more comprehensive in nature and often incorporate procedures for facilitating cognitive and affective change.

Fluency-shaping procedures are a little like physical therapy for the vocal tract. The techniques can be beneficial for any speaker (fluent or not) as they increase understanding of speech physiology, and speakers learn to use techniques that make the most efficient use of the speech production mechanism. Mastery of these techniques can result in smooth, flowing, easy respiratory, vocal and articulatory adjustments that may result in more efficient as well as more fluent speech. If done well and practiced diligently, it can also result in making a speaker considerably easier to, listen to even if some (easy) fluency breaks continue to be present.

A few final points about both stuttering- and fluency-modification techniques. I typically begin treatment using a stuttering-modification approach. As a client is able to identify and becomes somewhat desensitized to the features of stuttering, in general, and his own stuttering, in particular, I begin using a selection of fluency-modification techniques. On other occasions, when client's are having great difficulty producing any fluent speech and are demonstrating profound struggle behavior, I may begin with fluency-facilitating techniques in order to give them some immediate success in modifying their fluency. Once they have achieved some success, they can learn to identify, become desensitized to and modify specific features of their stuttering. Most adults who stutter need both sides of this therapeutic coin. They benefit from learning how to produce speech in a way that promotes fluency, and both the anatomical and physiological characteristics of speech production and the increased awareness of the distinctive features of sound production gives them information that is essential for analyzing and monitoring speech. But most also need to know what to do when caught in the middle of a stuttering event. Fortunately, if they can develop confidence in using techniques for repairing the stuttered moment, much of the helplessness that accompanies stuttering will begin to subside.

Both fluency- and stuttering-modification approaches tend to heighten a speaker's monitoring and self-evaluation abilities and development of the critical ability to self-monitor speech via proprioceptive feedback. As clients are able to take charge of their stuttering moments and achieve higher levels of fluency, there are fewer stuttering events left to modify. Voluntary stuttering, in which the person decides to stutter in an easy, open manner, is often useful at this point. It provides a good test of whether or not a client is still running from the stuttering. As treatment progresses and there are fewer stuttering moments available to modify, fluency-modification techniques, quite naturally, take precedence. These procedures can sometimes be used to smooth out any remaining unstable speech. And finally, fluency-modification techniques provide clients with helpful techniques for smoothly modifying stuttering moments, particularly during later stages of stuttering modification programs, when pre-event or preparatory sets are being mastered.

The Importance of Group Treatment

The support provided by group treatment sessions is often a valuable component of treatment. Group treatment can be especially helpful for student clinicians because the group setting provides them an opportunity to learn about other clients and see their own client in what can be a more stressful communication situation. A group setting also provides support for clients during the action stage of change, a time when they are likely to be in need of a helping relationship.[50] The diversity of a group setting provides the opportunity for a variety of role-playing and public speaking activities. It also enables clients to realize that they are not alone with their problem.

One surprising effect of a group treatment situation that combines stuttering clients and nonstuttering clinicians is that both clinicians and clients soon understand the common nature of most anxiety-producing situations. Many people who stutter are amazed to learn that some people who don't stutter may also be extremely afraid of public-speaking experiences and go to great lengths to avoid speaking in front of a group. Although the threshold of avoidance may be reached sooner if a person stutters, everyone shares the anxiety associated with many speaking situations (e.g., public speaking, making introductions, telephoning members of the opposite sex, speaking with a superior at work). As the group discusses negative and positive self-talk and takes both speech and nonspeech risks during therapy, student clinicians often express the idea that they feel as if they are also undergoing treatment as they experience the excitement and challenge of pushing the envelope of their speech and their lives.

Expected Outcomes

An ideal but often unrealistic view of treatment would have clients speaking with normal fluency that sounds natural in all situations. This is possible, of course, and it happens, but it is the exception. It may not even be desirable for all persons. Following treatment, some people are speaking with what I call "technical" fluency. Their speech is, in a technical sense, free from repetitions, prolongations, and obvious struggle behavior, which can certainly be interpreted as progress. But, on occasion, some are controlling their speech so carefully that they are speaking with strain and effort. They are not communicating with ease, even the ease that is possible for a person whose speech contains easy, tension-free fluency breaks. Being in grim pursuit of fluency can result in overcontrolled speech and, even in the absence of stuttering, results in less natural and less desirable communication.

I do NOT want clients to be speaking carefully. Like writing carefully, it is not likely to be spontaneous or creative or enjoyable for listeners. Speaking carefully reflects a narrow way of thinking about, but not a truly functional way of, communicating. As Perkins[47,52] commented, clients will not likely use techniques that feel or sound to them at least as abnormal as their stuttering; however, even traditional techniques of stuttering modification may result in adverse listener reactions. Recent findings by Manning, Thaxton, and Ells[53] speak to the challenges that clients face when using stuttering modification techniques outside the clinical setting. It was found that nonprofessional listeners consistently rated a stuttering-only video condition significantly more positively than a stuttering + cancellation or a stuttering + pullout speaking condition. This result was 180 degrees out of phase with our experimental hypotheses that naive listeners, like clinicians, would respond more favorably to forthright attempts by clients to modify a speech problem. If these preliminary findings are replicated in subsequent investigations, it appears that clients who use these techniques to modify stuttering should be prepared for some aversive (possibly verbal as well as nonverbal) reactions from listeners in extratreatment speaking situations. Clients not only must work against the momentum of their own long-standing reactions to the stuttering experience but also the expectations and reactions of others. In order to reduce the possibility of posttreatment relapse, clinicians may need to assist clients in preparing for such negative responses and inform those in clients' environments about appreciating and reinforcing their use of modification techniques.

Many clients leave treatment with relatively high levels of fluency; however, the maintenance of that fluency will continue to take considerable effort. Consistent effort and practice can lead to high levels of fluency which, in turn, may result in less practice when a problem is no longer prominent. Of course, what usually follows decreased practice is an increase in stuttering moments. This sequence of events is not unusual and should not be surprising, and both client and clinician should be prepared for this possibility. In addition, there will be many speaking situations when maintenance of fluency will not have the highest priority. This is apt to be the case in high-stimulus social situations, such as weddings, receptions, or parties, where there are many things to concentrate on other than fluency. For some speakers, it may not be worth the effort to monitor and modify all moments of stuttering. It may be more important on such occasions not to work so hard on speech and simply enjoy the situation. Of course, the "ideal" client would use such speaking situations as an opportunity to practice. However, if this was not the choice, clients should not berate themselves, for such decisions are natural and to be expected. Positive self-talk following either success or failure to maintain fluency are an important feature of clients' continued progress.[53,54]

The completion of formal treatment is actually the initial stage for years of further growth. Usually, it takes a long time for changes in the affective and cognitive features of stuttering to catch up to behavioral modifications. Even though clients may be able to demonstrate high levels of fluent speech in a number of speaking situations, it will take some time before they no longer view themselves primarily as a person who stutters in making many decisions.[55] Adults with the impairment of stuttering usually find that both the handicap, as well as the disorder, persist.

As I indicated earlier, my primary goal for formal treatment is to reduce the handicap associated with stuttering. This means that I am not as interested in achieving a complete absence of stuttering as a significantly decreased handicap. I want clients to demonstrate more open decision-making, expanded risk-taking behavior, and greater freedom in speaking to anyone, anywhere, at anytime about anything. In short, I want the quality of their life to improve across all communication and some noncommunication situations. I want them to feel better about themselves, have an internal locus of control, and self-efficacy scores that indicate near normal participation and fluency values. I want them to continue to challenge themselves with public-speaking opportunities if that's what they want to do. To the degree that that they may continue to stutter, I want them to stutter in an open and smooth manner. I am especially interested in having them stutter without shame; a change in attitude that is truly an example of progress. Not all clients want or even need to sound as fluent as the anchor person on the national news.

Throughout treatment, and especially following treatment, client involvement with a support group can be extremely important. DiClemente[4] indicates that support groups probably play a critical role for eliciting change and especially for maintaining it. There are several organizations that promote such groups, with the National Stuttering Project being the most prominent in the United States. The value of such support to people with similar challenges can hardly be underestimated. The nurturing provided by a well-run and active support group can facilitate continued growth during the maintenance stage of change. The support and information that support meetings can provide to spouses, parents, and other interested family members can be critical for continued success both during and following treatment. Support group experiences and professional treatment can be complementary and should be thought of as enhancing one another. There are also a number of electronic support networks available on the internet that are especially valuable for adolescents who might not want to reveal their stuttering in the presence of others.

Relapse is a common problem in the treatment of adult stuttering.[16,40,56,57] A regression to earlier stages of change are the rule, not the exception. Prins[58] reported that approximately 40% of clients experience some regression following intensive treatment; however, it should be noted that relapse is common for any long-standing, complex, multivariate human condition. For example, DiClemente's[4] summary of programs that assist people to quit smoking reported that 1-year success rates are, at best, 20%–40% for intensive smoking cessation programs and are considerably less than that for nonintensive interventions. Because relapse is likely to occur to some degree, clinicians should address this issue with their clients and develop strategies for working through such periods. The door for additional treatment should be open and thought of as an opportunity for future growth rather than a failure. Such cycles are a natural and normal aspect of the change process. Should people make the decision to seek additional help they should be rewarded for their wisdom.

An adult woman who has stuttered all of her life recently expressed her view of recovery from stuttering on one of the e-mail networks. She equated recovery with freedom—the freedom to talk gently, not hide her stuttering, and be comfortable in speaking situations. She described the outward manifestations of her freedom as being able to

- no longer chase the fluency god,
- seek treatment for her stuttering,
- live without constant fear of uncontrolled stuttering,
- use the telephone without fear,
- speak without anxiously scanning for feared words and situations,
- initiate conversations where before she was usually silent,
- speak for herself instead of relying on others,
- speak to people and enter speaking situations previously avoided,
- talk even if she knows she will stutter,
- choose leisure activities without worrying about stuttering,
- explore career options that require talking, and
- stutter gently without avoidance or shame.

Conclusion

Because stuttering is a complex, multidimensional problem that is bound together by fear and helplessness, it is no easy task to help an adult who has had practice negotiating in the nonfluent world for many years. Sometimes it takes several cycles of treatment, sometimes with different clinicians, before things begin to come together and real progress takes place. Treatment by one or more clinicians may set the stage for change. But growth is possible and it has been demonstrated that adults who stutter can become not only more fluent, but more importantly, much less handicapped as a result of the treatment process. They may still be a person who stutters to varying degrees, but they can also be extremely successful communicators, and, in some cases, adult clients can achieve spontaneous fluency that is indistinguishable from the speech of nonstuttering speakers. Successful treatment depends not so much on the overall treatment strategy and its associated clinical techniques, but on the relationship of the client and the clinician and the ability of the clinician to make wise and timely decisions in facilitating the client's change.

Suggested Readings

Jezer M: *Stuttering: A Life Bound Up in Words*. New York, Basic Books, 1997.
> This book provides instant connection to the world of a person who stutters. Filled with many humorous and entertaining anecdotes, it is the author's story of his attempts to adjust to a fluent world in spite of stuttering. It is a story of self-awareness and growth and a book that provides unique insight and warmth about the culture of stuttering. A highly recommended source for clinicians, clients, and the families.

Manning W: *Clinical Decision Making in the Diagnosis and Treatment of Fluency Disorders*. Albany, NY, Delmar Publishers, 1996.
> Two chapters in this book are uniquely useful for working with clients who stutter. Chapter 1 provides a description of clinician characteristics as well as an explanation of why it may be worthwhile to pay attention to the variable of humor both during and following the process of treatment. Chapter 7 concerns counseling strategies and techniques that are helpful with clients and their families.

Egan G: *The Skilled Helper: A Problem-management Approach to Helping*. Pacific Grove, CA, Brooks/Cole Publishing Company, 1994.
> This highly readable fifth edition text is internationally recognized as a practical resource for a problem-management approach for counseling. The emphasis of the strategies and techniques are on client's taking action and moving from their present conditions to preferred scenarios for their life.

References

1. Chmela K, Reardon N: The emotions of stuttering. Presentation to the annual conference on Stuttering Therapy: Practical Ideas for the School Clinician. Memphis, TN. 1997.
2. Jezer M: *Stuttering: A Life Bound Up in Words*. New York, Basic Books, 1997.
3. Maslow A: *Towards a Psychology of Being* (2nd ed). Princeton, NJ, Van Nostrand, 1968.
4. DiClemente CC: Changing addictive behaviors: A process perspective. *Current Directions Psychol Sci* 1993; 101–106.
5. Prochaska JO, DiClemente CC: Stages of Change in the Modification of Problem Behaviors, in Herson M, Eisler R, Miller P (eds): Sycamore, IL, Sycamore Publishing Company, 1992.
6. Egan G: *The Skilled Helper: A Problem-management Approach to Helping*. Pacific Grove, CA, Brooks/Cole Publishing, 1994.
7. Peck MS: *The Road Less Traveled*. New York, Simon and Schuster, 1978.
8. Manning W, Monte K: Fluency breaks in older speakers: Implications for a model of stuttering throughout the life cycle. *J Fluency Dis* 1981; 6:35–48.
9. Manning W, Shirkey E: Fluency and the Aging Process, in Beasley DS, Davis GA (eds): *Aging: Communication Processes and Disorders*. New York, Grune & Stratton, 1981.
10. Kimmel DC: *Adulthood and Aging*. New York, John Wiley and Sons, 1974.
11. Sheehy G: *Passages: Predictable Crises of Adult Life*. New York: Bantam, New York, 1974.

12. Valiant GE: *Adaptation to Life*. Boston, Little, Brown and Co., 1977.
13. Daly D, Hood S, Guitar B, Manning W, Murphy W, Nelson L, Quesal R, Ramig P, St. Louis K: Successful treatment of fluency disorders: Examples of long-term change. Presentation to the annual meeting of the American Speech-Language-Hearing Association, Seattle, November, 1996.
14. Luterman DM: *Counseling the Communicatively Disordered and Their Families* (2nd ed). Austin, Pro-Ed, 1991.
15. Cooper EB, Cooper CS: The Effective Clinician, in Cooper EB, Cooper CS (eds): *Personalized Fluency Control Therapy—revised* (handbook). Allen, TX, DLM, 1985.
16. Manning W: *Clinical Decision Making in the Diagnosis and Treatment of Fluency Disorders*. Albany, NY, Delmar Publishers, Albany, 1996.
17. Bloodstein O: *A Handbook on Stuttering* (4th ed). Chicago, National Easter Seal Society, 1987.
18. Yaruss JS: Clinical implications of situational variability in preschool children who stutter. *J Fluency Dis* 1997; 22:187–203.
19. Ingham RJ, Cordes AK: Self-measurement and Evaluating Stuttering Treatment Efficacy, in Curlee RF, Siegel GM (eds): *Nature and Treatment of Stuttering: New Directions* (2nd ed). Boston, Allyn and Bacon, 1997.
20. Craig A, Andrews G: The prediction and prevention of relapse in stuttering. The value of self-control techniques and locus of control measures. *Behav Mod* 1985; 9:427–442.
21. Ornstein A, Manning W: Self-efficacy scaling by adult stutterers. *J Commun Dis* 1985; 18: 313–320.
22. Manning WH: The SEA-Scale: Self-efficacy scaling for adolescents who stutter. Presentation to the annual meeting of the American Speech-Language-Hearing Association, New Orleans, 1994.
23. Riley J: The Subjective Stuttering Scale (SSS), 1997 (unpublished).
24. diNil LF, Kroll RM: The relationship between locus of control and long-term stuttering treatment outcome in adult stutterers. *J Fluency Dis* 1995; 20:345–364.
25. Ladouceur R, Caron C, Caron G: Stuttering severity and treatment outcome. *J Behav Ther Exp Psych* 1989; 20:49–56.
26. Bandura A: Toward a unifying theory of behavior change. *Psych Rev* 1977; 1:191–215.
27. Manning W, Perkins D, Winn S, Cole D: Self-efficacy changes during treatment and maintenance for adult stutterers. Paper presented to the annual meeting of the American Speech-Language-Hearing Association, San Francisco, 1984.
28. Hillis JW: Ongoing assessment in the management of stuttering: A clinical perspective. *Am J Speech-Language Pathol* 1993; 2(1):24–37.
29. Blood G: POWER 2: Relapse management with adolescents who stutter. *Lang Speech Hear Serv Schools* 1995; 26:169–179.
30. Hillis J, Manning WH: Extraclinical generalization of speech fluency: A social cognitive approach. Presentation to the annual meeting of the American Speech-Language-Hearing Association, Seattle 1996.
31. Hillis J, Manning W: Dimensions of oral-verbal communication and respective categories, a proposal for items in a multidimensional self-efficacy scale. Presented to the 2nd World Congress on Fluency Disorders, San Francisco, 1997.
32. Watson JB: A comparison of stutterers and nonstutterers affective, cognitive, and behavioral self reports. *J Speech Hearing Res* 1988; 31:377–385.
33. Ingham RJ: Stuttering treatment efficacy: Paradigm dependent or independent? *J Fluency Dis* 1993; 18:133–145.
34. Prins D: Improvement and regression in stutterers following short-term intensive therapy. *J Speech Hearing Dis* 1970; 35:123–135.
35. Curlee R: Evaluating treatment efficacy for adults: Assessment of stuttering disability. *J Fluency Dis* 1993; 18:319–331.
36. Prochaska JO, DiClemente CC, Norcross JC: In search of how people change: applications to addictive behaviors. *Am Psychol* 1992; 47(9):1102–1114.
37. Yaruss JS. Describing the consequences of disorders: Stuttering and the ICIDH. *J Speech Lang Hear Res* 1997, (*in press*).
38. Culatta R, Goldberg SA: *Stuttering Therapy: An Integrated Approach to Theory and Practice*. Boston, Allyn and Bacon, 1995.

39. Max L, Caruso A: Contemporary techniques for establishing fluency in the treatment of adults who stutter. *Contemp Issue Commun Sci Dis* 1997; 24:45–52.
40. Van Riper C: *The Treatment of Stuttering*. Englewood Cliffs, Prentice-Hall, 1973.
41. Van Riper C: Modifying the Stuttering, in Starkweather CW (ed). *Therapy for Stutterers.* Memphis, TN, Stuttering Foundation of America, 1989.
42. Van Riper C, Erickson RL: *Speech Correction: An Introduction to Speech Pathology and Audiology* (9th ed). Needham Heights, Allyn & Bacon, 1996.
43. Van Riper C: Adult Stuttering Therapy. A series of eight videotapes produced at Western Michigan University, Kalamazoo, MI. Distributed by The Stuttering Foundation of America, 1977.
44. Manning W, Beachy T: Humor as a Variable in the Treatment of Fluency Disorders, in Starkweather CW, Peters HFM (eds): *Stuttering: Proceedings of the First World Congress on Fluency Disorders*. Munich: International Fluency Association, 1995.
45. St. Louis KO, Westbrook JB: The Effectiveness of Treatment for Stuttering, in Rustin L, Purser H, Rowley D (eds): *Progress in the Treatment of Fluency Disorders*. London, Taylor & Francis, 1987.
46. Perkins WH: Techniques for Establishing Fluency, in Perkins WH (ed.): *Stuttering Disorders*. New York, Thieme-Stratton, 1984.
47. Neilsen M, Andrews G: Intensive Fluency Training of Chronic Stutters, in Curlee RF (ed): *Stuttering and Related Disorders of Fluency*. New York, Thieme Medical Publishers, 1993.
48. Shames GH, Florence CL: *Stutter Free Speech: A Goal for Therapy*. Columbus, Merrill, 1980.
49. Boberg E, Kully D: The Comprehensive Stuttering Program, in Starkweather CW, Peters HFM (eds): *Stuttering: Proceedings of the First World Congress on Fluency Disorders*. Munich, International Fluency Association, 1995.
50. Prochaska JO, DiClemente CC: Toward a Comprehensive Model of Change, in Miller WR, Heather N (eds): *Treating Addictive Behaviors, Process of Change*. New York, Plenum, 1986.
51. Perkins WH: From Psychoanalysis to Discoordination, in Gregory HH (ed): *Controversies About Stuttering Therapy*. Baltimore, University Park Press, 1979.
52. Manning W, Thaxton D, Ells A: Listener response to stuttering versus modification techniques. Paper presented to the 2nd World Congress on Fluency Disorders, San Francisco, 1997.
53. Emerick L: Counseling adults who stutter: A cognitive approach. *Semin Speech Lang* 1988; 9(3):257–267.
54. Maxwell D: Cognitive and behavioral self-control strategies: Applications for the clinical management of adult stutterers. *J Fluency Dis* 1982; 7:403–432.
55. Manning WH: Making progress during and after treatment. *Semin Speech Lang* 1991; 12: 349–354.
56. Kuhr A, Rustin L: The maintenance of fluency after intensive inpatient therapy: Long-term follow-up. *J Fluency Dis* 1985; 10:229–236.
57. Silverman FH. Relapse Following Stuttering Therapy, in Lass NJ (ed): *Speech and Language, Advances in Basic Research and Practice*, vol. 5. New York, Academic Press, 1981.
58. Prins D: Models for treatment efficacy studies of adult stutterers. *J Fluency Dis*, 1993; 18: 333–349.

Stuttering and Related Disorders of Fluency, 2nd edition.
Edited by Richard F. Curlee, Ph.D.
Thieme Medical Publishers, Inc., New York © 1999.

10

Cognitive–Behavioral Treatment of Adults Who Stutter: The Process and the Art

MEGAN D. NEILSON

This account of treatment for adults who stutter is based on an intensive group program offered at St. Vincent's Hospital, Sydney, Australia between 1986 and 1995. With little change in framework but with increasing attention to cognitive aspects of therapy, the St. Vincent's Program[1,2] succeeded the Prince Henry Program,[3–6] which, in turn, derived from the experimental treatment regimes of Ingham and Andrews,[7,8] now part of the history of behavior therapy for stuttering.[4,9,10] Since the 1960s well over 1000 adults who stutter have participated in these programs. Some 35 publications document the experimental foundations, the management procedures, and the clinical outcomes, from the developmental beginnings of the treatment to its full-service delivery implementation. A previous account[2] of the St. Vincent's Program gives complete information on pretreatment clinical evaluation and case selection criteria, as well as a detailed description of day-to-day treatment procedures for a nonresidential intensive group format. The present chapter complements that report. It sets out an account of the processes underlying the cognitive–behavioral approach to treating stuttering and offers the clinician a guide to the effective implementation of these processes. It does not endeavor to give a complete account of the running of the program; that is already available in the client's treatment manual[1] and in the aforementioned procedural information for clinicians.[2] Rather, it attempts the less certain task of communicating something of the "art" of treatment, the tips and the traps that facilitate or hinder the treatment process, yet easily go undocumented.

Treatment Format

The following brief overview will orient those unfamiliar with the program. Intensive group treatment takes place over 3 consecutive weeks, and clients attend on a day-patient basis. It commences on a Sunday, with a half-day introductory session, then runs Monday through Friday, with weekends free. The first week of treatment is devoted to the instatement and shaping of fluency. Procedures involve instruction in the technique of smooth speech,[2] a derivative of prolonged speech, followed by group conversations, or rating sessions, in which clients practice and shape their fluency at gradually increasing speeds. These rating sessions also provide a forum for improving pragmatic aspects of communication. In addition, some sessions are videotaped so that clients progressively learn to appraise and enhance their fluency skills and interactional behavior. The group starts at 8:00 each morning and concludes when every client has attained a goal of stutter-free speech at a specified speaking rate. Normal speech rates are reached on Thursday evening. With a group of four clients, the median duration of these daily sessions the first week is 11 hours, with a range of 9–14 hours.

The second week of treatment focuses on the transfer of fluency skills to everyday environments beyond the clinic. Clients complete a graded set of assignments which require smooth speech to be practiced in real-life situations of increasing difficulty. They continue to refine and consolidate their fluency skills during morning and evening rating sessions and learn cognitive and behavioral coping strategies to be used when fluency becomes unstable. Again, there is an 8:00 am start, with days lasting a median of 10 hours, although those who complete their assignments on target leave earlier.

During the third week of treatment, clients generalize fluency skills to the specific circumstances dictated by each one's needs and life-styles. They also complete tasks that are challenging to normal speakers, such as giving a formal presentation to an unknown audience and speaking on call-in radio shows. Rating sessions emphasize melding smooth-speech skills into natural-sounding speech, while instruction focuses on cognitive and behavioral strategies for self-management during maintenance. An evening meeting with family and friends allows a group discussion of the changes that have occurred and any important concerns and expectations that group members and their families have about the future. By formally assessing fluency skill, attitudes, and locus of control early in week 3, it is possible to evaluate each client's risk of relapse and intervene accordingly with an individual remedial program for the remaining time in therapy. Treatment days during week 3 last a median of 9 hours.

Clients are expected to return for follow-up sessions 1, 2, 3, 6, and 12 months after treatment so that their speech can be assessed and discussed. These follow-up sessions run once a month and are open to all who have completed the program at any time. They provide a forum for clients at various stages in their maintenance program to interact, exchange experiences, report on progress, and seek advice.

Treatment Process

Cognitive behavior therapy (CBT) is used by clinical psychologists and psychiatrists to treat a range of disorders including depression, schizophrenia, anxiety disorders, eating disorders, and sexual and marital dysfunction. Controlled trials have shown that it can be an effective and permanent method of treating otherwise chronic and incapacitating disorders.[11] Unlike the traditional medical model, in which the patient is a passive recipient, CBT requires a client and clinician to collaborate. The clinician teaches, guides, and supports when necessary. This requires an understanding and empathic approach if the relationship is to be therapeutic. The key lies in the client becoming actively involved in the treatment process. In CBT, client and clinician take a trip together, with the client gradually acquiring self-mastery and assuming greater self-responsibility as the journey progresses.

The process underlying comprehensive CBT can be divided into four elements: education, skill acquisition, graded exposure, and cognitive restructuring. In the treatment of stuttering these elements do not correspond directly to discrete phases in a program. Rather, they are woven interdependently throughout the treatment period, as the following sections on each component show.

Education

The educational component of CBT for stuttering begins with discussions of the nature of the disorder. Clients learn that stuttering is understood to be a physical rather than a psychological disorder; however, psychological factors are very important in how one copes with the problem. Fluency instatement is prefaced by a discussion of stuttering in terms of a demands and capacities formulation,[12–15] with disfluency seen as the result of speech control processes not having sufficient neural resources to work efficiently under all circumstances. Conditions conducive to fluency are contrasted, in terms of their linguistic, motor, situational, and emotional demands, with conditions that provoke stuttering. This provides clients with a rationale for the slow, simplified speech pattern they are about to learn, as well as for the initially restricted circumstances in which they will use their fluency skills. Their comprehension of why the program is as it is not only enhances compliance, but also begins the essential, collaborative partnership between client and clinician. In CBT the educational component allows clients to undertake tasks and to introspect, not simply because the clinician tells them to do it, but because they have sufficient understanding for each step to make sense.

Education, woven throughout the program, introduces and facilitates the companion components of CBT. The clinician presents information so that it best provides a rationale for what the client is about to attempt, giving a framework for troubleshooting and realistic assessment of performance. Concepts are reiterated and elaborated as appropriate at various stages of the client's progress. For example, in acquiring fluency skills, the notion of demands and capacities initially explicates the need for slowing and simplifying but is useful subsequently as a framework for the rationale of graded exposure. In analyzing the effect of cognitive, behavioral, and affective variables in terms of their intrinsic and extrinsic demands, a client gains an appreciation of the principles that guide the sequence of his transfer tasks. He later uses this learning to construct his own task hierarchies in preparation for self-management. Likewise, the same knowledge is drawn on in cognitive restructuring; clients interpret a fluency failure not as a matter of bad luck or cause for personal denigration, but rather as a misjudgment of the attention and control necessary in that particular circumstance.

Clients are also educated about the role of anxiety in relation to stuttering as the prospect of transfer nears. The clinician discusses the unwarranted association of stuttering with trait anxiety as a consequence of inferred stereotype.[16] This is followed by discussions of state versus trait anxiety, the physiological effects of the flight/fight response, the Yerkes–Dodson relationship between anxiety and performance, and the principles of approach/avoidance.[11,17] The positive effects of normal anxiety are contrasted to the debilitating effects of excessive anxiety. Clients in need of anxiety management skills, such as relaxation training and hyperventilation control, are directed to these interventions prior to fluency treatment when possible,[2] so such regimens are not a routine part of the program. However, by gaining a realistic appreciation of how anxiety operates, even the most taciturn clients find that they have a useful background for understanding performance limits.

As clients move through transfer and approach maintenance, the clinician actively begins to educate them about self-management. Each client has to leave the program equipped with the principles of constructing his own ad hoc graded exposure, self-control, and self-reinforcement procedures. The family and friends evening, which is scheduled early in the third week of the program, gives a special opportunity to educate clients, together with their family, friends, and perhaps work associates, about the progress already made and the longer-term expectations of treatment. It is an occasion to show and discuss the pretreatment videos, which most clients have not yet seen, for two educational purposes. First, it allows the clinician to illustrate the specific behaviors that compromised each client's fluency. These are tagged as "danger signals" to be watched for in the future. Second, it validates the client's progress of the past 2 weeks and endorses the worth of the effort involved for both clients and family. Cognitively, many clients find it a confronting, but salutary, experience to compare their past and present ability to communicate, which often increases their incentive to prepare well for maintenance. The meeting also gives the clinician a chance to address some possible behavior changes and role changes that may cause concern to clients and their associates during the posttreatment adjustment period.

In discussing long-term expectations, the clinician stresses the fact that what has occurred is not a cure. The gathering is especially warned about the false security of a posttreatment fluency "honeymoon"[18] (p. 101) and the temptation to abandon controlled speech when spontaneous speech seems relatively reliable. It is useful here to inform the group about recent work in adult primates[19] suggesting that performance of a novel sensory–motor task can be accompanied by quite rapid reorganization of cerebral representations, but such reorganization occurs and persists only so long as the task is attended. This suggests that the use of controlled speech produces neural changes that facilitate fluency. It also suggests that these changes are not sustained if speech becomes entirely spontaneous. This gives clients a rationale for regular formal practice and an incentive to use smooth speech on an everyday basis. Three weeks is a very short time considering that a minimum of 10 years of deliberate practice has recently been considered as being more relevant than innate talent to the acquisition of expert performance.[20]

Those close to the client are usually keen to offer support in maintaining fluency and often want to know about how to react at times of difficulty or carelessness. It is wise to recommend a positive approach with encouragement, praise, or gentle reminders, rather than nagging or criticism. Most associates of clients take their own fluency for granted and need to be aware of the perseverance involved during maintenance. Moreover, due to the ubiquitous principle of power law learning,[21] gains will lessen progressively as a client approaches various performance asymptotes, even though his effort and application remain the same. External support and recognition are, therefore, welcome and desirable at that later stage, perhaps even more so than during the program, when clients' gains are large and obvious, and other reinforcement is plentiful.

While repeatedly stressing the importance of consistent daily use of the smooth-speech technique, clinicians need to urge clients and family members to be realistic about everyday variations in fluency. This involves discussion of the fluency variations observable in people who do not stutter, demonstrated by a videotape of a professional speaker who becomes markedly disfluent when placed unexpectedly in an unusually demanding circumstance. The aim is to have everyone realize that variation in fluency is normal and occurs in all speakers. The principle of capacities and demands applies alike to people who do and do not stutter, although their fluency baselines are different. At the same time, the clinician cautions about the distinction between short-term variation due to circumstance and a longer-term decline which signals lapse or relapse. When everyday variation is super-imposed on a downward trend, it is time for concern. Lapses need attention before they turn into relapses, and those close to a client can encourage remedial action, sooner rather than later, if they have been taught the importance of doing so.

Educational preparation for maintenance is reiterated and individualized for each client on the final day of the program. Each person's progress and achievements are reviewed, and an honest appraisal is given of strengths and vulnerabilities. It is important to provide a realistic view of the effort involved in controlled rather than spontaneous speech. Already clients will have experienced a lessening of that effort with the practice acquired during the program. Optimistically, they can expect further decreases but, considering the long-term anecdotal experience of graduates of this and other fluency management programs,[22] they should be prepared for the likelihood that such effort will never become negligible.

After 3 weeks of directing their energies predominantly to speech, clients often express concern about how they can manage to focus adequately on fluency while getting on with their usual responsibilities. This is the time when clinicians need to contrast the goal of totally stutter-free speech during the program with the goals that clients will choose for themselves in everyday life. The lesson is that treatment has not delivered a cure; rather, it has given a choice about fluency, a choice that clients did not previously have but which is now within their control.

Acquisition of Skills

Learning to produce fluent, natural-sounding speech is the main and most obvious focus of skill acquisition in CBT for stuttering. Clients are taught a technique known as "smooth speech"[2] which incorporates objectives common to many fluency establishment procedures.[23] The learning of the smooth-speech technique is predicated on a basic understanding of the respiratory, phonatory, and articulatory components of speech production. The clinician introduces anatomical models, diagrams, and analogies to emphasize the complexity of the central and peripheral processes that underlie speech and language functions and their vulnerability to disruption. This leads to a discussion of stuttering behaviors, focusing individually on each client's pattern of stuttering, which usually has been well exhibited by this point. Again using demonstration material, the clinician shows how repetitions and blocks depend on laryngeal and/or articulatory constriction and stresses the importance of air flow and the respiratory patterns that control this behavior. This leads naturally to teaching the smooth-speech technique, which is described to clients as a simplified form of speech that allows them to speak fluently within their lowered capacity for reliable speech motor control. The clinician explains this simplification as resulting from a lessening of articulatory precision as well as from the slow speaking rate initially used, linking it with sleepy or drunk speech patterns, which also reflect lowered capacity for speech motor control.

Smooth speech is a derivative of prolonged speech. It was refined gradually from its predecessor to sound sufficiently natural at normal speeds for naïve listeners to remain unaware that a speaker is using a "technique." The fundamental skills comprising smooth speech are rate control, breathing, easy phrase initiation, phrase continuity, gentle vocal onset/offset, soft articulatory contact, appropriate phrasing and pausing, and naturalness of prosody and presentation. Only the first four skills are taught at instatement, the remainder are introduced during fluency shaping, then refined during rating sessions. Procedures are fully detailed elsewhere[1,2] and are addressed here only selectively to illustrate the process of skill acquisition that is of primary interest.

Rating sessions consist of interactive conversations in which each client's speech is evaluated on-line by a clinician. Each client has a target speaking rate and must keep within a given range of that rate while generating a specified number of fluent syllables within a session's set time limit. Speech rate in syllables per minute (SPM), number of syllables generated, and the elapsed speaking time for each client are displayed throughout the session on computer monitors visible to both clients and clinician. During fluency shaping, the target number of fluent syllables corresponds to 7 min of speech at the target rate. Thus, for initial rating sessions at 50 SPM, each client must generate 350 syllables of speech without a stutter. For final rating sessions during fluency shaping, the target rate is 200 SPM, so each client must generate 1400 syllables of perfectly fluent speech.

The rules for progressing through these rating sessions[1,2] ensure a skill acquisition process that is overtly behavioral.[5] Three behavioral management procedures are used— differential response contingent stimulation, successive approximation, and conditioning of replacement behavior.[23] The schedule establishes smooth-speech skills at a very slow speed, after which the technique is shaped and consolidated at gradually increasing speeds. When a client's skill is insufficient to remain stutter-free, the procedure requires as much further practice at a given rate as is necessary to achieve the skill to stay fluent. Only then does the client progress to the next speed. Each day all clients begin with the same target rate but, as the day progresses, some may fall behind. The rating sessions allow each participant to speak at a different rate, with those who are speaking slower required to say fewer syllables in their allocated 7 min. Clients are positively reinforced for maintaining fluent conversational speech within specified rate limits with small monetary rewards and with being allowed to increase their rate in the next session. Stuttering results in an immediate loss of credit for fluent syllables already spoken, and no reward or progression to the next rate until a fluent session is achieved.

Notwithstanding this clearly behavioral orientation, clients are encouraged not to view a stutter as a failure, but rather as an indicator that their level of skill, or the degree to which they are applying that skill, is inadequate. Likewise, a repeated rating session is not looked on as a punishment but as an opportunity for clients to consolidate the technique at the current rate rather than moving up to a faster rate and becoming even more vulnerable to stuttering. The token reward system which operated in early programs[7] has long been abandoned, but clients earn small monetary payments on a schedule[1] which reinforces good performance and consistency.[5] The principal reward in the open-ended, nonresidential program, however, is the opportunity to leave for home close to schedule. Leaving the clinic is contingent on clients' achieving the required number of successful rating sessions that day; good skill means early departure, whereas fragile skill ensures a late stay.

The rating session procedure facilitates the shaping of fluency skills by successive approximation in several respects. Most obvious is the gradual increase in speaking rate, taking 4 days of intensive practice to reach the normal range. Because overall speech rate governs the timing of respiratory, phonatory, and articulatory events, slower rates allow more flexibility in timing. In smooth speech, slow rate is also associated with reduced precision of articulatory movement. Likewise, the amount of information communicated in one breath phrase may be limited to only two or three syllables. Concomitantly, the linguistic complexity of utterances produced under such circumstances is low. There is also a reduction of customary prosody. Thus, in all these aspects, motoric and linguistic, the task of conversational speech is simplified. From a demands and capacities perspective, slow smooth speech proceeds fluently, because it consumes fewer cognitive and behavioral processing resources and demand stays within the speaker's capacity. The path to skill acquisition, therefore, requires the client to juggle a number of successive and interacting approximations, in both linguistic and motor domains, which are reinforced selectively according to the resulting effects on fluency. As speed of speech production increases across rating sessions, the client has to make successive approximations toward normal, in terms of motor timing and syllables produced, but can vary motoric precision and linguistic complexity to stay within his performance limits. Viewed in this light, the sequence of rating sessions is akin to the extended length and complexity of utterance procedures used in the treatment of children.[24,25]

In addition to being trained in a new speech production skill, clients are also required to show that they have the corresponding perceptual skills to self-evaluate their performance. Twice-daily video sessions during fluency shaping call for gradually increasing scrutiny of smooth-speech skills. Initial sessions focus only on rate control, breathing, easy phrase initiation, and phrase continuity. Later sessions introduce assessment of gentle vocal onsets and offsets, soft articulatory contacts, appropriate phrasing and pausing, and naturalness of prosody and presentation. Video sessions require clients to evaluate these aspects of smooth-speech skill, first while speaking on camera, then after viewing the replay. A major emphasis is placed on self-assessment, but clients also practice their observational abilities by assessing each other's performance. Clients compare their evaluations with those of the clinician who gives detailed, correctional feedback on both their perception and production skills. Rewards are given for good judgment rather than for the quality of their speech performance. The ability to be objectively critical of their performance puts clients in a better position to troubleshoot and correct difficulties. This, in turn, fosters the cognitive strategy of reality-focused coping, which is discussed in a later section. Building clients' skill in performance appraisal continues throughout transfer using audio recordings of assignments. Additional video sessions may also be scheduled during transfer in which further work on naturalness, interactional style, or presentation techniques can be meshed with cognitive restructuring.

Skill acquisition during intensive group treatment for stuttering can also extend into social and pragmatic domains. Abilities such as maintaining a conversation, keeping listeners' interest, interrupting, dealing with interruptions, and being verbally assertive are sometimes lacking, despite new fluency. This is more often the case in adults who have stuttered severely and have had less opportunity to develop and practice these skills. In tandem with fluency shaping, the clinician can help to build competence and confidence in these areas. Normal group interactions often provide clients appropriate reinforcement, but the clinician should also model targeted behaviors and reward them with praise. Likewise, undesirable behaviors, such as lack of eye contact, can be punished by not rating the client's speech during such behaviors, which deprives the client of hard-earned syllables.

When proceeding from fluency shaping to transfer, clients are required to learn another skill which is associated more often with stuttering modification than with the fluency training approach which characterizes this program. In the process of learning smooth speech, a client becomes more aware of the physical concomitants of his disfluencies, which will help him later to acquire the "coping technique."[2] Coping speech is taught immediately before transfer and captures the essentials of classic Van Riperian preparatory sets and pull-outs.[26] Unlike some treatment programs which accept occasional stuttering during fluency instatement and transfer,[27,28] this program, like its experimental predecessor,[7] requires clients to achieve perfect fluency throughout intensive treatment. The rationale is that, even with some relaxation of standards during maintenance, a client is still likely to stay within normal fluency limits. Nevertheless, it recognizes the importance of equipping clients with skills and strategies to deal with fluency failures. Clients quickly appreciate the intrinsic relationship between fluency and coping techniques. As Perkins remarked long ago when rapprochement between fluency shaping and stuttering modification had barely begun, the procedures are not that different: "in a sense, [in fluency shaping] all we have done is to refine the controls used in preparatory set and pull-out techniques and move them far enough ahead of moments of stuttering that the anticipatory anxieties and 'stickiness' of impending stuttering tend not to arise."[18] (p. 108)

Graded Exposure

Graded exposure procedures in CBT for stuttering have the client apply his newly acquired speech skills in circumstances of increasing difficulty. This principle has underpinned transfer of fluency from the clinic to the wider environment in all behaviorally oriented programs. The client begins by testing his skills with simple communication tasks in situations which are familiar and nonthreatening and which have been conducive to fluency in the past. On achieving success, he moves to a task that is slightly more challenging, and this process continues through to speaking circumstances of greatest difficulty. For a person who stutters, the degree of difficulty of a speaking task is determined by the nature of the task and his past experience of fluency (or otherwise) in that situation. The nature of the task is defined by many variables, which can be categorized broadly in terms of the following: who? what? when? where? and for how long? The answers to these questions allow tasks to be sequenced hierarchically, in the order of their composite level of cognitive, behavioral, and affective demand for a typical client. For some clients, however, that sequence may be inappropriate. Clients with neurogenic stuttering, or with dyslexia, are ready examples, but most of the variation is determined by a client's past experience. This may impose very different demands during task performance, especially in the cognitive and affective domains, thereby altering the typical difficulty of the task substantially.

When the effects of past experience have led to fear and avoidance, graded exposure procedures in the treatment of stuttering are employed just as they are in the behavioral treatment of anxiety disorders, where they have a long history. Graded exposure was reported to have been the basis of self-administered treatment for fear of heights, noise, darkness, and blood injury by Goethe in the 1770s.[11] As summarized recently by Andrews and colleagues:

> Graded exposure is perhaps the most powerful technique assisting patients to overcome feared situations. The roots of these procedures are firmly based in learning theory and have also been known as "graduated extinction." In short, the procedures involve the gradual reexposure of the individual to the fear or anxiety evoking stimuli. On the basis of information supplied by the patient, the therapist devises a series of exposure tasks arranged hierarchically, so that engagement in those behaviors can be performed without overwhelming anxiety. Progress through the hierarchy is systematic, commencing with behaviors that are minimally anxiety provoking. Although similarities in form and mechanism may be noted with systematic desensitization (which primarily involves exposure in imagination), the procedures involved in graded exposure differ in two important ways. First, as much as possible of the exposure is conducted "in vivo" rather than in

imagination. Second, no competing response such as relaxation is taught, and no response is designed to replace the anxiety response when the individual is exposed to the fear-evoking stimuli. Each person has to learn for themselves that the anxiety is groundless.[11] (p. 19)

Stuttering is not an anxiety disorder, but clients who harbor fears about particular speech situations, with or without avoidance, benefit from the anxiety-reducing effects of carefully graded exposure. High anxiety can degrade smooth-speech skill, just as it does other sensory–motor behavior requiring control and concentration. In a demands and capacities formulation, anxiety decreases capacity by waylaying cognitive resources as well as possibly decreasing the efficiency of neural processing. As arousal lessens, the client has more resources to devote to the cognitive and behavioral demands of the circumstance at hand. When fear subsides to normal apprehension, graded exposure no longer serves primarily to increase a client's available processing resources. Instead, it provides the framework for a client to test his performance in circumstances of gradually increasing demand, just as it does for clients whose emotional arousal is not an issue.

Clients who have not been subject to fears and avoidance benefit from graded exposure principally because it allows them to consolidate their new skills under conditions in which the demand for cognitive, behavioral, and affective resources increases slowly. As consolidation progresses, smooth speech makes fewer behavioral demands on available resources, and performance can be maintained in circumstances where competition for available resources is higher. As demands increase, the client gradually gains experience in finding his current capacity limit for keeping his smooth-speech skill intact. If that limit is surpassed, the breakdown in skill may lead to stuttering. Alternatively, he may choose to decrease the precision and/or rate of speech. In this case his fluency skills need fewer resources, but the technique will be more obvious.

Thus, seen in terms of demands and capacities, the process of graded exposure is a logical continuation of the skill acquisition process during fluency shaping. In both circumstances clients have the opportunity to verify by experiment what they have learned in the educational component of the program. With appropriate grading of tasks, they learn to exercise their fluency skills in circumstances where cognitive, behavioral, and/or affective demands formerly exceeded their capacity to be fluent. Together, this interplay of education and experiment is the basis for the process of cognitive restructuring.

Although graded exposure is usually associated with the transfer phase of intensive treatment programs, in fact, it begins during fluency shaping. By judicious direction of discussion topics during rating sessions, the clinician can manipulate the cognitive and affective load under which clients exercise their fluency skills. Similarly in video sessions, the topic, preparation time, and formality of the recording situation, all can be varied to create situations of appropriate difficulty. In addition, these sessions allow the clinician to provide learning experiences about anticipatory anxiety, task avoidance, and procrastination. Most clients experience some stress in performing on camera, which can be graded at the clinician's discretion by manipulating the order of performance and amount of forewarning given to each client. Word avoidance can also be addressed in a graded way in both rating and video sessions, for example, by requiring clients to give their name or speak on topics involving feared sounds and words.

Homework assignments during the first week of intensive nonresidential treatment are the initial step in exposing clients to speech tasks beyond the clinic. The first task requires clients to audiotape and review 3 min of stutter-free speech in conversation with a family member or close friend. If a stutter occurs, the conversation must not be "edited," and the task is repeated until successful. If the length of the task is a problem, clients are instructed to record separate, shorter conversations which do not have to be redone if a stutter occurs in a subsequent segment. Thus, this assignment can be decomposed into manageable steps if the task is not attainable initially as a whole. This principle is used as needed to modify the standard assignments which clients attempt during the second week of treatment and which are described in detail elsewhere.[1] They are designed to provide clients practice across a range of common speech situations, the ease of which fluent speakers take for granted, but which people who stutter frequently find difficult, and sometimes fear or avoid. Assignments are presented in order of their increasing difficulty for most clients. If a particular assignment is likely to pose problems for a client, the order is renegotiated.

Clients are encouraged to generate their own hierarchical steps within each assignment. In the task calling for conversation with female strangers, for example, a young male client might choose to commence his attempts by speaking with a kindly, older woman and work gradually toward conversing with an attractive younger woman. If a task is especially problematic, the clinician may need to prescribe a simplified version of the task as a prelude to the full assignment. Thus, a client with a history of severe difficulty when talking on the telephone may speak first into a disconnected telephone during rating sessions; then move to dialing and listening to recorded information, such as the weather forecast; then to talking to the recording; then to telephoning a real person with a well-rehearsed, one-line inquiry not requiring further conversation.

During the third week of treatment most clients tackle four set assignments which are difficult even for some fluent speakers. They involve conversing with workplace superiors, introducing guests at a large gathering, giving a prepared speech to an unfamiliar audience, and speaking on call-in radio programs. Clients also construct a series of personal assignments, which can address areas in need of extra practice and greater exposure. Those clients who are performing confidently and well in all areas often use this opportunity to present themselves special personal challenges. Those who have encountered problems in moving through the standard assignments, however, use whatever time is necessary to complete those earlier tasks, before tackling more challenging, personal assignments.

All clients leave the program knowing how to design their own graded exposure hierarchy for new tasks and for difficulties that rearise during maintenance. Their experiences during the program are complemented with a final-week tutorial. They learn that the difficulty of a task can be modified in terms of who, what, when, where, and for how long; that the number of steps depends on the difficulty of the task; that each step should have a reasonable (say, 75%) chance of success; and that additional steps should be inserted if success is less certain.[11] When faced with a daunting task after treatment, clients know that it will become manageable over time if they persevere with a suitably constructed hierarchy.

During completion of transfer assignments, reinforcement is deliberately made more intermittent than during fluency shaping. As noted by Andrews and Feyer,[5] intermittent schedules are known to resist extinction and allow reinforcement of complex goals rather than details. Thus, there is no monetary reward for each successful assignment but rather, an overall financial incentive is given if all of the second-week tasks are completed within that week. Progress toward that goal is reinforced by a tally on a treatment room chart of each client's attempts at each assignment, both successful and unsuccessful. Clients who maintain an average of three successful assignments per day are allowed to leave for home early and skip the evening rating session, which is another meaningful incentive. In the third week, in preparation for maintenance, there are no financial rewards other than a group reward for completing the radio call-in assignment. Clients are encouraged to design their own self-reinforcement for personal assignments and continue this process after the program ends.

A final example of graded exposure, and one of importance to the process of cognitive restructuring, is application of the coping technique for forestalling or recovering from a stutter. Unlike smooth speech, which sounds natural if acquired well, the coping technique involves the use of obvious fluency techniques and is likely to draw attention. Clients are often reluctant to use coping speech; therefore, the program provides a sequence of graded-exposure experiences for clients to accustom themselves to reactions to coping speech and ultimately to reactions to simulated stuttering followed by coping speech recovery. They first use the technique in rating sessions, then with family, then with a "safe" stranger to whom they explain the reason for their use of coping speech. In subsequent assignments they use coping optionally but are encouraged to employ it whenever they feel fragility in their fluency. Lastly, after role-play with the clinician, they complete an assignment which consists of brief inquiries to passersby in the street. During each inquiry they simulate their characteristic pattern of stuttered speech, then "recover" using coping. This is typically the most difficult assignment for clients and also the most illuminating in terms of their cognitive change.

Cognitive Restructuring

If presented with a treatment which incorporates the above three CBT processes, the client stands to achieve the following fundamental gains. Via the educational process he learns that the core of his stuttering lies with a compromised speech control system which fails to support fluency when competing cognitive, behavioral, and/or affective demands prevail. Via the skill acquisition process he learns that this compromise need not result in fluency failure. Using smooth-speech technique he can optimize the efficiency of his limited resources for speech control and, if necessary, reduce the speed and precision of speech production in circumstances of high demand. Via the graded-exposure process he demonstrates to himself that his fluency skills are successful in a range of circumstances. Moreover, the experience of success helps to reduce previous fears, avoidances, and negative self-perceptions. In short, these three processes combine to provide the basis for positive cognitive change.

The predication of cognitive change on behavioral change is well recognized[29] and comes about through the resolution of cognitive dissonance.[30] Historically, behavioral programs relied on this as the sole means of reconstructing the maladaptive cognitions often associated with chronic stuttering. Attitude therapy, intrinsic to the rival stuttering modification approach, was seen as unnecessary. This view was seemingly endorsed by conclusions from a metanalysis of stuttering therapies which found that attitude modification made only a minor contribution to treatment outcome,[31] although those conclusions have not been without criticism.[8,32] Today the situation is different; treatment is characterized by a more integrated approach.[25,26,33] With increased attention to cognitive processes, programs like the one just described are more accurately characterized as cognitive–behavioral.

The transition began at the end of the 1970s when rapprochement first became evident[34,35] between the opposing camps of behaviorally-oriented fluency management and cognitively-oriented stuttering management.[36] There was concern that, after apparently effective treatment, many adults remained vulnerable to relapse[3] and this paved the way for a more eclectic approach. Starkweather, writing in 1984, put it thus:

> *Stuttering has two major components*: feelings that arise from the experiences of being a stutterer, and overt stuttering behaviors.... Both the feelings and the overt behavior must be treated. If only the feelings are treated, the client is likely to relapse because many of his original overt behaviors remain intact, even though they may be much reduced in severity. When they occur, the stutterer is likely to react to them all over again and become resensitized. Desensitization alone is not enough. Conversely, if only the overt behaviors are treated, there is another danger of relapse. If the fear of being disfluent is still present, normal disfluencies can provoke the old reactions of struggle and avoidance and the relearning of the old overt behaviors. Furthermore, if old fears are left intact, minor setbacks, that is, transient stuttering, can lead to a total breakdown of treatment effects.[37] (pp. 129–130)

Curlee, in the same volume, gave an influential account of cognitive restructuring techniques used in conjunction with behavioral intervention:

> I use counseling to supplement behavioral techniques for establishing, transferring, and maintaining fluency. This approach presumes that changes in stutterers' speech and cognitive systems may be important complementary factors in determining their long-term treatment outcomes. It is my impression that adjunctive counseling is most successful with stutterers who are inclined to be introspective and reflective regarding their thoughts and subjective experiences.[38] (p. 153)

Likewise, Howie and Andrews responded to the problem of relapse, drawing on findings[39–41] from adults treated at Prince Henry:

> ... in prolonged speech treatments, long-term prognosis may be poorer for clients who begin treatment with highly negative attitudes to speech[39] or with external locus of personal control.[40] Negative attitudes may not cause stuttering, but in some individuals, at least, the attitudinal consequences of stuttering may interfere with treatment.... If we can develop valid measures of attitude which predict outcome, then the clinician may be able to select for special attention any clients whose pre- or post-treatment attitudes put them at risk of relapse.[4] (p. 441)

Accordingly, the St. Vincent's program incorporates cognitive as well as behavioral intervention and includes branch procedures to potentiate cognitive restructuring in clients who are identified specifically as at risk. Techniques for active cognitive intervention stem from the work of Ellis[42,43] and Beck[44] but, as recounted by Andrews and colleagues,[11] the underlying premise goes back to the Greek philosopher Epictetus who asserted that we are not affected by events per se, but by our interpretation of those happenings. Cognitive methods, therefore, seek to change the way a client is influenced by events by changing their interpretation. In stuttering, as in other disorders,[11] behavioral change without cognitive change is likely to be short-lived.[45] Thus, throughout intensive treatment the clinician takes the opportunity, both formally and informally, to monitor each client's evolving thoughts and feelings and appraise their resilience or vulnerability to relapse.

Formal information comes from scores on a set of questionnaires: the S24 Modified Erickson Scale of communication attitudes[46]; an Australian derivative[47] of the Iowa Stutterer's Self-Ratings of Reactions to Speech Situations[48]; the Locus of Control of Behaviour Scale (LCB)[40]; the Eysenck Personality Inventory[49]; and the General Health Questionnaire (GHQ-12).[50] Clients also list 10 speaking situations, from easiest to hardest. This information is obtained at initial assessment and again immediately before treatment. At this time clients also complete the Defense Style Questionnaire.[51,52] Repeat measures of the S24 and the LCB are taken when the client has successfully completed the standard set of transfer assignments, at the end of treatment, and at selected times during maintenance. Additionally, if phobic behavior is suspected at any time, the Fear of Negative Evaluation Scale (FNE)[53] is administered.

At the outset of treatment, scores on the EPI familiarize the clinician with a client's likely level of arousal under stress, and those on the LCB, and DSQ point to probable ways that he will choose to cope. Derivative versions of these three scales have recently been used to establish a measure of personality vulnerability as an index of a person's resilience, or otherwise, in the face of stressful experience.[54] The three underlying constructs of this measure are compatible with an instructive model of anxiety which relates adversity, personality, arousal, coping, and symptoms.[11,55] Even though stuttering is not an anxiety disorder, the model is relevant to how people who stutter perceive themselves and deal with the threats that can lead to fears and avoidances.

The model sets out two basic coping mechanisms, reality-focused coping, assessed by the LCB, and emotion-focused coping, assessed by the DSQ. Reality-focused coping means "accurate and considered appraisal of the problem, rehearsal and then implementation of possible solutions, and finally, continual reassessment after any such attempts, much like the steps in structured problem solving."[11] (p. 8) In other words, a client who applies reality-focused coping is able to implement a practical solution to a threatening event and feels in control of the situation; i.e., the client has an internalized locus of control. This differs from emotion-focused coping used to maintain equanimity in the face of a threatening event. The DSQ taps mature, neurotic, and immature defense styles, which were originally shown to be important by Vaillant.[56] As summarized by Andrews and colleagues,[11] a client with mature defenses is able to acknowledge the nature and extent of the threat but is also able to limit the consequent anxiety directly. Humor is one such defense, recently discussed as an important aspect of cognitive intervention in stuttering.[33] In contrast, a client with neurotic defenses acknowledges that a threat has occurred, but distorts its personal meaning to limit anxiety. An example is the disfluent speaker who avoids a particular situation and attempts to convince himself (and perhaps others) that he has no need or desire to communicate in that circumstance. This differs from the client with immature defenses who lowers anxiety by distorting both the occurrence of the event and the salience of the threat[11]; daydreaming or acting out are common examples of such coping.

Reality-focused coping and emotion-focused coping with mature defenses are both desirable ways of lessening the arousing effects of stress and the consequent debilitating symptoms of anxiety. Neurotic and immature defenses also reduce symptoms, but in the process foster the development of fears, avoidances, and negative self-perceptions. Thus, the cognitive component of therapy seeks to move the client away from the latter defense styles by demonstrating the effectiveness of the former, more desirable ways of coping with adversity. By being alert to maladaptive ways that a client may use to cope with problems encountered during treatment, the experienced clinician can begin to facilitate change, even in the early stages of the treatment program.

During introductory sessions with a group it is both confronting and revealing for some clients to be part of a matter-of-fact discussion about stuttering. Openness and objectivity, in particular about a client's own disfluencies, is important and is encouraged in other programs.[25,26] By learning to perceive stuttering as an explicable consequence of competing demands, rather than a capricious signal of personal inadequacy, the client can begin to see himself differently. He also comes to see stuttering as something he does, rather than something that happens to him.[33,38] The clinician can encourage this realization by offering on-the-spot interpretations of the likely sources of fluency breaks that occur. As a client begins to acquire fluency skills, together with skill in troubleshooting problems with the smooth-speech technique, the clinician can actively encourage reality-focused coping. Individual feedback in video sessions is a good opportunity for this. The same applies to individual discussions of audiotaped transfer assignments, where the client must assess his performance before the clinician reviews the tape. The assessment sheet asks the client to delineate objective ways of overcoming problems he may have encountered in the assignment. The clinician can praise and encourage sensible suggestions or steer the client's focus toward more productive solutions. Explicit discussion of a client's increasing control, even when that control is still imperfect, helps foster feelings of self-achievement and self-responsibility.

With judicious guidance, rating session discussions can be used productively to tap group members' perceptions and attitudes and have them speak candidly about fears and avoidances. Again, other programs foster similar disclosure.[18,33] Early in fluency shaping it is necessary to keep discussion topics pedestrian and nonemotive, simply to allow maximum focus on skill acquisition. Gradual introduction of more complex topics allows clients to gauge the fragility of their skill, still within the clinic but with real-world connotations. Talking about oneself is sometimes a special challenge, but one which many groups progress to without encouragement from the clinician. General reminiscences can move on naturally to those involving stuttering, and the experiences revealed often are opportunities for reinterpretation and cognitive restructuring. Almost always this can be done within group discussions. Clients usually identify with another's maladaptive perceptions and feelings, if not share them, and resilient clients often communicate helpful strategies from their own experience. The clinician can note which matters are better explored individually and use this growing knowledge of each client to provide suitable cognitive challenges in transfer assignments. Rating sessions can also be a useful forum for discussing anticipated difficulties in assignments. Clients can be rehearsed in rational versus irrational thinking which can be followed through when debriefing clients about their ensuing difficulties or triumphs.

During the first 2 weeks of the program, the large behavioral changes ordinarily bring about the implicit cognitive changes previously discussed, so explicit cognitive restructuring proceeds largely on an ad hoc basis, interspersed wherever and whenever appropriate in the full schedule of tasks which all clients are expected to complete. In the third week, clients move to an individual program, planned according to each one's needs. This gives the clinician an opportunity to facilitate those cognitive changes that are lacking and reinforce those which have already occurred. Clinician and client collaborate in designing an individual's program, taking account of current fluency skills and retest scores on the S24 and the LCB. If the client has natural-sounding, stutter-free speech when speaking on the telephone to strangers, has normalized his speech attitudes, and has internalized his locus of control, he is considered to be on track for successful, long-term maintenance of fluency. The clinician encourages these clients to stretch their wings and deliberately challenge their fluency with ambitious personal assignments. By deliberately seeking difficulty, such clients maximize their opportunity for effective troubleshooting while free of ordinary responsibilities and while the guidance and support of the clinician and group are at hand. Active cognitive intervention is usually limited to interpreting and endorsing the changes that an on-track client has already made and reinforcing his self-responsibility.

Clients who still have residual stuttering, or whose fluency sounds unnatural, undertake extra rating session practice in their personal programs. This gives them additional opportunities for individual skill building and feedback. Such behavioral bolstering can be accompanied by cognitive probing which may reveal that the client is not comfortable or satisfied with his current level of skill and/or the attention required to maintain it. If so, the clinician needs to help him to develop rational expectations and consider the alternatives to his not persevering with skill consolidation. Concern about how others perceive his speech is frequently an issue. This may be a reasonable concern if his fluency depends on obvious use of technique or slower speed, and a rational approach again is appropriate. The clinician should always be honest and never try to cajole a client that his speech sounds fine if that is not true. The clinician should also acknowledge a client's right to reject a treatment technique he is unhappy with as a viable alternative to other solutions.

Clients who have not yet normalized their speech attitudes undertake a personal program that incorporates extra work on the standard transfer assignments, concentrating on those they previously completed with difficulty or found it necessary to limit the task in some way. This behavioral strategy ensures increased practice and greater exposure in areas where the client is less competent and/or resilient. If persisting negative self-perceptions stem from the client's accurate assessment of his current capabilities, these stand to normalize once full competence is achieved. Likewise, clients who have not yet enhanced their perceived sense of control undertake an individual self-management program like that described by Craig and Andrews.[41] The experience of carefully monitoring unwanted behavior and reducing it in achievable steps is extremely helpful in convincing clients that the seemingly unmanageable is manageable. In fact, sometimes this is demonstrated simply by the process of monitoring. But such additional behavioral intervention will not be sufficient for some. Negative self-perceptions can be profound in adults who have stuttered chronically for the majority of their lives. These perceptions are well-documented[17,26,38] and may respond only to active cognitive challenging. Similarly, clients who maintain an external locus of control may require parallel cognitive intervention in which maladaptive defenses are addressed and the power of reality-focused coping is endorsed.

Strategies for cognitive intervention in stuttering translate readily from those used in other disorders.[11] An important part of the armory lies in the clinician's ability to challenge irrational thinking and work with the client to develop rational thoughts to use when coping with difficulty. Webster and Poulos[17] provide excellent material on what they call ineffective and effective "self-talk," directed specifically at problems encountered by adults who stutter, however, in adapting the general techniques of cognitive therapy, it is wise to remember the following important point recognized by Curlee.[38] Unlike people with psychiatric disorders, where irrational thoughts lead to outright cognitive distortions, most adults who stutter, do not harbor unsound *beliefs*. Rather, their faulty thinking results in "assumptions that can be characterized as relatively arbitrary or extreme, or which reflect broad, absolute standards. [Therapy helps] them consider how such assumptions may function as self-fulfilling prophecies that contribute to their transfer problems and relapse."[38] (p. 155, 156) Curlee goes on to describe four common types of faulty thinking which the clinician may need to challenge. Some clients generalize isolated failures to the broad conclusion that "it doesn't work." Some exaggerate the significance of failure into catastrophe or of success into triumph. Some operate with a filter that screens out positive input leaving them with mostly negative perceptions. And some are so preoccupied with speech-related fears that they are unable to cope rationally and objectively, leaving them prone to misperceive or misinterpret events. Indeed, Curlee's account of this last category encapsulates perfectly the seesaw between reality-focused coping and emotion-focused coping, with the eventual development of cognitive distortion if the latter prevails.

In active cognitive restructuring clinician and client first must work cooperatively in the clinic to identify, challenge, and dispute maladaptive thoughts. The client is then encouraged to take every opportunity to apply these cognitive techniques when encountering problems in real-life situations. Specific cognitive experiments are often useful here. Once this process is underway successfully, the clinician can move to a more provocative role, raising the stakes by deliberately finding weaknesses in the client's belief system. Andrews and colleagues,[11] writing about this process in the treatment of phobic disorders, point out that for this process to be therapeutic, the client must come to the point of floundering. Then, rather than provide the client resolution, the clinician encourages the development of new understanding via a careful Socratic approach. If a client is handed the resolution, he may acquire the adaptive cognition, but if he is helped to discover it for himself, he gains the means to do likewise in the future. Challenging the client often requires the clinician to be resourceful, creative, and perceptive, always trying to judge the client's limits and pushing hard, but not too hard. As Manning says: "Challenging another person signifies that you take him seriously enough to respond when his choices are not in his best interests. It also indicates the clinician's belief in the client's potential."[33] (p. 194)

Expected Outcomes and Conclusions

Each client should leave intensive cognitive–behavioral treatment equipped with sufficient knowledge, richly illustrated by experience, to understand the cognitive, behavioral, and affective demands of a situation, balance these with an appropriate level of control to maintain fluency, and troubleshoot problems with realistic, objective strategies rather than with maladaptive defenses that feed old negative attitudes. In responding to an episode of disfluency the client needs to be able to say, not "I stuttered, I've failed, this is a disaster, and the like" but rather, "I know what led to my stuttering, it was reasonable under the circumstances, and I know the steps to take to reduce the likelihood of stuttering when I encounter that situation again."

Suggested Readings

Neilson M, Andrews G: Intensive Fluency Training of Chronic Stutterers, in Curlee R (ed): *Stuttering and Related Disorders of Fluency*. Current Therapy of Communication Disorders Series. New York, Thieme, 1992.
    This companion to the present chapter gives a detailed description of day-to-day treatment procedures for a nonresidential intensive group format. It also contains complete information on pretreatment clinical evaluation and case selection criteria.
Andrews G, Neilson M, Cassar M: Informing stutterers about treatment, in Rustin L, Purser H, Rowley D (eds): *Progress in the Treatment of Fluency Disorders*. Progress in Clinical Science Series. London, Taylor and Francis, 1987.
    A step-by-step account of the program in the form of a client treatment manual.

Andrews G, Craig A: Prediction of outcome after treatment for stuttering. *Br J Psychiatry* 1988; 153:236–240.

This study gives the background to the determination of individual program components in the third week of intensive treatment.

Andrews G, Crino R, Hunt C, et al.: *The Treatment of Anxiety Disorders: Clinician's Guide and Patient Manuals.* Cambridge, Cambridge University Press, 1994.

Guide to principles and practice of cognitive–behavioral treatment of anxiety, as implemented in the companion programs at St. Vincent's Hospital.

References

1. Andrews G, Neilson M, Cassar M.: Informing stutterers about treatment, in Rustin L, Purser H, Rowley D (eds): *Progress in the Treatment of Fluency Disorders.* Progress in Clinical Science Series. London, Taylor and Francis, 1987.
2. Neilson M, Andrews G: Intensive Fluency Training of Chronic Stutterers, in Curlee R (ed): *Stuttering and Related Disorders of Fluency.* Current Therapy of Communication Disorders Series. New York, Thieme, 1992.
3. Howie PM, Tanner S, Andrews G: Short and long term outcome in an intensive treatment program for adult stutterers. *J Speech Hear Disord* 1981; 46:104–109.
4. Howie P, Andrews G: Treatment of Adults: Managing Fluency, in Curlee RF, Perkins, WH (eds): *Nature and Treatment of Stuttering: New Directions.* San Diego, College-Hill Press, 1984.
5. Andrews G, Feyer A-M: Does behavior therapy still work when the experimenters depart: an analysis of a behavioral treatment program for stuttering. *Behav Mod* 1985; 9:443–457.
6. Craig A, Feyer A-M, Andrews G: An overview of a behavioural treatment for stuttering. *Austral Psychol* 1987; 22:53–62.
7. Ingham RJ, Andrews G: An analysis of a token economy in stuttering therapy. *J Appl Behav Anal* 1973; 6:219–229.
8. Ingham RJ, Andrews, G: Behavior therapy and stuttering: A review. *J Speech Hear Disord* 1973; 38:405–411.
9. Ingham RJ: *Stuttering and Behavior Therapy. Current Status and Experimental Foundations.* San Diego, College-Hill Press, 1984.
10. Siegel GM (ed): Richard R. Martin symposium on behavior modification and stuttering. *J Fluency Disord* 1993; 18:1–114.
11. Andrews G, Crino R, Hunt C, et al.: *The Treatment of Anxiety Disorders: Clinician's Guide and Patient Manuals.* Cambridge, Cambridge University Press, 1994.
12. Andrews G, Craig A, Feyer A-M, et al.: Stuttering: A review of research findings and theories circa 1982. *J Speech Hear Disord* 1983; 48:226–246.
13. Neilson MD, Neilson PD: Speech motor control and stuttering: A computational model of adaptive sensory-motor processing. *Speech Commun* 1987; 6:325–333.
14. Starkweather CW: *Fluency and Stuttering.* Englewood Cliffs, NJ, Prentice-Hall, 1987.
15. Adams MR: The demands and capacities model I: Theoretical elaborations. *J Fluency Disord* 1990; 15:135–141.
16. White PA, Collins SR: Stereotype formation by inference: A possible explanation for the 'stutterer' stereotype. *J Speech Hear Res* 1984; 27:567–570.
17. Webster WG, Poulos MG: *Facilitating Fluency: Transfer Strategies for Adult Stuttering Treatment Programs.* Tucson, AZ, Communication Skill Builders, 1989.
18. Perkins WH: From Psychoanalysis to Discoordination, in Gregory HH (ed): *Controversies about Stuttering Therapy.* Baltimore, University Park Press, 1979.
19. Merzenich MM, Jenkins WM: Cortical Representation of Learned Behaviors, in Andersen P, Hvalby Ø, Paulsen O, et al. (eds): *Memory Concepts—1993: Basic and Clinical Aspects* (Proceedings of the 7th Novo Nordisk Foundation Symposium, Copenhagen, Denmark, 28–30 June 1993). Amsterdam, Elsevier, 1993.
20. Ericsson KA, Krampe RT, Tesch-Römer C: The role of deliberate practice in the acquisition of expert performance. *Psych Rev* 1993; 100:363–406.
21. Newell A, Rosenbloom PS: Mechanisms of Skill Acquisition and the Law of Practice, in

Anderson JR (ed): *Cognitive Skills and Their Acquisition*. Hillsdale, NJ, Lawrence Erlbaum Associates, 1981.

22. Perkins WH, Fluency controls and automatic fluency. *Am J Speech-Lang Pathol* 1992; 1:9–10.
23. Curlee RF: The early history of the behavior modification of stuttering: from laboratory to clinic. *J Fluency Disord* 1993; 18:13–25.
24. Ryan B: *Programmed Therapy for Stuttering in Children and Adults*. Springfield, IL, Thomas, 1974.
25. Costello JM: Current Behavioral Treatments for Children, in Prins D, Ingham RJ (eds): *Treatment of Stuttering in Early Childhood: Methods and Issues*. San Diego, College-Hill Press, 1983.
26. Van Riper C: *The Treatment of Stuttering*. Englewood Cliffs, NJ, Prentice-Hall, 1973.
27. Boberg E, Kully D: *Comprehensive Stuttering Program*. San Diego, College-Hill Press, 1985.
28. Peters TJ, Guitar B: *Stuttering: An Integrated Approach to Its Nature and Treatment*. Baltimore, Williams & Wilkins, 1991.
29. Regan DT, Fazio RH: On the consistency between attitudes and behavior: Look to the method of attitude formation. *J Exp Soc Psychol* 1977; 13:28–45.
30. Festinger L: *A Theory of Cognitive Dissonance*. Stanford, CA, Stanford University Press, 1957.
31. Andrews G, Guitar B, Howie P: Meta-analysis of the effects of stuttering treatment. *J Speech Hear Disord* 1980; 45:287–307.
32. Sheehan J: Problems in the Evaluation of Progress and Outcome, in Perkins WH (ed): *Current Therapy of Communication Disorders: Stuttering Disorders*. San Diego, College-Hill Press, 1984.
33. Manning WH: *Clinical Decision Making in the Diagnosis and Treatment of Fluency Disorders*. Albany, NY, Delmar, 1996.
34. Boberg E (ed): *Maintenance of Fluency: Proceedings of the Banff Conference*. New York, Elsevier, 1981.
35. Gregory HH (ed): *Controversies about Stuttering Therapy*. Baltimore, University Park Press, 1979.
36. Curlee RF, Perkins WH: Preface, in Curlee RF, Perkins, WH (eds): *Nature and Treatment of Stuttering: New Directions*. San Diego, College-Hill Press, 1984.
37. Starkweather CW: A Multiprocess Behavioral Approach to Stuttering Therapy, in Perkins WH (ed): *Current Therapy of Communication Disorders: Stuttering Disorders*. San Diego, College-Hill Press, 1984.
38. Curlee RF: Counseling with Adults Who Stutter, in Perkins WH (ed): *Current Therapy of Communication Disorders: Stuttering Disorders*. San Diego, College-Hill Press, 1984.
39. Guitar B: Pretreatment factors associated with the outcome of stuttering therapy. *J Speech Hear Res* 1976; 19:590–600.
40. Craig A, Andrews G: The prediction and prevention of relapse in stuttering: The value of self-control techniques and locus of control measures. *Behav Mod* 1985; 9:427–442.
41. Craig A, Franklin J, Andrews G: A scale to measure locus of control of behaviour. *Br J Med Psychol* 1984; 57:173–180.
42. Ellis A: Outcome of employing three techniques of psychotherapy. *J Clin Psychol* 1957; 13:344–350.
43. Ellis A: *Reason and Emotion in Psychotherapy*. New York, Lyle Stuart, 1962.
44. Beck AT: *Cognitive Therapy and the Emotional Disorders*. New York, International Universities Press, 1976.
45. Andrews G, Craig A: Prediction of outcome after treatment for stuttering. *Br J Psychiatry* 1988; 153:236–240.
46. Andrews G, Cutler J: Stuttering therapy: The relation between changes in symptom level and attitudes. *J Speech Hear Res* 1974; 39:312–319.
47. Andrews G: Evaluation of the Benefits of Treatment, in Perkins WH (ed): *Current Therapy of Communication Disorders: Stuttering Disorders*. San Diego, College-Hill Press, 1984.
48. Johnson W, Darley FL, Spriestersbach DC: *Diagnostic Methods in Speech Pathology*. New York, Harper and Row, 1963.
49. Eysenck HJ, Eysenck SBG: *Manual of the Eysenck Personality Inventory*. London, University of London Press, 1964.
50. Goldberg DP: *The Detection of Psychiatric Illness by Questionnaire*. London, Oxford University Press, 1972.

51. Andrews G, Pollock C, Stewart G: The determination of defense style by questionnaire. *Arch Gen Psychiatry* 1989; 46:455–460.
52. Andrews G, Singh M, Bond M: The Defense Style Questionnaire. *J Nerv Ment Dis* 1993; 181:245–256.
53. Watson D, Friend R. Measurement of social-evaluative anxiety. *J Consult Clin Psychol* 1969; 33:448–457.
54. Andrews G, Page AC, Neilson MD: Sending your teenagers away: controlled stress decreases neurotic vulnerability. *Arch Gen Psychiatry* 1993; 50:585–589.
55. Andrews G: Anxiety, personality and anxiety disorders. *Int Rev Psychiatry* 1991; 3:293–302.
56. Vaillant G: Theoretical hierarchy of adaptive ego mechanisms. *Arch Gen Psychiatry* 1971; 24:107–118.

Stuttering and Related Disorders of Fluency, 2nd edition.
Edited by Richard F. Curlee, Ph.D.
Thieme Medical Publishers, Inc., New York © 1999.

11

Performance-Contingent Management of Stuttering in Adolescents and Adults

Roger J. Ingham

This chapter describes the procedures that are currently used in experimental therapy studies at the University of California, Santa Barbara. These therapy studies are designed to implement some of the critical elements of "prolonged speech" within group and, more recently, individualized therapy formats that utilize performance-contingent* schedules. These schedules, which are managed in conjunction with speech models, computer systems, and self-recording strategies, are also designed to aid the transfer and maintenance of within-clinic therapy gains. For the most part, the procedures that are described are end products of experimental treatments designed to improve the durability of gains from behaviorally oriented stuttering therapy procedures.[1] The therapy programs using these procedures have been conducted with both adult and adolescent clients.

These therapy programs follow the now-familiar establishment–transfer–maintenance format, a format that was developed originally from attempts to train speakers to achieve a new and durable stutter-free speech pattern via delayed-auditory-feedback-instated "prolonged speech." The goal of the establishment phase is to train the speaker to be able to produce stutter-free and natural-sounding speech within clinic settings. The goal of the transfer and maintenance phases is to train the speaker to produce stutter-free and natural-sounding speech in beyond-clinic settings; especially those settings that represent, as much as possible, a client's customary speaking environment. The transfer and maintenance phases incorporate self-managed schedules which have been developed, in part, from studies of individual therapy,[2,3] but primarily from therapy studies that involved intensive group programs conducted in residential settings[4] in which the establishment and transfer phases are completed over 9–28 days. Transfer procedures are introduced during the residential period of the program, then gradually blended with maintenance procedures. Thus, maintenance procedures are actually introduced prior to the cessation of a client's residential treatment period and continue, with scheduled decreases in frequency of contact

---

*The term "performance-contingent" is used here in preference to "response-contingent." Performance-contingent indicates that consequences have been arranged to occur contingent on the production of a target level of performance (e.g., 700 syllables that are stutter-free and spoken at a speech rate of 80–120 syllables per minute), rather than a particular response. It is the overall performance level that generates a consequence (i.e., progression to a next stage in the program), rather than any single response.

between client and clinician, over 2 or 3 years. In short, the aim of the maintenance phase is to decrease contact between client and clinician contingent on the client demonstrating normal-sounding speech that has been sustained in routine speaking situations. An integral feature of the entire treatment program is that it is embedded within a framework of audio recordings that are made routinely in clinic and nonclinic conditions. These recordings are used to obtain all performance measures and are scored by either the clinician or the client.

Current behavioral or cognitive–behavioral stuttering therapy programs appear to have at least four general, though not always compatible, objectives.[5] These objectives are supposed to be reflected in therapy benefits which are sustained across situations and over time:

1. to have the client use therapy-trained skills which continue to reduce or eliminate stuttering in the absence of formal therapy,
2. to have the client demonstrate that factors associated with therapy (e.g., situations and/ or people) are not necessary for the client to continue to evidence therapy benefits,
3. to have others regard the client as a normally fluent speaker, and
4. to have the client no longer "do things with his or her speech" to sound fluent.

A principal difficulty in characterizing most current therapy procedures is that it is far from clear how it can be determined which of those objectives has been, or will be, achieved. As a result, much of recent research has been as concerned with measurement of stuttering and its treatment to ensure that any clinical validity that these procedures may have is not compromised by inadequate measurement methodology. Unfortunately, present measurement methods do not appear to be sufficiently valid to determine which objective is reached by any procedure. Objective 1 may be demonstrated satisfactorily, but attainment of the others is more difficult to demonstrate. The two therapy programs that are described next were developed in an effort to fulfill objectives 2 through 4.

The current residential or intensive treatment program[4] is outlined first. This is a "core" program which has been used routinely and investigated in a number of treatment research studies. An experimental program, known as the Modifying Phonation Interval (MPI) program,[6] which was derived from the core program, is then outlined. It is an individualized and a less intensive therapy program which is suitable for use with customized software.

The Core Performance-Contingent Therapy Program

The core therapy program I employ emerged from a token economy therapy program that was developed some years ago.[7] That program now relies on what has been termed "hierarchy control"[4]; the token system is rarely used. The current program continues to be constructed around a stepwise hierarchy of generic speaking tasks, or stages, that must be completed at criterion levels of speech performance, in a prescribed number of trials, prior to progressing to another stage; otherwise the client must return to the tasks of the previous stage. Thus, the core program relies on a performance-contingent schedule, one that typifies many behaviorally oriented therapies; the difference in this case is that the schedule combines task and time-completion criteria in the maintenance phase.

Increasingly, it is recognized that the setting in which therapy is conducted may also provide some essential or necessary conditions for effective therapy. These conditions are probably crucial to ensuring a client's continued participation in a demanding therapy schedule. For instance, clients are seldom admitted to therapy unless the following contractual arrangement has been agreed upon: All treatment phases must be attempted and are changed only if the client continues to fail after four attempts at a hierarchy stage, and informal sampling of the client's speech must be permitted at any time throughout the course of therapy. (All recordings made are returned for the client's decision whether or not to erase them.) This is far less contentious than it may seem, because most clients, especially adults, appreciate that informed covert assessment may yield very different speech performance data from that collected overtly or at times known to the subject.[8,9] Finally, most clients are admitted to intensive therapy only after it has been determined that they have not responded to less intensive therapy for their disorder.

The Core Establishment Phase

The initial or establishment phase is the most intensive phase of the program. All speaking tasks are completed during rating sessions which are usually conducted once every hour (except for meal hours) during an 8- to 12-hour treatment day. The goal of this phase, which may take up to 9 days, is to train the client to complete a hierarchy of six successive speaking stages with zero stutterings, at specified speech rates and speech naturalness ratings. In the first three stages of the hierarchy, the client is required to be stutter-free throughout a schedule that requires gradual increments in speech rate; in the last three stages, speech rate targets are replaced by incremental changes in speech naturalness targets. If two successive attempts at the first step of a hierarchy stage are failed, the client returns to the beginning of the preceding step. Prolonged speech target characteristics are provided via tape-recorded models that the client and clinician practice between rating sessions. These target characteristics are now being replaced by phonation interval control using a computerized biofeedback procedures (see below). The current schedule, based on target models, is outlined in Tables 11-1a and 11-1b.

Table 11-1a.   Summary of Establishment
Phase Stages and Target Behaviors.

Stage	Target Range	Minimum Syllables
40*	20–60 SPM	300
70	50–90 SPM	500
100	80–120 SPM	700
NA**	As calculated	900
NB	As calculated	1100
NC	<3.0	1300

*An audio recording of the target speech pattern characteristics for stages 40, 70, and 100 is available for clients to use as a model. This recording should be used to practice the target speech pattern prior to each rating session.

**NA is the first stage in which speech naturalness ratings are used. These ratings are made for each minute of speaking time on the 1–9 rating scale where 1 = highly natural sounding speech and 9 = highly unnatural sounding speech. The target NA range is derived from NA ratings also made during stages 100/4-6 (see Table 11-1b). The average naturalness rating (per minute) for stages 100/4-6 is obtained first and is then used to calculate the target maximum rating per minute for stages NA and NB. For example, if the average naturalness rating per minute for stage 100 is 8, then there are 6 units between stage 100 and stage NC where the target value is 2. Thus the target rate for NA is 6 (or <7 per min) and for NB it is 4 (or <5 per min).

The client talks on most any topic during rating sessions while speech is rated in real time by a clinician using an electronic button-press counter.[10] Clinicians are trained to count syllables and stutterings on previously recorded samples of stutterers and nonstutterers. Their accuracy is then checked against a criterion test of unfamiliar stutterers' speech samples.[11] They are also trained to record speech naturalness ratings at 1-min intervals during rating sessions using the procedure described by Martin, Haroldson, and Triden.[12]

Table 11-1b. Establishment Phase Rating Sessions Schedule

Establishment Phase Schedule		
*Stage Attempted**	*Failed: Return to*	*Success: Progress to*
40/1	40/1	40/2
40/2	40/1	40/3
40/3	40/1	40/4
40/4	40/1	40/5
40/5	40/1	40/6
40/6	40/1	70/1
70/R	40/1	70/2
70/1	70/R	70/2
70/2	70/1	70/3
70/3	70/1	70/4
70/4	70/1	70/5
70/5	70/1	70/6
70/6	70/1	100/1
100/R	70/1	100/2
100/1	100/R	100/2
100/2	100/1	100/3
100/3	100/1	100/4
100/4	100/1	100/5
100/5	100/1	100/6
100/6	100/1	NA/1
NA/R	100/1	NA/2
NA/1	NA/R	NA/2
NA/2	NA/1	NA/3
NA/3	NA/1	NA/4
NA/4	NA/1	NA/5
NA/5	NA/1	NA/6
NA/6	NA/1	NB/1
NB/R	NA/1	NB/2
NB/1	NB/R	NB/2
NB/2	NB/1	NB/3
NB/3	NB/1	NB/4
NB/4	NB/1	NB/5
NB/5	NB/1	NB/6
NB/6	NB/1	NC/1
NC/R	NB/1	NC/2
NC/1	NC/R	NC/2
NC/2	NC/1	NC/3
NC/3	NC/1	NC/4
NC/4	NC/1	NC/5
NC/5	NC/1	NC/6
NC/6	NC/1	

Progression Schedule: *Progress* if no stuttering and syllables correct and rate correct. *Repeat* if no stuttering but syllables or rate incorrect. *Return* if any stuttering.

Between rating sessions, the client's speech is informally monitored by other clinicians; any stuttering observed during these intervals causes the client to repeat the preceding rating session. The client may then receive guidance or may choose self-directed practice speaking with or without the clinician.

When the establishment phase is completed, the client is expected to speak spontaneously and stutter-free in six consecutive rating sessions of 1300 syllables with mean ratings of less than 3 (per 60 sec) on the 9-point speech naturalness scale; this is also the target behavior for all subsequent therapy phases.

The Core Transfer Phase

The transfer procedures are logically connected to the format of the previously described establishment phase. The principal assumption underlying the design of these procedures is that, if target behavior can be consistently demonstrated in settings that constitute the client's routine speaking situations, then the target behavior has been transferred to those settings. Of course, the fact that the target behavior appears across speaking settings does not mean it is maintained consistently in those settings. That is the principal reason why most current transfer and maintenance procedures are necessarily integrated.

A feature of this program is the effort to ensure that each client is fully aware of the rationale for the program's structure and the purpose of each speaking task. I am also increasingly persuaded that the most powerful therapy effects might be linked to a client's judgment of self-efficacy[13]; that is, the client comes to recognize that normal-sounding speech is effectively and essentially achieved by self-managed practices. For this reason every effort is made to ensure that a client achieves the target behavior in the most personally relevant and routine speaking situations. I suspect that this feature is common to many current stuttering treatments, but one that is greatly in need of research to delineate its functional components.

The core transfer phase is built around a hierarchy of six to seven speaking tasks or stages. Clients nominate the order in which they will complete these stages, all of which involve self-formulated conversations. Each stage requires the client to make six 1300-syllable recordings that are stutter-free and yield mean speech naturalness ratings of less than 3 (speech naturalness is rated at 1-min intervals). A typical transfer phase might be as follows: 1. conversing with a male stranger in the institution; 2. conversing with a female stranger in the institution; 3. conversing on the telephone (we permit only two conversations with familiar persons and at least two must be calls received from strangers); 4. conversing with salespersons in a local shopping center; 5. conversing with family members; 6. conversing with peers at the client's workplace or school; and 7. making speeches before an unfamiliar audience. Recordings are made on a voice-activated microcassette recorder that is concealed during conversation with strangers. Throughout this phase, the clinician intermittently monitors the client covertly when possible; any observed stuttering means that the client must repeat that step in the hierarchy stage. By the end of the hierarchy, frequency of contact between the clinician and client is decreased to reduce as much as possible any contrast between the transfer and maintenance phases.

The Core Maintenance Phase

After completing the transfer phase during the residential period of therapy, the maintenance phase is initiated 1 week after the client leaves the institution. The maintenance procedure schedule is shown in Table 11-2. The client must obtain six recordings, each of 1300 syllables of conversational speech, on occasions that are systematically separated in time contingent on the client achieving the target behavior. These recordings are given to the clinician during scheduled visits to the clinic, at which time visual and auditory recordings are also made. It should be apparent from this table that the requirements for completing the maintenance phase hierarchy is more demanding than are the requirements in the establishment and transfer phases. For instance, the client may reach MP32(1) and still be returned to MP1(1) if stuttering or a departure from the target range of speech naturalness ratings is recorded.

Between-session monitoring of a client is conducted in several different ways. The most useful appears to be at least one unscheduled telephone conversation between each visit to the clinic. This is supplemented by "surprise" meetings arranged through the client's parents, teachers, or peers. If any stuttering is identified, the client is informed immediately and returned to MP1(1), the first step of the hierarchy.

Throughout the maintenance phase, the clinician is expected to tap relevant sources of information to estimate, informally, the client's beyond-clinic performance. Three sources of information are commonly used for this purpose: the office staff's contact with the client (usually through telephone conversations), the client's parents, and the client's peers or teachers. This information is used to determine whether additional recording procedures should be integrated with core maintenance phase assessments. For example, if parents have indicated that stuttering still occurs at home, then home conditions are specified as a task and the client must obtain at least two recordings in this setting for assessment at the next clinic session. This requirement continues until the target behaviors are achieved on the recordings and the sources report that stuttering has ceased. At each session, the client is also questioned, and if stuttering is reported, then the same procedure is followed.

The effectiveness of the maintenance phase schedule in sustaining durable improve-

Table 11-2. The Core Maintenance Procedure

Weeks Between Stages	Stage Attempted	Failed Criterion Performance* Return to	Passed with Criterion Performance* Proceed to
1	MP1(1)	MP1(1) R	MP1(2)
1	MP1(2)	MP1(1)	MP2(1)
2	MP2(1)	MP1(1)	MP2(2)
2	MP2(2)	MP1(1)	MP4(1)
4	MP4(1)	MP1(1)	MP4(2)
4	MP4(2)	MP1(1)	MP8(1)
8	MP8(1)	MP1(1)	MP8(2)
8	MP8(2)	MP1(1)	MP16(1)
16	MP16(1)	MP1(1)	MP16(2)
16	MP16(2)	MP1(1)	MP32(1)
32	MP32(1)	MP1(1)	MP32(2)
32	MP32(2)	MP1(1)	Finish

*Criterion Performance: Zero percent syllables stuttered and mean ratings <3 on the speech naturalness scale on three 1300-syllable conversations and three 1300-syllable telephone conversations. Four weeks on maintenance session week 1 results in cessation of maintenance stage schedule, because it is concluded that the client is not benefiting from the schedule, and it is necessary to introduce alternative procedures.

ments in speech performance was demonstrated in a group study that was conducted with nine subjects (9–56 years of age).[8] A modified version of this schedule, which was used with one subject, was also reported by the author.[2] This schedule has also been employed in recent treatment studies reported by Onslow and colleagues.[14,15]

Self-Managed Maintenance

Subsequently, I developed a self-managed variation of the performance-contingent schedule, which is based on self-evaluation training.[9] This variation in maintenance is introduced while clients are still in residence during the last three stages of the transfer phase. It requires them to estimate their speech performance during specified rating sessions in terms of stuttering frequency and speech naturalness (i.e., above, below, or at a mean rating of 3 on the naturalness scale). If the client's scores agree with the clinician's (within +1 unit on the naturalness scale), then the client's scores are used to score performance in the clinic. Intermittent checks ensure that agreement is maintained; if not, clinician–client agreement training is reintroduced. The client's transfer phase is not complete until six consecutive self-evaluation checks are passed, with the client's scores on the final six rating sessions meeting target behavior requirements.

When the residential portion of treatment is completed, the client returns to the clinic for a series of weekly sessions which form a further self-evaluation training phase. This phase precedes initiation of the maintenance schedule outlined in Table 11-2 and is used to verify that the client accurately evaluates relevant speech behaviors and is ready to begin self-managed maintenance. The procedure is summarized in Table 11-3.

It can be seen from this that a client obtains two 1300-syllable recordings in three conditions: telephoning, at home, and at work or school. Each sample is scored by the client before being checked by the clinician. When two consecutive weeks of recordings are matched (SEMI and SEM2), intermittent checks are made of some by the clinician (two of six per week). After six successive checks confirm that the client's recordings are accurate, the client scores all samples without these checks. The self-evaluation training phase is completed when the client scores two consecutive weeks of recordings (a total of 12 1300-syllable recordings), while achieving target behavior.

At this point, the client initiates the performance-contingent schedule shown in Table 11-2 and performs the same speech tasks, but moves through the hierarchy solely on the

Table 11-3.   Self-Evaluation Phase Schedule
Preceding Client-managed Core Maintenance Procedure

Weeks Between Stages	Stage Attempted	Failed, Retreat to Success, Progress to	Success, Progress to
1	SEMI	SEM1R	SEM2
1	SEM2	SEMI	SENT
1	SENT	SEMI	SEN2
1	SEN2	SEMI	SEN3
1	SEN3	SEMI	SEN4
1	SEN4	SEMI	MP1(1)

*At each stage the client must provide two 1300-syllable recordings in each of three conditions: telephoning, home, and work or school. In SEMI and SEM2, all six 1300-syllable assignment recordings must be scored by the client and must match the scores of the clinicians.

basis of self-recorded data. When MP4(1) is reached, or if MP(1) is failed on two con-secutive occasions, the client must return to the clinic. At MP4(1) the client brings the recordings of all the samples to the clinic, and the clinician randomly selects six samples. If any sample fails to match the client's ratings, which usually means departures from the target behavior, then the client begins self-evaluation training once more. These clinician verification checks are also carried out again at MP32(2). If the client fails two successive attempts at MP1(1) at any time after completing the self-evaluation phase, the clinician-controlled performance-contingent schedule is introduced.

This self-evaluation procedure has been effective with some adult clients,[8] but others have needed the clinician-controlled performance-contingent schedule.[2] Informal checks on clients using this system are conducted in exactly the same way as those in the clinician-controlled program: If a client stutters during any contact, he or she returns to the beginning of the self-evaluation phase. The most immediate advantage of this procedure is that it reduces the frequency of a client's contact with the clinician and, not unimportantly, the amount of management time. At present, I am reasonably confident that this method of managing maintenance procedures produces a faster rate of passage through this phase, which usually means the client's speech shows better evidence of maintained fluency.

Alternatives to the Core Transfer-Maintenance Procedures

Several alternatives have been developed to supplement the clinician-controlled performance-contingent schedule if MP1(1) is failed on successive occasions. They are introduced after careful investigation of the perceived difficulties reported by the client and significant others. Such difficulties, ordinarily, are of two types: difficulties in producing stutter-free speech regardless of circumstances or continuing evidence of situation-specific stuttering.

If the former difficulty is in evidence, then the client's speech is assessed during a criterion period following an instructional session. Usually, this session determines whether the client can sustain the target behaviors during 5 min each of oral reading, monologue, and conversation in the clinic. Then, increasingly complex-speaking conditions, as rated by the client, are introduced over two 8-hour treatment days. In effect, another hierarchy control schedule is instituted. Thereafter, the clinician-controlled performance-contingent schedule is reintroduced. To date, however, that has not been very successful. Two clients with whom this procedure was used have served only to identify either the inadequacy of the initial fluency-inducing treatment method or the situations that repeatedly produce stutterings.

In the case of situation-specific stuttering, alternative treatment procedures have been carefully constructed around the situation. The situation is analyzed until its critical features appear to be identified. The alternative procedures used are best described by examples. One of the more useful procedural principles is to pair fluency-associated conditions with a problem situation; for example, arranging for a clinician to enter the problem situation with the client, then systematically withdrawing the clinician's presence. This has been most effective with clients at home or using the telephone. Another alternative has been to role-play an event shortly before it occurs, such as speaking before a particular audience, which was effective with one client but failed with another. I have also used paired stimuli in certain situations, particularly the microrecorder (stimulus) used to record a client's speech. In the course of treatment, the recorder appears to achieve considerable stimulus control properties. Consequently, some clients have simply carried the recorder in some problematic speaking situations. The most useful techniques have been frequent telephone contact with the client or arranging to accompany the client during the problem-causing task. Both of these techniques are then systematically faded using variations of the core maintenance schedule.

For the most part, these treatment programs involve formalized data-recording procedures coupled with tight success criteria. These same procedures can be used with less formal data collection methods and more liberal criteria; however, my experience with less stringent variations is essentially vicarious. I could present examples of clinicians who have liberalized this procedure and reported poor outcome, but that would not be useful without examples from those who have used this approach successfully. For the most part, though, such examples serve to vindicate the continued use of a schedule with stringent performance criteria.

The Modifying Phonation Interval (MPI) Program

Currently I am investigating the use and effectiveness of a Modifying Phonation Interval (MPI) Stuttering Treatment Program which was developed by myself and colleagues[6] from a series of experiments on phonation interval modification and stuttering. These studies[16-18] demonstrated that adult and adolescents who stutter can learn to control the frequency of relatively short intervals of phonation (e.g., 10–150 or 10–200 msec) during spontaneous speaking tasks. More specifically, when the frequency of those phonation intervals (PIs) is reduced by at least 50%, stuttering is also reduced or eliminated, often without reducing the rate or naturalness of speech.

The MPI program is a computer-aided, biofeedback program that requires appropriate hardware and software. The hardware requires a Pentium series PC computer equipped with an A/D card plus an amplifier and oscilloscope (the full specifications for this system may be obtained on application to the author). The PIs are recorded from the surface of a speaker's throat via either an accelerometer or an electroglottograph. Software has been developed which records all PIs as well as clinician-judged stuttered intervals, syllables spoken per minute, and speech naturalness ratings. All PIs falling within a specified millisecond range are fedback in real time to the speaker via a computer terminal display or an audio signal. The speaker uses this PI feedback to learn to reduce the frequency of PIs in the target range which, in turn, is associated with reduced occurrences of stuttering.

The MPI Stuttering Treatment Schedule is divided into four phases: Preestablishment, Establishment, Transfer, and Maintenance. The Preestablishment phase is directed by the clinician. Subsequent phases are largely self-managed, but require intermittent performance verification by the clinician in charge of the program.

Preestablishment Phase

PURPOSE

The Preestablishment Phase includes *Beyond-clinic speaking tasks* and *Within-clinic speaking tasks*. The principal purpose of these tasks is to 1. collect base rate beyond- and within-clinic recordings of the client's speech performance and 2. identify the client's *Functional PI range.*

Beyond-clinic Speaking Tasks.   Each week clients are required to obtain at least two 15-min recordings of their speech in routine speaking conditions. These recordings include one recording of their conversing with a friend or relative, and one speaking on the telephone to a friend or relative. The same communication partner cannot be used for the conversation and telephone task. Additional speaking tasks in self-identified problematic speaking situations are selected by the client, but they can be integrated with the program only if the client can obtain weekly recordings in these situations.

The data are collected from 3-min recordings of the client's speaking time using the Stuttering Treatment Rating Recorder (STRR) program[10] which is set to record the following:

• Number of 5-sec stuttered intervals.
• Number of syllables spoken during stutter-free intervals.
• Speech naturalness ratings (of 1–9) every 30 sec.

The STRR program is then set with a pause interval of 1.3 sec and the accelerometer positioned to display maximum signal activation during voicing. Signal activation is recorded via an oscilloscope that is linked to the hardware. The details of the procedure for establishing satisfactory signal activation are contained in the full specifications for this system which, as previously stated, may be obtained on application to the author.

Within-clinic Speaking Tasks.   The purpose of within-clinic speaking tasks is to obtain base rate speech performance and PI frequency data. There are at least three once-a-week sessions in this phase. During each session, the client's speech performance is assessed during three 3-min periods each of oral reading, three 3-min monologues, and three 3-min telephone monologues. During these sessions the client's PIs are recorded via an accelerometer taped on the client's throat.

Data collected during these sessions consist of stuttering frequency (number of 5-sec intervals containing stuttering), syllables spoken per minute (during nonstuttered intervals), speech naturalness ratings (a 1–9 rating each 30 sec), and PI frequency.

Identifying the Functional PI Range.   A client's PI frequency is the number and duration of all PIs > 10 msec. Program software categorizes these PIs into selected duration ranges, which are ranked in order of PI durations to identify the duration ranges (in milliseconds) that contain each individual's percentage of PIs. A client's *Functional PI Range* is identified in two steps as follows:

Step 1. A software program (PISYS) retrieves the total distribution of PIs across the nine 3-min recordings for a particular speaking task (i.e., oral reading, monologue, or telephone) and ranks them from the shortest to the longest millisecond duration. The program then identifies the millisecond range that contains the lowest 20% of PIs, then the lowest 40%, etc., for each speaking task. A typical distribution might be a 10- to 60-msec range for the Lowest 20% of PIs, a 10- to 150-msec range for the Lowest 40%, and a 10- to 290-msec for the Lowest 60%, etc.

Step 2. The client's *Functional PI Range* is identified empirically with the assistance of a second customized software program (PITRG). Past research has suggested that clients who reduce the frequency of PIs in the Lowest 20% or Lowest 40% range over a number of 1- to 3-min trials, also show a reduction in stuttering. Hence, the initial PI range target is the Lowest 20% range. The PITRG software provides training to help the client achieve a 50% reduction in the PIs produced in the shortest quintile (or combined quintile) range identified in the Preestablishment Phase tasks. Thus, if a client produced an average of 16 PIs per minute in the Lowest 20% range, the target frequency would be eight or fewer PIs per minute.

The PITRG program provides real-time visual and auditory feedback of PIs that the client produces in the target PI range. If the target PI count is exceeded before 1 min has elapsed, then the program signals the client and restarts the training trial. The criterion for completing this phase is for a client not to exceed a target PI frequency for three, 1-min trials while showing at least a 90% reduction in stuttering. Stuttering should return when the target PI frequency is restored to the base rate level. This ABA sequence of trials is used to establish that modifying the target PI frequency does control the frequency of stuttering. If the criterion of a 50% reduction in the target PI frequency and a 90% reduction in stuttering frequency is not achieved, then the target PI range is shifted to the lower 40% range. To date, no subject has failed to achieve functional control over the lower 40% range.

Training PI control is achieved by carefully instructing clients how the PI feedback system operates and providing them oral reading practice. During practice, a client is instructed to pause immediately after each feedback signal and repeat the word in a way that does *not* produce the signal. Such practice proceeds until the client achieves the target frequency during a sequence of three 1-min trials.

Functional control of the PIs is demonstrated when the client 1. reduces the frequency of PIs in the target range by at least 50%, relative to base rate, which is accompanied by a cessation of stuttering, and 2. increases the target range PIs to the base rate level and stuttering increases to base rate level also.

When 1. and 2. are completed successfully, the client's *Functional PI Range* has been established, and the Establishment Phase of treatment begins.

Establishment Phase

PURPOSE

The purpose of this phase is to establish stutter-free, natural sounding speech within the clinic. This purpose is met by training a client to meet self-rated, clinician-verified speech performance criteria on a series of speaking tasks. Throughout this phase, the client speaks for 1–3 min while PIs are recorded via an accelerometer positioned to display maximum signal activation during voicing. The client records whether or not stuttering occurred and rates speech naturalness.

Speech Performance Criteria.   At the beginning of the Establishment Phase, the client is trained to make the following measures for each speaking task and must score all speaking tasks except those marked with an asterisk (*) in Appendix A. These tasks with an asterisk (*) must be scored as "passed" by the clinician. The minimal criteria for scoring a speech task as "passed" are

1.   reduced functional PI frequency $< 50\%$ base rate frequency,
2.   zero self-judged stuttering, and
3. < 3 self-judged naturalness ratings.

Speaking Tasks   Each speaking task is identified in the following way. The first task is labeled "1min/F/Read alone/1." This means that it is a 1-min task, with PI feedback (F) presented auditorially and visually, while reading aloud with nobody in the room, and is the first task.

When the client completes a speaking task step (i.e., ORAL READING, MONO-LOGUE, ETC) he or she chooses whether or not to proceed directly to the 3-min stage in the next task. These options are highlighted in bold print in Appendix A, which lists the schedule of speaking tasks that form the Establishment Phase.

Transfer Phase

PURPOSE

The purpose of this phase is to demonstrate that treatment gains achieved within the clinic (i.e., during the Establishment Phase) can be transferred to beyond-clinic speaking conditions. During this phase, the client is required to obtain recordings of both telephone and normal conversations while using the target behavior. The schedule of tasks followed is shown in Appendix B. These tasks with an asterisk (*) must scored as "passed" by the clinician.

Maintenance Phase

PURPOSE

The purpose of this phase is to demonstrate that treatment gains achieved during the Transfer Phase can be maintained. This phase is designed as a performance-contingent maintenance schedule. The effectiveness of this schedule has been demonstrated in two studies.[8,9] During this phase, the client completes the Transfer Speaking Tasks on the week dates shown in Appendix C. The 3-min Telephone Conversation, 3-min Conversation, and 3-min Self-selected tasks must be completed while meeting the speech performance criteria in order to pass to the next step in this phase. All tasks completed after week number 6 must be scored as "passed" by the clinician.

Some Additional Considerations

An overarching consideration when using these treatment programs is the continuing problem with stuttering event judgments. Like others, I am now increasingly concerned about the reliability of perceptual judgments of stuttering events, especially when such judgments form the basis for this type of treatment. It is obvious that clients and clinicians may vary greatly in the consistency with which they are able to make perceptual judgments of stuttering events. Despite the use of training tapes to improve the reliability of those judgments, it is an imperfect measure at best and is subject to the vagaries of judgments made under various circumstances. At worst, the measure may be completely misleading: It bypasses visual features when audio recordings are used, and does not address the problem of word avoidance. Our research has confirmed that groups of judges from different training institutions make very different event counts on both audio and on audiovisual samples of stutterers.[19,20] Similar findings by other researchers raise serious questions about the utility of clinic programs that are structured around this measure. It is, of course, entirely possible that, the programs described here will still produce satisfactory clinical changes, even when relying on this imperfect measure. At present, however, there are no obvious alternatives to frequency counts of stuttering events that are suitable for such treatment. Many clinical researchers are now devoting their energies to remedying this situation and searching for measurement procedures that are sufficiently reliable to provide valid accounts of therapy effects. The use of intervals of speech that are judged to be stuttered or nonstuttered is one option that colleagues and I are exploring.[21]

Assuming that stuttering event judgments still prove to be useful in a clinical context, some clinicians may rightly complain that the transfer and maintenance schedules I've described depend on questionable sources of information for determining the presence or absence of stuttering, speech rate, and speech naturalness. These data do not measure how natural a client feels or experiences speech. Recently, several colleagues and I have been investigating the use of clinically viable methods for assessing and training clients to judge how natural speech feels. These investigations[22] have been based upon findings that listeners or clinicians are able to use a 9-point scale to rate naturalness with exceptional reliability.[11] As a result, we have been working to develop procedures that will use this scale to measure how natural speech feels to the speaker and the use of this measure in a performance-contingent schedule. For the present, though, every endeavor is being focused on training clients to use measures of speech naturalness to measure and manage their therapy progress.[23]

There are other ways of assessing normalcy, including ratings made by relatives or associates of a client. The difficulty with such measures is the uncertainty of how to use them in the clinical process, other than describing the extent to which a client's speech may resemble normal speech. Ideally, the critical dimensions of normalcy would be incorporated in the performance-contingent schedule. Some clinicians believe it is possible to use ratings of breathiness, phrasing, gentle contact, and so forth, in the clinical process, but neither the reliability nor the functional value of such measures has yet been adequately demonstrated.

Some Final Comments

Finally, some mention should be made about follow-up assessments in the absence of a maintenance schedule. This still requires extensive research; however, it should be clear that by the time clients reach MP32(2) in a performance-contingent schedule, periodic checks of their fluency have been sustained over virtually 2 years. This evaluation process also includes informal and covert assessments that are used to verify that a client's improved speech is reasonably durable. If follow-up data reveal otherwise, revisions are made on the performance-contingent schedule.

At present, I am unable to identify critical factors associated with sustained fluency in the performance-contingent schedule. I know only that clients usually succeed in opening a number of gates, which provide entry to decreasing amounts of assessment. It may be that this extended period of fluency depends on the client's exploitation of speech tactics, which, of course, may not be sustained during follow-up. All that can be claimed is that a start has been made on devising a generalization technology that offers some promise of improving the transfer and maintenance of therapy benefits.[24] I hope it is a technology that will encourage other clinicians to investigate its efficacy.

Suggested Readings

Ingham RJ: The effects of self-evaluation training on maintenance and generalization during stuttering treatment. *J Speech Hear Disord* 1982; 47:271–280.
> This article describes an experimental investigation of the use of self-evaluation training for maintenance and generalization. The procedures can be applied in a conventional clinic setting.

Ingham RJ: Generalization and Maintenance of Treatment, in Curlee R, Perkins W (eds): *Nature and Treatment of New Directions*. San Diego, College-Hill Press, 1984.
> This chapter reviews and critically evaluates generalization and maintenance procedures in the treatment of children and adults who stutter.

Ingham RJ, Cordes AK: Self measurement and evaluating treatment efficacy, in Curlee R, Siegel G (eds): *Nature and Treatment of Stuttering: New Directions*. Boston, Allyn and Bacon, 1997. This chapter reviews the use of self-management procedures in the treatment of children and adults who stutter.

References

1. Ingham RJ: The experimental analysis and evolution of a stuttering therapy. *Semin Speech Lang* 1991; 12:336–348.
2. Ingham RJ: Evaluation and Maintenance in Stuttering Treatment: A Search for Ecstasy with Nothing but Agony, in Boberg E (ed): *Maintenance of Fluency*. New York, Elsevier, 1981.
3. Ingham RJ, Packman A: Treatment and generalization effects in an experimental treatment for a stutterer using contingency management and speech rate control. *J Speech Hear Dis* 1977; 42:394–407.
4. Ingham RJ: *A Residential Prolonged Speech Stuttering Therapy Manual*. Santa Barbara, University of California, Santa Barbara, 1987.
5. Ingham RJ: Current status of stuttering and behavior modification II: Principal issues and practices in stuttering therapy. *J Fluency Dis* 1993; 18:57–79.
6. Ingham RJ, Moglia R, Kilgo M: *Modifying Phonation Interval (MPI) Stuttering Treatment Program*, Santa Barbara, University of California, Santa Barbara, 1997.
7. Ingham RJ, Andrews G: Details of a token economy stuttering therapy programme for adults. *Aust J Human Commun Disord* 1973; 1:13–20.
8. Ingham RJ: Modification of maintenance and generalization during stuttering treatment. *J Speech Hear Res* 1980; 23:732–735.
9. Ingham RJ: The effects of self-evaluation training on maintenance and generalization during stuttering treatment. *J Speech Hear Disord* 1982; 47:271–280.
10. Fowler SC, Ingham RJ: *Stuttering Treatment Rating Recorder*. Santa Barbara, University of California, Santa Barbara, 1986.
11. Ingham JC, Ingham RJ: *Stuttering Measurement Training* (Video). Santa Barbara, University of California, Santa Barbara, 1987.
12. Martin RR, Haroldson SK, Triden KA: Stuttering and speech naturalness. *J Speech Hear Disord* 1984; 49:53–58.
13. Bandura A: Self-efficacy: Toward a unifying theory of behavioral change. *Psychol Rev* 1977; 84:191–215.
14. Lincoln M, Onslow M, Lewis C, Wilson L: A clinical trial of an operant treatment for school-age children who stutter. *Am J Speech-Lang Path* 1996; 5(2):73–85.
15. Onslow M, Costa L, Andrews C, Harrison E, Packman A: Speech outcomes of a prolonged-speech treatment for stuttering. *J Speech Hear Res* 1996; 39:734–749.
16. Gow ML, Ingham RJ: The effect of modifying electroglottograph identified intervals of phonation on stuttering. *J Speech Hear Dis* 1992; 35:495–511.
17. Ingham RJ, Devan D: Phonated and nonphonated interval modifications in the speech of stutterers. Paper read to Annual Convention of the American Speech-Language-Hearing Association, New Orleans, November 1987.
18. Ingham RJ, Montgomery J, Ulliana L: The effect of manipulating phonation duration on stuttering. *J Speech Hear Res* 1983; 26:579–587.
19. Cordes AK, Ingham RJ: Judgments of stuttered and nonstuttered intervals by recognized authorities in stuttering research. *J Speech Hear Res* 1995; 38:33–41.
20. Ingham RJ, Cordes AK: Identifying the authoritative judgments of stuttering: Comparisons of self-judgments and observer judgments. *J Speech Lang Hear Res* 1997; 40:581–594.
21. Cordes AK, Ingham RJ: Time-interval measurement of stuttering: Establishing and modifying judgment accuracy. *J Speech Hear Res* 1996; 39:298–310.
22. Ingham RJ, Ingham JC, Onslow M, Finn P: (1989). Stutterers' self-ratings of speech naturalness: Assessing effects and reliability. *J Speech Hear Res* 1989; 32:419–431.
23. Ingham RJ, Cordes AK: Self measurement and evaluating treatment efficacy, in Curlee R, Siegel G (eds): *Nature and Treatment of Stuttering: New Directions*. Boston, Allyn and Bacon, 1997.
24. Ingham RJ: Generalization and Maintenance of Treatment, in Curlee R, Perkins W (eds): *Nature and Treatment of Stuttering: New Directions*. San Diego, College-Hill Press, 1984.

Appendix A: MPI Establishment Phase Speaking Tasks

ORAL READING

Stage Attempted	Failed: Retreat to	Passed: Progress to
1min/F/Read alone/1	1min/F/Read alone/1	1min/F/Read alone/2
1min/F/Read alone/2	1min/F/Read alone/1	1min/F/Read alone/3
1min/F/Read alone/3	1min/F/Read alone/1	1min/NF/Read alone/1
1min/NF/Read alone/1	1min/NF/Read alone/1R	1min/NF/Read alone/2
1min/NF/Read alone/1R	1min/NF/Read alone/1	1min/NF/Read alone/2
1min/NF/Read alone/2	1min/NF/Read alone/1	1min/NF/Read alone/3
1min/NF/Read alone/3	1min/NF/Read alone/1	2min/F/Read alone/1
2min/F/Read alone/1	2min/F/Read alone/1R	2min/F/Read alone/2
2min/F/Read alone/1R	1min/NF/Read alone/1	2min/F/Read alone/2
2min/F/Read alone/2	2min/F/Read alone/1	2min/F/Read alone/3
2min/F/Read alone/3	2min/F/Read alone/1	2min/NF/Read alone/1
2min/NF/Read alone/1	2min/NF/Read alone/1R	2min/NF/Read alone/2
2min/NF/Read alone/1R	2min/F/Read alone/1	2min/NF/Read alone/2
2min/NF/Read alone/2	2min/NF/Read alone/1	2min/NF/Read alone/3
2min/NF/Read alone/3	2min/NF/Read alone/1	3min/F/Read alone/1
3min/F/Read alone/1	3min/F/Read alone/1R	3min/F/Read alone/2
3min/F/Read alone/1R	2min/NF/Read alone/1	3min/F/Read alone/2
3min/F/Read alone/2	3min/F/Read alone/1	3min/F/Read alone/3
3min/F/Read alone/3	3min/F/Read alone/1	3min/NF/Read alone/1
3min/NF/Read alone/1	3min/NF/Read alone/1R	3min/NF/Read alone/2
3min/NF/Read alone/1R	3min/F/Read alone/1	3min/NF/Read alone/2
3min/NF/Read alone/2	3min/NF/Read alone/1	3min/NF/Read alone/3
3min/NF/Read alone/3	3min/NF/Read alone/1	**3min/F/Read not alone/1**

1min/F/Read not alone/1
1min/F/Read not alone/1R
1min/F/Read not alone/2
1min/F/Read not alone/3
1min/NF/Read not alone/1
1min/NF/Read not alone/1R
1min/NF/Read not alone/2
1min/NF/Read not alone/3
2min/F/Read not alone/1
2min/F/Read not alone/1R
2min/F/Read not alone/2
2min/F/Read not alone/3
2min/NF/Read not alone/1
2min/NF/Read not alone/1R
2min/NF/Read not alone/2
2min/NF/Read not alone/3
3min/F/Read not alone/1
3min/F/Read not alone/2
3min/F/Read not alone/3
3min/NF/Read not alone/1
3min/NF/Read not alone/1R
3min/NF/Read not alone/2
3min/NF/Read not alone/3*

1min/F/Read not alone/1R
3min/F/Read alone/1
1min/F/Read not alone/1
1min/NF/Read not alone/1R
1min/NF/Read not alone/1
1min/NF/Read not alone/1R
1min/F/Read not alone/1
2min/NF/Read not alone/1
2min/NF/Read not alone/1R
2min/NF/Read not alone/1
1min/F/Read not alone/1R
2min/NF/Read not alone/1
2min/NF/Read not alone/1
2min/F/Read not alone/1R
2min/F/Read not alone/1
3min/F/Read not alone/1
3min/F/Read not alone/1
2min/NF/Read not alone/1R
3min/NF/Read not alone/1
3min/F/Read not alone/1
3min/NF/Read not alone/1
3min/NF/Read not alone/1R
3min/NF/Read not alone/2
3min/NF/Read not alone/1

1min/F/Read not alone/2
1min/F/Read not alone/2
1min/F/Read not alone/3
1min/F/Read not alone/1
1min/NF/Read not alone/1R
1min/NF/Read not alone/2
1min/NF/Read not alone/3
2min/F/Read not alone/1
2min/F/Read not alone/1R
2min/F/Read not alone/2
2min/F/Read not alone/3
2min/NF/Read not alone/1
2min/NF/Read not alone/2
2min/NF/Read not alone/1R
2min/NF/Read not alone/2
3min/F/Read not alone/1
3min/F/Read not alone/2
3min/F/Read not alone/3
3min/NF/Read not alone/1
3min/NF/Read not alone/2
3min/NF/Read not alone/1R
3min/NF/Read not alone/2
3min/NF/Read not alone/3
3min/F/Monologue alone/1

MONOLOGUE

Stage Attempted	Failed: Retreat to	Passed: Progress to
1min/F/Monologue alone/1	1min/F/Monologue alone/1R	1min/F/Monologue alone/2
1min/F/Monologue alone/1R	**3min/F/Read not alone/1**	1min/F/Monologue alone/2
1min/F/Monologue alone/2	1min/F/Monologue alone/1	1min/F/Monologue alone/3
1min/F/Monologue alone/3	1min/F/Monologue alone/1	1min/NF/Monologue alone/1
1min/NF/Monologue alone/1	1min/NF/Monologue alone/1R	1min/NF/Monologue alone/2
1min/NF/Monologue alone/1R	1min/NF/Monologue alone/1	1min/NF/Monologue alone/2
1min/NF/Monologue alone/2	1min/NF/Monologue alone/1	1min/NF/Monologue alone/3
1min/NF/Monologue alone/3	1min/NF/Monologue alone/1	2min/F/Monologue alone/1
2min/F/Monologue alone/1	2min/F/Monologue alone/1R	2min/F/Monologue alone/2
2min/F/Monologue alone/1R	2min/F/Monologue alone/1	2min/F/Monologue alone/2
2min/F/Monologue alone/2	2min/F/Monologue alone/1	2min/F/Monologue alone/3
2min/F/Monologue alone/3	2min/F/Monologue alone/1	2min/NF/Monologue alone/1
2min/NF/Monologue alone/1	2min/NF/Monologue alone/1R	2min/NF/Monologue alone/2
2min/NF/Monologue alone/1R	2min/NF/Monologue alone/1	2min/NF/Monologue alone/2
2min/NF/Monologue alone/2	2min/NF/Monologue alone/1	2min/NF/Monologue alone/3
2min/NF/Monologue alone/3	2min/NF/Monologue alone/1	3min/F/Monologue alone/1
3min/F/Monologue alone/1	3min/F/Monologue alone/1R	3min/F/Monologue alone/2
3min/F/Monologue alone/1R	3min/F/Monologue alone/1	3min/F/Monologue alone/2
3min/F/Monologue alone/2	3min/F/Monologue alone/1	3min/F/Monologue alone/3
3min/F/Monologue alone/3	3min/F/Monologue alone/1	3min/NF/Monologue alone/1
3min/NF/Monologue alone/1	3min/NF/Monologue alone/1R	3min/NF/Monologue alone/2
3min/NF/Monologue alone/1R	3min/NF/Monologue alone/1	3min/NF/Monologue alone/2
3min/NF/Monologue alone/2	3min/NF/Monologue alone/1	3min/NF/Monologue alone/3
3min/NF/Monologue alone/3*	3min/NF/Monologue alone/1	**3min/F/Monologue not alone/1**

1min/F/Monologue not alone/1
1min/F/Monologue not alone/1R
1min/F/Monologue not alone/2
1min/F/Monologue not alone/3
1min/NF/Monologue not alone/1
1min/NF/Monologue not alone/1R
1min/NF/Monologue not alone/2
1min/NF/Monologue not alone/3
2min/F/Monologue not alone/1
2min/F/Monologue not alone/1R
2min/F/Monologue not alone/2
2min/F/Monologue not alone/3
2min/NF/Monologue not alone/1
2min/NF/Monologue not alone/1R
2min/NF/Monologue not alone/2
2min/NF/Monologue not alone/3
3min/F/Monologue not alone/1
3min/F/Monologue not alone/1R
3min/F/Monologue not alone/2
3min/F/Monologue not alone/3
3min/NF/Monologue not alone/1
3min/NF/Monologue not alone/1R
3min/NF/Monologue not alone/2
3min/NF/Monologue not alone/3*

1min/F/Monologue not alone/1R
3min/F/Monologue alone/1
1min/F/Monologue not alone/1
1min/F/Monologue not alone/1
1min/NF/Monologue not alone/1
1min/NF/Monologue not alone/1R
1min/NF/Monologue not alone/1
2min/F/Monologue not alone/1
2min/F/Monologue not alone/1
2min/F/Monologue not alone/1R
2min/NF/Monologue not alone/1
2min/NF/Monologue not alone/1
2min/NF/Monologue not alone/1
3min/F/Monologue not alone/1
3min/F/Monologue not alone/1R
3min/NF/Monologue not alone/1
3min/NF/Monologue not alone/1
3min/F/Monologue not alone/1
3min/F/Monologue not alone/1
3min/F/Monologue not alone/1R
3min/F/Monologue not alone/1
3min/NF/Monologue not alone/1
3min/NF/Monologue not alone/1
3min/NF/Monologue not alone/1
3min/NF/Conversation/1

1min/F/Monologue not alone/2
1min/F/Monologue not alone/2
1min/F/Monologue not alone/3
1min/NF/Monologue not alone/1
1min/NF/Monologue not alone/2
1min/F/Monologue not alone/3
2min/F/Monologue not alone/1
2min/F/Monologue not alone/2
2min/F/Monologue not alone/3
2min/NF/Monologue not alone/1
2min/NF/Monologue not alone/2
2min/NF/Monologue not alone/3
2min/F/Monologue not alone/1
2min/F/Monologue not alone/2
2min/F/Monologue not alone/3
3min/F/Monologue not alone/1
3min/F/Monologue not alone/2
3min/F/Monologue not alone/3
3min/NF/Monologue not alone/1
3min/NF/Monologue not alone/2
3min/NF/Monologue not alone/1
3min/NF/Monologue not alone/2
3min/NF/Monologue not alone/3

CONVERSATION

Stage attempted	Failed: Retreat to	Passed: Progress to
1min/NF/Conversation/1	1min/NF/Conversation/1R	1min/NF/Conversation/2
1min/NF/Conversation/1R	**3min/F/Monologue not alone/1**	1min/NF/Conversation/2
1min/NF/Conversation/2	1min/NF/Conversation/1	1min/NF/Conversation/3
1min/NF/Conversation/3	2min/NF/Conversation/1	2min/NF/Conversation/1
2min/NF/Conversation/1	1min/NF/Conversation/1R	2min/NF/Conversation/2
2min/NF/Conversation/1R	2min/NF/Conversation/1	2min/NF/Conversation/2
2min/NF/Conversation/2	2min/NF/Conversation/1	2min/NF/Conversation/3
2min/NF/Conversation/3	2min/NF/Conversation/1	3min/NF/Conversation/1
3min/NF/Conversation/1	3min/NF/Conversation/1R	3min/NF/Conversation/1
3min/NF/Conversation/1R	3min/NF/Conversation/1	3min/NF/Conversation/2
3min/NF/Conversation/2	3min/NF/Conversation/1	3min/NF/Conversation/3
3min/NF/Conversation/3*	3min/NF/Conversation/1	**3min/F/Telephone monologue/1**

TELEPHONE MONOLOGUE

Stage attempted	Failed: Retreat to	Passed: Progress to
1min/F/Telephone monologue/1	1min/F/Telephone monologue/1R	1min/F/Telephone monologue/2
1min/F/Telephone monologue/1R	3min/F/Conversation/1	1min/F/Telephone monologue/2
1min/F/Telephone monologue/2	1min/F/Telephone monologue/1	1min/F/Telephone monologue/3
1min/F/Telephone monologue/3	1min/F/Telephone monologue/1	1min/NF/Telephone monologue/1
1min/NF/Telephone monologue/1	1min/F/Telephone monologue/1	1min/NF/Telephone monologue/2
1min/NF/Telephone monologue/1R	1min/NF/Telephone monologue/1R	1min/NF/Telephone monologue/2
1min/NF/Telephone monologue/2	1min/F/Telephone monologue/1	1min/NF/Telephone monologue/3
1min/NF/Telephone monologue/3	1min/NF/Telephone monologue/1	2min/F/Telephone monologue/1
2min/F/Telephone monologue/1	1min/NF/Telephone monologue/1	2min/F/Telephone monologue/2
2min/F/Telephone monologue/2	2min/NF/Telephone monologue/1R	2min/F/Telephone monologue/2
2min/F/Telephone monologue/3	1min/NF/Telephone monologue/1	2min/F/Telephone monologue/3
2min/F/Telephone monologue/1R	1min/NF/Telephone monologue/1	2min/NF/Telephone monologue/2
2min/F/Telephone monologue/2	2min/F/Telephone monologue/1	2min/NF/Telephone monologue/3

Telephone monologue (continued)

Stage Attempted	Failed: Retreat to	Passed: Progress to
2min/F/Telephone monologue/3	2min/F/Telephone monologue/1	2min/NF/Telephone monologue/1
2min/NF/Telephone monologue/1	2min/NF/Telephone monologue/1R	2min/NF/Telephone monologue/2
2min/NF/Telephone monologue/1R	2min/F/Telephone monologue/2	2min/NF/Telephone monologue/2
2min/NF/Telephone monologue/2	2min/NF/Telephone monologue/1	2min/NF/Telephone monologue/3
2min/NF/Telephone monologue/3	2min/NF/Telephone monologue/1	3min/F/Telephone monologue/1
3min/F/Telephone monologue/1	3min/F/Telephone monologue/1R	3min/F/Telephone monologue/2
3min/F/Telephone monologue/1R	3min/F/Telephone monologue/1	3min/F/Telephone monologue/2
3min/F/Telephone monologue/2	3min/F/Telephone monologue/1	3min/F/Telephone monologue/3
3min/F/Telephone monologue/3	3min/F/Telephone monologue/1	3min/NF/Telephone monologue/1
3min/NF/Telephone monologue/1	3min/NF/Telephone monologue/1	3min/NF/Telephone monologue/2
3min/NF/Telephone monologue/1R	3min/NF/Telephone monologue/1R	3min/NF/Telephone monologue/2
3min/NF/Telephone monologue/2	3min/NF/Telephone monologue/1	3min/NF/Telephone monologue/1
3min/NF/Telephone monologue/3	3min/NF/Telephone monologue/1	**3min/NF/Telephone conversation/1**
3min/NF/Telephone monologue/3*	3min/NF/Telephone monologue/1	

TELEPHONE CONVERSATION

Stage Attempted	Failed: Retreat to	Passed: Progress to
1min/NF/Telephone conversation/1	1min/NF/Telephone conversation/1R	1min/NF/Telephone conversation/2
1min/NF/Telephone conversation/1R	**3min/F/Telephone monologue/1**	1min/NF/Telephone conversation/2
1min/NF/Telephone conversation/2	1min/NF/Telephone conversation/1	1min/NF/Telephone conversation/3
1min/NF/Telephone conversation/3	1min/NF/Telephone conversation/1	2min/NF/Telephone conversation/1
2min/NF/Telephone conversation/1	1min/NF/Telephone conversation/1R	2min/NF/Telephone conversation/2
2min/NF/Telephone conversation/1R	2min/NF/Telephone conversation/1	2min/NF/Telephone conversation/2
2min/NF/Telephone conversation/2	2min/NF/Telephone conversation/1	2min/NF/Telephone conversation/3
2min/NF/Telephone conversation/3	2min/NF/Telephone conversation/1	3min/NF/Telephone conversation/1
3min/NF/Telephone conversation/1	3min/NF/Telephone conversation/1R	3min/NF/Telephone conversation/2
3min/NF/Telephone conversation/1R	3min/NF/Telephone conversation/1	3min/NF/Telephone conversation/2
3min/NF/Telephone conversation/2	3min/NF/Telephone conversation/1	3min/NF/Telephone conversation/3
3min/NF/Telephone conversation/3*	3min/NF/Telephone conversation/1	TRANSFER

Appendix B: MPI Transfer Phase Speaking Tasks

Stage Attempted	Failed: Retreat to	Passed: Progress to
3min/Telephone conversation/1	3min/Telephone conversation/1R	3min/Telephone conversation/2
3min/Telephone conversation/1R	3min/NF/Telephone conversation/1 (Est)	3min/Telephone conversation/2
3min/Telephone conversation/2	3min/Telephone conversation/1	3min/Telephone conversation/3
3min/Telephone conversation/3*	3min/Telephone conversation/1	**3min/Conversation/1**
3min/Conversation/1	3min/Conversation/1R	3min/Conversation/2
3min/Conversation/1R	3min/Conversation/1	3min/Conversation/2
3min/Conversation/2	3min/Conversation/1	3min/Conversation/3
3min/Conversation/3*	3min/Conversation/1	**3min/Self-selected task/1**
3min/Self-selected task/1	3min/Self-selected task/1R	3min/Self-selected task/2
3min/Self-selected task/1R	3min/Self-selected task/1	3min/Self-selected task/2
3min/Self-selected task/2	3min/Self-selected task/1	3min/Self-selected task/3
3min/Self selected task/3*	3min/Self selected task/1	**Maintenance 1**

Appendix C: MPI Maintenance Phase Speaking Task Schedule

Maintenance Session Week Number: Week for Completing Speech Tasks	Failed Criterion Speech Performance: Complete Next Speech Tasks on Week Number	Passed with Criterion Speech Performance: Complete Next Speech Tasks on Week Number
1	1R	2
1R	**3min/NF/Self selected task/1**	
2	1	4
4	1	6
6	1	10
10	1	14
14	1	22
22	1	30
30	1	46
46	1	62
62	1	Completed program

Stuttering and Related Disorders of Fluency, 2nd edition.
Edited by Richard F. Curlee, Ph.D.
Thieme Medical Publishers, Inc., New York © 1999.

12

Cluttering: Traditional Views and New Perspectives

David A. Daly, Ed.D.
Michelle L. Burnett

Overview and Traditional Perspectives

Traditionally, cluttering has been viewed as a fluency disorder. It is thought to be congenital in nature and is often called a syndrome because of the myriad of symptoms reported to characterize it. Cluttering is an elusive disorder that has puzzled professionals for decades. Despite sincere interest by physicians, such as Froeschels,[1] Weiss,[2] and Luchsinger and Arnold,[3] and by speech pathologists, such as Tiger, Irvine, and Reis,[4] St. Louis,[5] Myers,[6] Diedrich,[7] and Daly,[8] cluttering has been ignored by the speech-language pathology profession. More than four decades ago, Weiss[2] called cluttering the "orphan" in the family of speech-language pathology, because he believed that it had been neglected and treated as an illegitimate relative of stuttering by most speech–language pathologists.

We agree that cluttering presents as a syndrome, which may manifest itself differently in different individuals; however, we do not necessarily view cluttering as an offspring of stuttering, but more as a "fraternal twin." Like fraternal twins, cluttering and stuttering are similar in some ways, but vastly different in others. The perspectives presented in this chapter highlight these differences.

Physicians, including those cited above, described this unique language-fluency disorder decades before speech–language pathologists seriously began to conceptualize cluttering as a separate or co-occurring disability. Of these physicians, Weiss,[2] perhaps more than any other single person, familiarized speech-language pathologists with cluttering. He thought that Hippocrates' theory, which described *stuttering* as an improper balance between thought and speech was more applicable to *cluttering*. In 1964, Weiss authored a book, *Cluttering*, which many clinicians consider to be a classic. This text gave speech–language pathologists one source, written in English, devoted specifically to cluttering. At that time, Weiss listed but three obligatory symptoms that were pathognomonic and essential for diagnosis: 1. excessive repetitions of speech, 2. short attention span and poor concentration, and 3. lack of complete awareness of the problem. He also listed over a dozen faculative symptoms that are often present but not mandatory.

Three years later, Weiss[9] published a report that described the history, symptomatology, and therapy efforts of that time. In this article, he reminded readers that "cluttering has always been with us" and identified landmark contributions of others published in the 1960s. Included were Luchsinger's 1963 book,[10] a German text that was the first book devoted solely to cluttering; Luchsinger and Arnold's[3] book, which included a special section on cluttering and tachyphemia; and, of course, Weiss' own text.[2]

In 1968, Weiss[11] presented a revised list of 21 symptoms of cluttering. Speech–language pathologists will find his 1967 and 1968 articles highly informative. He synthesized many years of investigations in these two articles and provided information that is still of practical and theoretical interest. Additional information can be gleaned from a series of descriptive and experimental articles on cluttering published in *Logos* in the 1960s and in a special 1970 issue of *Folia Phoniatrica* dedicated to Deso Weiss. It should be noted that physicians usually described the symptoms associated with cluttering from a medical perspective.

More recent viewpoints on the etiology, symptomatology, and treatment of cluttering have been presented by speech–language pathologists such as, Tiger and colleagues,[4] Diedrich,[7] Burk,[12] St. Louis and Hinzman,[13] and Daly.[14] In 1989, Dalton and Hardcastle[15] devoted three chapters to the disorder of cluttering. Another book that focused exclusively on the multifaceted aspects of cluttering was published by Myers and St. Louis[16] in 1992. It rekindled researchers' and clinicians' interests in individuals who present with this challenging communication disorder. Then, in 1996, St. Louis[17] edited a double issue of the *Journal of Fluency Disorders* which was dedicated exclusively to cluttering. This issue of the journal contains an excellent annotated bibliography of works completed between 1964 and 1996, as well as current reports from investigators around the world.

Definitions and Characteristics of Cluttering

Like stuttering, cluttering is difficult to define. To borrow a phrase coined by Winston Churchill in a 1939 speech, cluttering is "a riddle wrapped in a mystery inside an enigma." Its varied and inconsistent symptomatology has led to numerous definitions and diverse etiological perspectives.

If cluttering is related to stuttering but is not stuttering, what is it? We agree with Weiss,[9] who asserted that cluttering is not a specific, isolated disturbance of speech. He[2] maintained that "cluttering is the verbal manifestation of central language imbalance in the area of verbal utterance" (p. 6). Others, however, define cluttering primarily as a speech defect. For example, *Webster's Third New International Dictionary*[18] defined cluttering as "a speech defect in which phonetic units are dropped, condensed, or otherwise distorted as a result of overly rapid, agitated speech utterance" (p. 431). The College of Speech Therapists in London[19] reported that cluttering is characterized by uncontrollable speed, which results in truncated, dysrhythmic, and incoherent sentences. St. Louis[20] sees cluttering as a speech–language disorder whose chief characteristics are 1. abnormal fluency that is not stuttering and 2. a rapid and/or irregular speech rate. Diedrich,[7] writing in a text about articulation disorders, stated that "cluttering is a problem in maintaining sequential articulatory units with little self-consciousness about the difficulty" (p. 315) and added that cluttering should be regarded as a problem in self-monitoring speech output. Although these proposed definitions focus on *speech*, they also allude to additional difficulties in other skills, such as prosody, language, and self-monitoring.

In 1970, de Hirsch[21] proposed that cluttering results from disturbances in a child's basic developmental pattern which operate at all levels of central integration. Moreover, she believed that the perceptual, motor, and verbal problems attributed to cluttering were due to an immature or impaired central nervous system.

Luchsinger and Arnold[3] proposed that cluttering is a disability in formulating language, which results in confused, hurried (tachyphemia), and slurred diction. They maintained that tachyphemia stemmed from a congenital, inheritable, and constitutional limitation of one's total psychosomatic personality structure. They also claimed that "this concept of an organic, familial, and dysphasia-like syndrome of disturbed language function is shared by all recent authors" (p. 599). Even though this view was accepted by many medical authorities interested in cluttering, other views persisted as well.

Freund[22] proposed that cluttering was a psychosyndrome, with concomitant, constitutional speech and language inadequacies. He postulated that cluttering was sometimes the underlying basis for stuttering. Froeschels,[23] on the other hand, believed that cluttering was caused by an incongruity between thinking and speaking. Op't Hof and Uys[24] hypothesized that it was a complex disorder which comprised deficits in articulation, receptive and expressive language, and perceptual–motor problems in addition to a disorder of fluency.

Tiger, Irvine, and Reis[4] argued that cluttering should be conceptualized as a constellation of learning disabilities (LD) and described the striking similarities between symptoms of cluttering and LD. A review of the literature revealed that both clutterers and individuals with LD may exhibit a wide range of similar impairments. The two populations are also similar in that the specific symptoms comprising each disorder may not necessarily be the same from one individual to the next. However, we believe that people who clutter and those who have learning disabilities likely comprise overlapping populations. Some individuals who clutter may also demonstrate a complex of learning disabilities, but individuals with learning disabilities may or may not clutter. For example, a child with impaired reading skills (relative to other cognitive or academic abilities) could be considered to exhibit LD with respect to reading; yet may not demonstrate cluttering. Nevertheless, the characteristics of these two populations are remarkably similar, thus lending themselves to ample research opportunities.

Daly[25] defined cluttering as a disorder of both speech and language processing which manifests itself as rapid, dysrhythmic, sporadic, disorganized, and frequently inarticulate speech by a person who is largely unaware of or unconcerned about these difficulties. He noted that accelerated speech is not always present but that an impairment in formulating language almost always is.

Years ago, Perkins[26] identified rate and erratic rhythm problems as central features of cluttering. He also noted general language disability with grammatical deficiency, impaired reading, bizarre handwriting, poor musical ability, and poor coordination as common difficulties. Perkins asserted that cluttering comprises a "microcosm" of speech therapies, because clinicians can find nearly every prominent speech and language disorder represented in the cluttering population.

Each of these definitions describes additional features that may be present with cluttering; thereby providing a broader view of how the disorder may manifest itself. It would seem, from these various definitions and descriptions, that cluttering involves many features and that its symptoms are variable.

Following a thorough review of the literature, in conjunction with our own clinical experience, we have come to appreciate Perkins' viewpoint and agree with those researchers who recognize the multifaceted nature of cluttering. The definitions and descriptions reviewed above reflect researchers' attempts to examine the specific characteristics they believe to represent cluttering. Each definition is distinguished by each author's perception of the salient characteristics of cluttering and colored slightly by his or her theoretical and therapeutic frameworks.

Weiss' thinking[2,9,11] evolved from his 1964 book to the ideas expressed in his 1967 and 1968 articles. Similarly, speech–language pathologists' reports on cluttering in recent years have gradually incorporated ideas and findings that were generated through the evolution and expansion of the field of speech–language pathology. During the last two decades the impact of studies focusing on language and cognition has been especially influential. Investigators and clinicians have learned more about linguistic and pragmatic concepts and skills, as well as learning disabilities and attention deficit disorders. This information has influenced their perceptions of cluttering and stuttering.

Likewise, we are continually developing and refining our conceptualization of cluttering. We have stepped back to view a bigger picture; to look at the syndrome, rather than focus upon the specific features or characteristics that individuals may exhibit. We now believe it is advantageous to view cluttering through a large window instead of through a microscope. The model that follows reflects our current thinking about cluttering. It deviates substantially from our earlier views as well as from perspectives that suggest cluttering is a type of fluency disorder. While keeping in mind the specific characteristics commonly associated with cluttering, we have broadened our perspective and classified these characteristics into five more widely applicable categories of impairment.

Reframing of Perspectives

Differentiating Cluttering from Stuttering

Although *stuttering* is not defined in a universally accepted manner, most clinicians agree that its central feature is "abnormal disfluency." The ability to describe speech disfluencies fairly accurately and consistently assists clinicians in the identification of stuttering. Assessment of severity, frequency, duration, and the types of disfluencies included may vary from one clinician to another as may judgments of the presence, absence, and severity of secondary characteristics. Philosophical differences regarding etiology and treatment may vary, too. Despite these differences, abnormal speech fluency can be identified with acceptable reliability.

Speech–language pathologists identify stuttering based on judgments of discontinuities in speech being atypical or abnormal. Fluent speech production results when the motor skills to produce a desired verbal message occur sequentially and synchronously in a smooth manner. The respiratory, phonatory, resonatory, and articulatory systems must function interdependently to produce fluent speech. When there is an aberration in the timing, synchronicity, valving, or sequencing of these systems, disfluency results. When such disruptions occur with excessive frequency and/or with notable tension, stuttering occurs.

With *cluttering*, there are even more variables to consider. Identification of cluttering should be based upon what is known about normal verbal output and communicative interaction. In the most basic terms, human communicative interactions require the ability to perceive messages (through looking and/or listening), assign meaning to them, and interpret them within the given context. This must be followed by the ability to formulate an appropriate response or request for clarification and deliver that response or request in a coherent, meaningful, socially acceptable manner. In order to do this, one must be able to translate concepts and ideas into words accurately and quickly; link these words in an appropriate sequence to form meaningful phrases and sentences; organize phrases and sentences appropriately to convey the ideas intended; and produce the message intelligibly and fluently. All of this must be done within the social-situational parameters dictated by the context, which the speaker must continually superimpose upon the formulation and delivery of the message. Therefore, normal communicative interactions require high levels of cognitive, linguistic, articulatory, and motoric agility within the constraints of social situations and cultural norms. When the precise orchestration of all of these interrelated skills and systems does not occur, cluttering may result. Thus, in comparing the two disorders, cluttering is to language expression as stuttering is to speech production.

Clinicians who have worked with children and adults who clutter readily acknowledge that speech output is almost always disfluent. Just as stuttering interrupts the ongoing, fluent production of sounds or words in sentences, cluttering interferes with the ongoing fluent expression of thoughts and ideas. Such *linguistic disfluency* is evidenced by the clutterer's frequent verbal revisions and interjections, excessive repetitions of words or phrases, poorly organized thoughts, lack of cohesion in discourse, and prosodic irregularities. This may be why many clutterers are referred for treatment of fluency, yet may or may not actually exhibit stuttering. Although cluttering often has been compared with stuttering and referred to as a fluency disorder, the similarity is largely limited to the disfluent verbal output common to both, but cluttering clearly appears to involve more than speech production difficulties. Individuals who clutter may, in fact, also stutter. Conversely, those who stutter may exhibit other concomitant speech and language problems, but the presence of these other difficulties may not be indicative of cluttering.

Several authors (e.g., Weiss,[9] Luchsinger and Arnold,[3] VanRiper,[27] Preus,[28] Daly and Burnett-Stolnack,[29] and Daly[30]) have provided comparative contrasts between cluttering and stuttering. Tables 12-1 and 12-2 display our current inventories of significant differences and similarities between cluttering and stuttering.

Note that the features listed in Table 12-1 are not considered to be exclusive to either cluttering or stuttering, but are designated as more typical (or atypical) of one disorder than the other. Features common to both disorders are shown in Table 12-2. When these features are considered in such a manner, cluttering and stuttering appear to be more different than similar.

The Linguistic Disfluency Model of Cluttering

Cluttering exists when an individual presents with one or more impairment(s) in each of five broad communicative dimensions reflecting cognitive, linguistic, pragmatic, speech, and motor abilities. Figure 12-1 illustrates this conceptualization of cluttering. In our combined clinical experience, we have not evaluated a clutterer who did not exhibit at least one disturbance in each dimension. The weakness(es) noted in these abilities may be subtle or profound, but at least one difficulty within each dimension is observed.

Further examination of Figure 12-1 reveals an overlap in the symptoms listed in each dimension. Throughout the evolution of our profession, these dimensions have become more clearly defined, but some degree of overlap, or ambiguity, between these areas exists. Recognizing that a given symptom may result from differing causes, we made no attempt to assign particular impairments to one specific category. An individual's verbal output inherently reflects components of his/her thinking, linguistic knowledge, awareness of

Table 12-1. Inventory of Significant Differences Between Cluttering and Stuttering

Feature	Cluttering	Stuttering
Started talking late; language delay	**Typical**	Atypical
Slurred articulation; telescope/condense/omit sounds or syllables	**Typical**	Atypical
Baby talk/lalling	**Typical**	Atypical
No remissions of fluency disruptions; never very fluent	**Typical**	Atypical
Clumsy, uncoordinated; hasty motor activities	**Typical**	Atypical
Poor rhythm/musical ability	**Typical**	Atypical
Poor penmanship; disintegrated writing	**Typical**	Atypical
Repeats longer words and/or phrases	**Typical**	Atypical
Clonic-type disfluencies	**Typical**	Atypical
Speaks better under pressure or on demand	**Typical**	Atypical
Prosodic deviances; irregular rate, rhythm	**Typical**	Atypical
Initial loud voice trailing off to a murmur; mumbles	**Typical**	Atypical
Language formulation difficulties	**Typical**	Atypical
Disorganized discourse; poor sequencing/story telling	**Typical**	Atypical
Word finding difficulties	**Typical**	Atypical
Improper linguistic structure/syntax; grammatical errors	**Typical**	Atypical
Improper pronoun referents	**Typical**	Atypical
Reading disability	**Typical**	Atypical
Poor written expression; parallels verbal errors	**Typical**	Atypical
Inappropriate topic introduction/maintenance/termination	**Typical**	Atypical
Tangentiality and verbosity	**Typical**	Atypical
Poor listening skills; impatient listener	**Typical**	Atypical
Insufficient processing of nonverbal signals	**Typical**	Atypical
Impulsivity; carelessness	**Typical**	Atypical
Lacks awareness of communication difficulty	**Typical**	Atypical
Attention deficits	More frequent	Less frequent
Excels in math and science	More frequent	Less frequent
Fluent episodes	Atypical	**Typical**
Secondary characteristics	Atypical	**Typical**
Repeats sounds and short words	Atypical	**Typical**
Starter sounds and words used	Atypical	**Typical**
Tonic-type disfluencies	Atypical	**Typical**
Sound prolongations	Atypical	**Typical**
Tension/struggle behaviors	Atypical	**Typical**
Pitch changes	Atypical	**Typical**
Word substitutions and circumlocutions	Atypical	**Typical**
Fearful about speech; shy and anxious	Atypical	**Typical**
Heightened awareness of disfluencies	Atypical	**Typical**

Table 12-2. Similarities Between Cluttering and Stuttering

Feature	Cluttering	Stuttering
Rapid rate of speech	**Typical**	**Typical**
Breathing dysrhythmia	**Typical**	**Typical**
Silent pauses; hesitations	**Typical**	**Typical**
Interjections; revisions; filler words	**Typical**	**Typical**
Poor oral coordination	**Typical**	**Typical**
Poor eye contact	**Typical**	**Typical**
Familial history	**Typical**	**Typical**

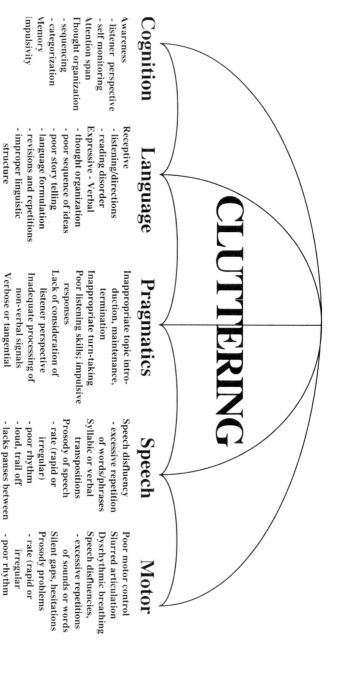

CLUTTERING

Cognition

Awareness
- listener perspective
- self monitoring
Attention span
Thought organization
- sequencing
- categorization
Memory
Impulsivity

Language

Receptive
- listening/directions
- reading disorder
Expressive - Verbal
- thought organization
- poor sequence of ideas
- poor story telling
- language formulation
- revisions and repetitions
- improper linguistic
    structure
- syllabic or verbal
    transpositions
- improper pronoun use
- dysnomia/word finding
- filler words, empty words
Expressive - Written
- run on sentences
- omissions and trans-
    positions of letters,
    syllables and words
- sentence fragments

Pragmatics

Inappropriate topic intro-
    duction, maintenance,
    termination
Inappropriate turn-taking
Poor listening skills; impulsive
    responses
Lack of consideration of
    listener perspective
Inadequate processing of
    non-verbal signals
Verbose or tangential
Poor eye contact

Speech

Speech disfluency
- excessive repetition
    of words/phrases
Syllabic or verbal
    transpositions
Prosody of speech
- rate (rapid or
    irregular)
- poor rhythm
- loud, trail off
- lacks pauses between
    words
- vocal monotony
Slurred articulation
- omit sound(s)
- omit syllable(s)
- /r/ and /l/
Dysrhythmic breathing
Silent gaps/hesitations

Motor

Poor motor control
Slurred articulation
Dysrhythmic breathing
Speech disfluencies,
- excessive repetitions
    of sounds or words
Silent gaps, hesitations
Prosody problems
- rate (rapid or
    irregular
- poor rhythm
Clumsy, uncoordinated
Poor penmanship
Impulsivity

Figure 12.1. Linguistic disfluency model illustrating possible impairment(s) within five broad communicative dimensions.

social norms, as well as the person's speech production and motor capabilities. Said another way, speaking is a complex cognitive-linguistic-motor act that occurs within a given context or social situation. Each component of the speech act impacts the final production. The specific categorization of symptoms should be determined on an individual basis.

Cognition: Impairments in certain cognitive skills are commonly reported in the cluttering literature, but are seldom described as cognitive deficits. Such impairments include lack of awareness of the disorder(s), poor self-monitoring, inadequate thought organization, poor attention span, impulsivity (verbal and nonverbal), and/or perceptual deficits, such as auditory or visual processing, or poor auditory memory.

An important cognitive feature of cluttering is the speaker's apparent lack of awareness of the deficit(s). This is a subjective variable that is difficult to quantify. Some cluttering clients occasionally acknowledge partial awareness of their dysrhythmic, rapid, unintelligible speech. Others seem indifferent that their speech deviates from normal. And still others deny that a problem exists. Clutterers often claim that the listener was not paying attention, rather than recognizing their own confused wording or the inarticulate nature of their speech. Weiss[2] considered this lack of awareness as an obligatory feature.

Weiss also included short attention span among his obligatory features for identifying cluttering. Pearson[31] agreed that attention span is a skill area that should be considered and objectively assessed. Attention skills can be evaluated informally by obtaining measures of time on task or the frequency with which a client needs to be redirected to a task within a given time period. Similarly, auditory memory, which reflects attention skills, is another area that can be objectively evaluated. A number of auditory and visual memory tests are commercially available. Daly et al.[32] developed a sentence imitation test for measuring auditory memory skills which provides norms for persons between 4 and 18 years of age.

Froeschels[1] remarked on another aspect of the relationship between thinking and speaking. He contended that many clutterers do not think faster than they can speak, but speak quickly, before they have thought their ideas through. Their verbalizations often appear disorganized and confused, as if they "get ahead of themselves." This observation may reflect problems with thought formulation or translating thoughts into words, possibly related to word-finding impairments.

Language: Language impairments, expressive and/or receptive, are frequently reported components of cluttering. Receptively, difficulty listening or following directions may relate to poor auditory memory, attention and concentration, or comprehension of language. Weiss[11] noted that clutterers are notoriously poor readers and believed that a reading disability could be a decisive diagnostic sign of cluttering when a client's classification was uncertain. The presence of a reading difficulty is not surprising since reading requires the ability to sustain concentration, reauditorize and assign meaning to words, and recall and integrate information on an ongoing basis. With respect to oral reading, some clients read well initially but begin making mistakes as they continue. This may be analogous to the deterioration of speech intelligibility following initially clear utterances during some clutterers' spontaneous discourse.

Although some stutterers are poor readers also, Conture and Van Naerssen[33] contended that most stutterers' reading skills are well within normal limits. Nippold and Schwartz[34] found inconsistent research findings in a literature review of stutterers' reading skills, suggesting that further research into the reading abilities of both stutterers and clutterers is needed. Clinicians are reminded that an individual who stutters and has a concomitant reading disability is not necessarily a clutterer.

It is through assessment of expressive language that disorders of formulation and thought organization are most evident in clutterers. Common linguistic deficits include narrative discourse with inappropriate syntax or word order or poor sequencing of ideas; frequent revisions, interjections or repetitions; syllabic or verbal transpositions; improper pronoun referents or overuse of pronouns; and/or excessive use of empty words or filler words. As is true with cognitive skills or receptive language abilities, each individual is likely to have different strengths and weaknesses with regard to expression, and one's performance can vary with the type of linguistic task. For example, weaknesses may not be evident in highly structured tasks, such as answering wh-questions, in which specific responses are elicited. Such activities and responses give an inflated estimate of a speaker's ability more often than do less structured tasks, such as story telling/writing or spontaneous discourse.

Written-expression abilities of clutterers often are revealing. Roman[35] described the unique impairments in written expression as follows:

> Disintegrated writing is the hallmark of the clutterer, who spills out the written word in headlong haste, clipping letters, omitting syllables, slurring substitutes, transposing words, hence producing in his almost illegible hand the counterpart of his inarticulate speech. (p. 29)

Deviant writing among persons who clutter has been reported by numerous authors (e.g., Orton,[36] Spadino,[37] and Sheperd[38]). de Hirsch[39] agreed and added that clutterers' writing demonstrates poor integration of ideas and space. Roman-Goldzieher[40] presented further evidence that clutterers' writing samples were characterized as uninhibited, sprawling, disorderly, and replete with repetitions and deletions. Whenever cluttering is suspected during an assessment, obtaining a writing sample is strongly recommended. Typically, the written sample parallels the client's verbal output. Written language contains similar types of omissions, transpositions, and disorganization. Also, there is a tendency to use run-on sentences with little punctuation, which is consistent with the clutterers' commonly noted tangentiality and inability to generate a cohesive story line or train of thought. We believe that reading and writing disorders are fruitful areas of investigation for differentiating clutterers and should be considered in treatment paradigms as well. Written assignments can be helpful to cluttering clients as a means of building awareness. Both children and adults often seem to benefit from the concrete feedback they receive from a thoughtfully corrected assignment.

Pragmatics: Individuals who clutter often display inappropriate language use. They frequently demonstrate inappropriate turn-taking, as well as inappropriate topic introduction, maintenance, and/or termination, which only adds to the linguistic confusion during conversation. In a study comparing the pragmatic skills of clutterers with age-matched controls, Teigland[41] reported fewer requests for clarification and fewer spontaneous repairs on the part of clutterers during dialogue. She also stated that clutterers produced "mazes," which she defined as "sequences of turns with ungrammatical structure" (p. 207), two to three times more frequently than noncluttering subjects did.

Prutting and Kirchner[42] studied 30 communicative acts included in their pragmatic protocol and found that clutterers violated one or more features in at least 50% of the acts analyzed. Severe clutterers were found to violate verbal and paralinguistic aspects of conversation, including speech acts; topic selection, introduction, maintenance, and change; turn-taking; lexical selection; stylistic variations; as well as intelligibility and prosodic features. Perhaps this is why Myers[43] referred to cluttering as a pragmatic problem. In order to use speech and language effectively, one must utilize appropriately the components that make up the whole.

In addition, clutterers frequently appear oblivious to nonverbal behaviors. They do not respond to quizzical looks from listeners nor do they acknowledge subtle nonverbal signs reflecting a lack of interest or attention on the part of the listener. Turn-taking also can be problematic due to some clutterers' tendency to interrupt or seemingly ignore another person's comments by replying with an unrelated remark.

Speech: Since cluttering has been viewed as a fluency disorder for such a long time, clinicians frequently focus on speech disfluencies; however, the disfluencies noted may or may not be stuttering. Stuttering can coexist with cluttering, but may be a separate impaired symptom. We view stuttering as a motor-speech disorder, which may or may not co-occur with cluttering. Irregularities in prosody are also reported and may include rapid or irregular rate, sporadic bursts of speech, variable vocal intensity, vocal monotony, and overall poor rhythm of speech. It is possible for combinations of these prosodic deviations to produce a generalized disfluency of speech without the presence of stuttering per se.

Rapid rate is one of the more frequently reported symptoms associated with cluttering. Martin and associates[44] analyzed cluttered speech spectrographically and verified the occurrence of rapid and variable rate, rushes of compressed speech, and articulatory inadequacy. Seeman and Novak[45] and Seeman[46] referred to clutterers' "interverbal acceleration," and Luchsinger[10] to the clutterers' "intraverbal acceleration." Both types of acceleration occur, and this increase in rate between and within words is a discriminating sign of cluttering. Wyatt[47] has also described the clutterer's propulsive impulse to speak with increasing speed. Tachylalia is common in cluttering, and Wohl[48] labeled the tendency for clutterer's speech to become faster and faster as it proceeds as "festination." However, rapid speech, in and of itself, is not necessarily indicative of cluttering. In fact, Weiss[2] argued that excessive speed should not be used as a prime indicator of cluttering, adding that signs of faulty integration may be better criteria.

Another verbal error typical of many clutterers is frequent "slips of the tongue." Bakwin and Bakwin[49] and Arnold[50] presented examples of such transpositions as "The Lord is a shoving leopard," and Daly[51] commented on the tendency for clutterers to make numerous verbal faux pas. For example, an adult cluttering client asked Daly to attend an important business meeting. Although several treatment sessions were devoted to practicing this brief presentation, several substitutions and transpositions were observed during the meeting. For example, the client said, "At this plant in time," thinking he had said, "At this point in time" and mis-spoke four other times during the 5-min presentation, including substitutions of "interrupted" for "interpreted" and "taking" for "talking." Throughout his presentation, this executive seemed oblivious to the mistakes he made. The listeners were confused, and his proposal was tabled for further discussion. More importantly, he did not receive the promotion he had expected. Although everyone has some slips of the tongue, the greater frequency of this type of error, coupled with a lack of awareness and an absence of spontaneous repair, may be indicative of cluttering. Norms for these types of transpositions and substitutions currently are not available, but repeated measures of their frequency of occurrence may be helpful in determining improvement during treatment.

Other speech errors reported in the literature include immature or imprecise articulation and sound or syllable transpositions or omissions. With respect to articulation errors, difficulty with /r/ and /l/ are common and Froeschels[1] reported that up to 50% of clutterers show dyslalias. Many clutterers tend to reduce consonant clusters into single consonant productions and show some signs of oral dyspraxia. It is common for polysyllabic words to be condensed or telescoped. This simplification process may be a function of accelerated rate, poor oral-motor skills, or both. Sheperd[38] and Arnold[50] observed that articulation errors may persist into adulthood. Although Bloodstein[52] concluded that functional difficulties in articulation and immature speech are unusually common among the stuttering population, a stutterer with concomitant articulation errors is not necessarily a clutterer. Thus, articulation errors alone are not diagnostically conclusive but may be another indicator of the clutterer's inability to integrate and execute multistep, complex tasks.

Motor: Speech is a motor act which involves precise execution of a sequence of motor movements. Since clutterers have been reported to demonstrate motor deficits in both gross and fine motor activities, errors in speech may reflect poor motor coordination in some cases. Clutterers are often described as clumsy, uncoordinated, physically immature, or as demonstrating impulsive motor movements. de Hirsch[39] documented clutterers' maturational delays in sitting, walking, and talking, which indicates less than optimal gross motor development. It is not uncommon for clutterers to look, act, and sound much younger than their age.

Fine motor skills may be problematic, also. With respect to motor-speech, repetitions are prominent in cluttering; characterized by excessively frequent repetitions of syllables, words, and phrases. Six, eight, or 10 units of effortless repetitions, with no apparent concern, are typical. Daly[25] noted that the repetitions in cluttering are often on larger linguistic units and are more clonic in nature, whereas the repetitions in stuttering are tense and occur on smaller linguistic units. While repetitions may represent a motoric deficit, they are commonly observed in clutterers during episodes of word retrieval problems and/or as a result of insufficient sentence formulation.

Frequently, in the literature, cluttering is likened to dyspraxia of speech. Arnold[50] and de Hirsch[21] suggested that clutterers' poor articulation may be related to possible dyspraxia, and Frick[53] proposed that some of the clutterer's difficulties might stem from problems with motor planning. On the other hand, Diedrich[7] pointed out that volitional speech is generally better than automatic speech for the clutterer, which is not consistent with that of dyspraxic individuals. Other signs of motor incoordination could be dysrhythmic breathing or inability to effectively coordinate breathing and speaking for some clutterers. Additionally, certain prosodic problems may be the result of motoric incoordination.

Another possible indicator of fine motor deficits in persons who clutter is poor penmanship. Legibility of writing often disintegrates from initially discernible print or script. Another commonly mentioned deficit for clutterers is a weakness in rhythm and musical ability (e.g., Luchsinger and Arnold[3]; Grewel[54]). Daly[8] found that many of his clients could not imitate a simple rhythmic pattern. Some clutterers report not liking music of any kind; others say they cannot sing. Such symptoms may reflect deficits in auditory attention and perception, timing or motor sequencing ability, or both. Musical ability, like writing, requires a high level of integration of several abilities and systems. An individual must draw on perceptual abilities as well as production skills in order to be successful in these activities. Similarly, conversation between two or more individuals is a verbal activity that also requires a high level of multiskill integration.

In summary, when assessing conversational skills of an individual suspected of cluttering, evaluations should be made of the person's thinking, thought organization and perspective; verbal proficiency, lexical, semantic, and syntactic knowledge; ability to produce intelligible speech, including proper use of suprasegmental features; fine motor precision as it pertains to speaking; awareness of and ability to self-monitor verbal and nonverbal feedback; ability to make appropriate adjustments and revisions based on such feedback; and acknowledgment of appropriate application of contextual, social, and cultural norms.

Comparing Cluttering with Other Disorders

Cluttering may be quite difficult to differentiate from language delay or disorder, learning disabilities, or attention deficit disorder (ADD/ADHD). We concur with Luchsinger and Arnold[3] and Diedrich[7] that cluttering is often difficult to differentiate until the age of 9 or 10 years; however, this may be achieved more easily using the linguistic disfluency model we presented earlier. For example, cluttering would be an appropriate diagnosis if the language delayed or disordered individual exhibited co-occurring deficits in cognitive, pragmatic, speech, and motor skills. Individuals who have a specific language impairment, a language disorder, or a language delay with co-occurring articulation disorder with stuttering would not be considered clutterers.

Tiger et al.[4] described the striking resemblance between cluttering and LD; however, a youngster with LD, by definition, must exhibit a deficit (or deficits) in a given area (or areas) significant enough to qualify for special education. A clutterer, on the other hand, may demonstrate more subtle difficulties across the five dimensions, which would not be significant individually but which could result in a significant impairment as a group. Another difference between LD and cluttering may be the tendency for individuals with LD to exhibit disorders in mathematics and reasoning, whereas clutterers often display strengths in these areas.

Similarly, individuals diagnosed as ADD or ADHD may present many of the same symptoms as clutterers. Clutterers are often described as inattentive, restless, impulsive, hyperactive, impatient, and short-tempered. Even though such reports are based on clinical observation, the traits reported by different researchers are remarkably similar. Naming such personality traits may not have strong diagnostic value with respect to differentiation of cluttering, but it may still provide a useful description of the clutterer. Moreover, while these traits are not exclusive to cluttering, neither are they exclusive to attention deficit disorders or learning disabilities, and it is entirely possible that two such disorders can co-exist in a given individual. However, based on the model we proposed earlier, an ADD/ADHD individual would have to present deficits or differences in each of the five dimensions in order to be classified as a clutterer.

Clinical Evaluation

Assessment of fluency problems in children and adults who stutter has been expertly described by other authors in this book and will not be reiterated here. For clients suspected of cluttering or stuttering clients who present with atypical features during the fluency assessment, more comprehensive evaluations are warranted. We agree with colleagues such as Hood,[55] Gregory and Hill,[56] and Riley and Riley[57] who recommend more in-depth speech and language evaluations including attention, auditory processing, motor, and educational aspects. The challenge is to differentiate stutterers with concomitant problems (see Bloodstein,[58] Blood and Seider,[59] Daly,[60] Nippold,[61] and Preus[62]) from those clients who more appropriately fit the cluttering classification.

In 1992, Daly, Myers, and St. Louis[63] supported the idea of a more comprehensive evaluation by delineating an assessment protocol for clients suspected of cluttering. This protocol included measures of fluency, rate, language, articulation, hearing, psychoeducational and academic skills, auditory and visual perception, fine motor control (including handwriting), and cognitive function. This type of comprehensive assessment may well require an interdisciplinary team, which may not be practical or available in some settings. Also, time constraints and fiscal realities may not allow such extensive testing. Therefore, clinicians must determine when it is important to probe further during a speech assessment in order to gather all the pertinent data.

Certain client behaviors indicate the need to expand the parameters of a typical fluency evaluation. Daly and Burnett-Stolnack[29] highlighted seven of these responses. For example, during an evaluation of a client referred for stuttering, observations of disorganized language, prosodic deviances, lack of awareness, and improvement of speech on demand may signal concomitant deficits. Assessment data should facilitate a clinical decision of whether or not the client demonstrates stuttering, cluttering, or stuttering with coexisting impairment(s). The presence of one or two deficits in addition to stuttering does not constitute cluttering based on the model we have proposed. Only when a client presents with disabilities in *each* of the five dimensions is cluttering identified. Therefore, speech disfluencies (i.e., stuttering) may be but one impaired feature among the constellation of symptoms that may be exhibited. The noted disfluencies may be just the tip of the iceberg. Thus, it is of the utmost importance for speech–language pathologists to obtain accurate historical information to support clinical observations made during an evaluation.

History and Background Information

Obtaining a detailed developmental history during a child's evaluation is especially important. Much of the literature refers to cluttering as a "congenital"[49,64] or "inheritable"[2,3] disorder, and a familial factor frequently is present. Weiss[2] maintained that, even though shifting symptomatology may make cluttering appear to be a functional disorder, he believed it to be hereditary. He argued that the hereditary nature of cluttering would be demonstrated in a definitive manner in the future. To date, this prediction has not been fulfilled.

Several studies (e.g., Kidd,[65] Luchsinger and Arnold[3]) have investigated the genetic transmission of stuttering, however, it is not clear if the data are accurately reflecting origins of stuttering or cluttering or both because the speech–language pathology profession has yet to distinguish the two disorders. Seeman,[66] in fact, proposed that cluttering and stuttering were not distinguishable on the basis of origin, and that a fluency disorder could manifest itself differently from one generation to the next. Some family members might stutter while others might exhibit speech and language more closely resembling cluttering. Therefore, it is important to inquire about the speech and language history of other family members and note any features similar to those exhibited by the client.

When reviewing the developmental history of an individual referred for fluency evaluation, there are several factors that may be useful for distinguishing cluttering. For example, parents of children who stutter often report episodes of disfluency alternating with episodes of fluency. Conversely, parents of children later identified as clutterers may indicate that their child was always disfluent or difficult to understand. Many children often have delays in the development of other speech and language skills as well. Likewise, attainment of other developmental milestones may be delayed.

It is important to gather information about motor development and abilities. Reports that clutterers tend to be clumsy, careless, or immature relative to peers may reflect subtle delays or deviations in motor coordination and control. Slight differences may not be considered impairments in and of themselves; however, when coordination or integration of more than one subtly deviant skill is required for a complex task, breakdown in performance may occur.

With respect to intellectual development, stutterers and clutterers may appear similar. Arnold[50] noted that a low I.Q. was not part of the tachyphemia syndrome. Many clutterers have average or above average intelligence; others may score in the superior range. School-aged clutterers often favor certain subjects such as mathematics or science; they seldom prefer English, social studies, or other language-based classes. Similarly, adult cluttering clients are often employed as engineers, mathematicians, or computer programmers. Luchsinger and Arnold[3] noted that clutterers tend to have a one-sided concentration or talent in exact disciplines of knowledge. They added that clutterers often become good scientists but usually remain poor speakers. Our clinical experience supports this observation, and it is our contention that clutterers' and stutterers' affinity for scientific or exacting occupations may be related to two different attributes. First is an individual's possession of high-level reasoning or mathematical skills necessary for these occupations. Second is the relatively low demand on communication skills required in some of these occupations.

Not infrequently, adult clutterers are referred for treatment because of employers' or coworkers' complaints about intelligibility of speech or difficulty presenting information to others. More than one executive has been referred by their employer to our practice. Following evaluation and diagnosis of cluttering in two such individuals, treatment was initiated. Unfortunately, after only a few sessions, both clients terminated treatment, indicating that they had no problem and would rather seek alternate employment than continue therapy. This behavior is consistent with Van Riper's[67] observation that clutterers deny their speech abnormalities and often do not cooperate with clinicians' efforts to improve communication skills.

Clinical Interview

Gathering the history and background information mentioned above is facilitated by asking a series of salient questions, e.g., "Does anyone in the family stutter?," "Does anyone in the family stammer?," "Does anyone in the family clutter?" Since some individuals may not be familiar with these terms, it is especially important to ask if the client's speech or behavior resembles anyone else's in the family. Quite frequently, parents may respond, "He talks (or acts) like Uncle Charley. That's why we brought him here in the first place. Can you do anything to help him?" Speech–language pathologists need to ask these kinds of questions because cluttering and stuttering often occur within the same families.

Clinical observations of communicative strengths and weaknesses are essential and should be confirmed with questions to complete the picture of the individual's abilities and insights. The questions asked, of course, influence the responses received. For example, many clutterers are unaware of their communication difficulties and may say "No" if asked "Do you have any trouble getting your point across?" or "Do you see the need for speech therapy?" However, if asked more concrete questions such as, "Do people ask you to repeat what you have just said?" or "Do you ever repeat yourself so much that other people ask you to slow down?" or for a younger client, "Does anyone ever tease you about your speech?," their responses may be more revealing. Asking both sets of questions (abstract and concrete) can be particularly informative with respect to an individual's awareness of his or her disorder(s). It is important to ask questions directly and probe deeply enough to gather relevant data.

In addition to noticing whether or not a client exhibits tension or struggle behaviors during disfluencies, it may be helpful to inquire about frustration with speech and about avoidance of speaking. Responses to such questions may assist in determining if the pattern of diagnostic signs is more typical of cluttering or of stuttering. Most often, stutterers become frustrated with their inability to fluently articulate a well-formulated thought. They are aware of stuttering to the point that they often can predict when they will stutter, which may lead to avoidance of certain words or, more dramatically, of certain speaking situations. Clutterers, on the other hand, do not express frustration with speaking difficulties, but they express frustration that listeners do not listen carefully enough. In addition, people who clutter often will indicate that they forgot what they intended to say, cannot find the right word(s), or they may continue talking tangentially without arriving at a specific point.

In summary, asking questions about the client's development, family history, specific communication abilities and disabilities, awareness of speaking difficulties, and fears or frustrations about communication will supplement the behavioral observations made during the evaluation. Asking the same questions of a client and family members can be enlightening as the responses are likely to vary. If information obtained from the client differs from that received from family member(s), this does not indicate that one person is wrong. Such discrepancies only indicate differences in the perceptions or levels of awareness of the individuals answering the questions.

Communication Skills Assessment

Questions elicit useful information from clients of all ages and should be woven into the clinical interview and objective data collection process during an evaluation. Other important components of the evaluation include assessment of speech, motor, pragmatic, linguistic and cognitive skills. Some of these abilities can be evaluated formally with standardized instruments, while others may have to be assessed more informally.

To explore a client's awareness of a problem, Woolf's[68] Perceptions of Stuttering Inventory (PSI) can be utilized. When the disfluency exhibited is not characteristic of stuttering or when an individual is notably unaware of his or her disfluency, the clinician may choose The Perceptions of Speech Communication (PSC) inventory (see Appendix A). This is a 60-item inventory which Daly[51] adapted from Woolf's PSI by substituting the words "speaking difficulty" for "stuttering." The altered inventory does not mention stuttering in its title or items, which permits its use with clutterers and other communicatively disordered clients.

The PSC has proven useful with adolescent and adult clients for determining how much they were aware of or worried about their speaking ability. Daly and colleagues[69] compared nonstuttering high school students' scores on Woolf's PSI form with those on the adapted PSC form and found that they checked an average of 10 items on either inventory. Daly and Darnton[70] administered Woolf's PSI to adolescent stuttering clients and found an average of 27 items were checked. Our clinical experience using the perceptions of speech communication (PSC) inventory with adolescents and adults suspected of cluttering has revealed that they usually check fewer than six items. This suggests that many clutterers may be only partially aware of their speaking difficulty. Conversely, some individuals with a number of cluttering symptoms check many items on the PSC, indicating that they are more aware of or perhaps apprehensive about their speech than most clutterers. This type of client may demonstrate features of both cluttering and stuttering.

When assessing a client's disfluency, it is important to make note of the *nature* of the disfluencies. Stuttering disfluencies are typically more tense, with evidence of struggle to produce a sound or word. Repetitions in confirmed stutterers are often described as tonic and usually occur on smaller linguistic units (sounds and syllables). Secondary characteristics are frequently present. In contrast, disfluencies in cluttering (without stuttering) are typically not tense. Repetitions are easy, more clonic in nature, and occur on relatively larger linguistic units (whole words and phrases). A clutterer's disfluencies often can be associated with word finding or language formulation problems. Secondary characteristics are usually not observed.

When assessing other speech skills, it is important to evaluate the client's oral motor coordination abilities. Fletcher's[71] normative data for diadochokinetic rates are useful in evaluating the speaker's ability to perform rapidly alternating oral movements with the articulators. Clutterers usually perform these exercises quickly, within the age-appropriate range, however, closer observation of the client's rate and rhythm on this task may show prosody which deviates from normal. Sometimes, rate of production becomes increasingly fast rather than remaining at a steady pace or a client may repeat syllables sporadically, without a discernible rhythm. Deficits are more apparent when a client attempts bisyllablic and trisyllablic productions. When difficulties are noted, the clinician should consider incorporating oral-motor exercises in therapy (see Riley and Riley,[72–74] Daly[30]).

In addition to oral-motor skills, the clinician should carefully observe other motor abilities and movements of the client. Noting an individual's movement in the environment, spatial awareness in activity, and fine motor skills, such as in writing, may be informative. Motor movements may not be seriously impaired, but often are hasty, impulsive, jerky, or uncoordinated.

Assessment of writing is important not only to the evaluation of motor skills, but also to the linguistic abilities of a client. Standardized language test scores can be supplemented by a few written language samples. To gather writing samples, we ask clients to write sentences to dictation. Next, we encourage them to write a one-page, descriptive narrative that describes a favorite movie or recent vacation. We note whether the client has difficulty initiating or organizing thoughts on one subject, as clutterers often do. A person's ability to organize, sequence, and describe such topics reveals a great deal about his or her cognitive and linguistic skills. Comparisons of dictated and spontaneous writing may highlight difficulties due to thought formulation problems.

To obtain a useful synopsis of the client's verbal expression, we recommend recording three or more 1-min monologues under different speaking conditions. For example, recording the client answering personally relevant wh-questions followed by samples of spontaneous monologues often reveals important discrepancies in linguistic skills, including formulation, organization, grammatical structure, and word finding.

It is important to note that comparing a client's performance across three or four samples may yield seemingly different abilities. Although performance will vary with the type of verbal task, it may also change as the client gets more comfortable being recorded. That is, clutterers often perform better initially when under pressure or on demand. When the recorder is first turned on, the client's attention to speech and language may be heightened and, for a clutterer, this may result in speech being better than usual. Some parents who sit in on their child's evaluation have told us, "We can never understand him this well at home!" or "This is not his usual speech; this is not what we are concerned about."

As the session continues, a deterioration in the clutterer's verbal output may be observed.

Signals of such deterioration may manifest themselves in both language and speech performance. Linguistic examples include off-topic, rambling remarks; difficulty sequencing ideas; use of empty words or circumlocutions; and inappropriate grammatical structure. Speech examples include irregular, sporadic rate or rhythm; loud bursts of speech trailing off to a murmur; and less precise articulation. All of these behaviors are typical of cluttering.

The language samples obtained must be representative of the client's typical speech and language performance to be of diagnostic value. Sometimes, it is only near the end of a session, when the client is less concerned about verbal performance, that a more typical speech pattern is evident. Leaving the tape recorder on during closing comments at the end of the evaluation and while the client (and a child's family) is preparing to leave may often capture an individual's more typical speech pattern. Casual speaking situations more often elicit the clutterer's typical communicative style and abilities.

To informally assess receptive language during an evaluation, clinicians should note the client's ability to follow directions and the need for repetition of instructions. Reading comprehension can be evaluated similarly. For example, oral reading of a passage is often used during fluency assessments. Upon completion, the clinician can ask content-related questions to determine the client's comprehension. Additional observations to note during oral readings include visual scanning abilities, prosody of speech, and reading miscues reflecting letter or word transpositions, omissions, or additions.

Throughout the evaluation process, clinical judgments of cognitive abilities, such as attention and concentration, self-monitoring, and awareness, can take place. Similarly, pragmatic skills can be observed and evaluated during the entire evaluation. Closely examining social and verbal behavior during structured and unstructured aspects of the session and asking questions that draw upon the client's knowledge of social skills can provide useful information.

Gathering and Interpreting the Data

All of the above information is essential to accurate diagnosis. Daly's Checklist for Possible Cluttering[75] was revised to aid in the identification and examination of the presence and severity of 36 features which a number of clinical researchers have reported to be indicative of cluttering. The revised checklist corresponds to the conceptual model described earlier. Compared to the previous version, the revised checklist omits features that have not been diagnostically important and includes other symptoms we have found to be more salient to clinical judgments. A copy of the revised checklist, now called the Checklist for Identification of Cluttering-Revised, appears in Appendix B.

To use the checklist, the clinician questions the client or parent to obtain certain information and ranks other items upon completion of the evaluation. The clinician records the extent to which each statement is judged to be true for the client. Each of the 36 items is rated on a four-point scale, ranking the feature from "not true" for the client (score of zero) to "very much true" (score of 3). Thus, a total score of 108 is possible. When the examiner's observations or objective findings differ from the rankings given by the parent or client, the scores should reflect the clinician's findings. Clinicians are reminded that the checklist is not a scientific instrument, but a tool that allows them to succinctly rank pertinent information on one page.

Previously reported clinical data,[76] using the experimental version of the checklist, proposed that a score of 55 or higher strongly suggested a diagnosis of cluttering. At present, the revised checklist has been utilized for only a few months making it difficult to determine the impact of the changes, if any, on the previously suggested score. When sufficient data are collected and analyzed, objective ratings and a recommended cutoff score for identifying cluttering may be reported. Data on a large number of clients suspected of cluttering would allow the 36-items to be weighted for diagnostic significance. We contend that a representation of impairments in all dimensions may be of greater diagnostic utility than a specific score.

Clinical Management

To examine the nature and severity of an individual's symptoms and deficits, an experimental profile analysis form for treatment planning was designed.[76] That profile analysis was reorganized in 1996[29] and was further revised for this chapter. The current profile analysis form (see Appendix C) organizes information by categorizing checklist items into areas consistent with those described in Figure 12-1.

To utilize the profile analysis form, scores are transferred from the checklist to the profile analysis. A score of three (3) on a certain checklist item corresponds to a negative three (−3) on the profile analysis. The negative sign indicates that a particular symptom is *undesirably different from normal*. Similarly, a score of two (2) on a checklist item is scored as negative two (−2), and a score of one corresponds to a negative one (−1) on the profile. A score of zero indicates that performance on a given item is within normal limits or better. Thus, the presence of a certain behavior or skill marked zero is considered normal or *desirably different from normal* (as may be the case with high-level math or reasoning abilities). After all scores are transferred, the clinician can connect the points to obtain a graphic display of the individual's communicative profile. The profile analysis highlights an individual's pattern of deficits and displays the extent of deviancy from normal for each item. Whether or not an individual exhibits deficits in each of the five dimensions is easily viewed. The profile analysis form combines the language and cognition dimensions as well as the speech and motor dimensions. While some items in the cognition and language section have a more linguistic basis and others reflect a more cognitive foundation, the basis for a given feature may not be distinguishable. The same is true for some items in the speech and motor section.

The completed profile can guide the clinician in diagnosing cluttering and designing an overall treatment plan. In terms of diagnosis, we have found that the profiles of stutterers and clutterers differ. Most stutterers' profiles reveal more items in the speech and motor and developmental dimensions scored as negative one's, two's, or three's with the majority of remaining items to be scored zero. In contrast, most clutterers' profiles reveal relatively few scores of zero, and negative scores in each of the four sections of the profile analysis form. This would be expected because the items were selected as indicators of cluttering. To be consistent with the model we have proposed, an individual would have to exhibit at least one deficit in each of the five dimensions.

Another diagnostic use of the profile analysis results from the visual display of deficits in each of the five dimensions. For example, we evaluated a 51-year-old adult who referred himself to our center following the threat of dismissal from a high-level administrative position. Subordinates had complained that his communication style was inconsistent, confusing, and inadequate. They reported difficulty understanding both his oral and written communication. Their complaints were substantiated when the evaluation was not completed after 90 min due to this gentleman's disorganized speech, compulsive talking, and difficulty with story telling and topic maintenance. Only three items were checked by this client on the 60-item PSC, indicating significant lack of awareness. Once the evaluation was completed, analysis of the data on the original 33-item checklist yielded a score of 45. While this score was below the previously suggested criterion for cluttering, this client exhibited at least mild difficulty with two-thirds of the 33 items. Upon transferring his scores to the profile analysis, it was clear that he did, in fact, demonstrate deficits in each of the five dimensions illustrated in Figure 12-1.

The profile analysis also facilitates individualized treatment planning. Before discussing treatment planning and specific treatment activities, some guiding principles for the treatment of cluttering are offered.

Principles of Treatment

We believe that treatment need not progress through a specific hierarchy of skills but may include a gradual progression in task difficulty. We also believe that specific skills in each of the dimensions should be addressed simultaneously. This can occur by utilizing activities that incorporate multiple skills or sequencing individual tasks within a session so that each task adds to the skill required by the previous activity and results in the use of multiple communicative skills in the final activity of the session. Ultimately, of course, the specific plan ought to be tailored to the particular strengths and weaknesses of the client. Additionally, there are three principles that we consider to be essential to treatment in general.

The first principle involves frequent repetition of therapy goals and rationale. As with any client, it is important for the clutterer to be well aware of specific goals. Knowing why a goal is being addressed as well as the expected outcome facilitates remediation. Since many clutterers are notoriously unaware of their communication behavior and its impact on their interactions with others, frequent reminders are necessary for client progress.

The second principle also relates to the clutterer's lack of awareness and promotes self-monitoring. Providing immediate, direct feedback is exceedingly important in assisting the clutterer with more effective communication. Due to many clutterers' tendency to deny communication difficulties, it is important to point out communication failures promptly and directly. It is equally, if not more important, however, to reinforce any and all appropriate communication behaviors. Use of audio- and videotape replays are effective in this regard; however, echoing or parroting a client's utterances (immediately restating what was said, exactly the way it was said) has been helpful when recording is not possible. Provision of feedback can gradually incorporate guiding the client in self-assessment.

The third principle regarding the treatment of cluttering applies more specifically to youngsters, but pertains to the significant others of adult clients as well. Parental involvement throughout the child's treatment is of the utmost importance. In addition to assisting with homework exercises, parents need to understand the goals of treatment. They may need to be trained to model appropriate communication behaviors and provide proper reinforcement of the child's output. Parents need to know what should not be done, but more importantly, they must be educated about what should be done during communicative interactions with their child. Knowledge of both desirable and undesirable performance facilitates more effective parent–child interaction. Parents may also require training with respect to appropriate means of feedback, correction, and reinforcement. Our experience indicates that off-target home practice is worse than no practice. Generalization is promoted when parents provide accurate models and feedback during homework exercises and in spontaneous interactions.

Treatment Planning

St. Louis and Myers[77] suggest a synergistic approach to treatment. We agree with this overall concept and its constructs; that is, a treatment program should address the multifaceted disorder of cluttering in all dimensions. However, given the multitude of concomitant deficits that may be present, determining a starting point can be quite difficult. Which deficit should be addressed first? Which difficulty most significantly impairs communication? The profile analysis form helps to ascertain answers to these and similar questions by highlighting which skills are more undesirably different from normal.

Effective communication is a dynamic, complex, highly interactive activity. Thus, the treatment program must be designed to enable a clutterer to execute and monitor multiple behaviors simultaneously. We recommend, therefore, that each of the five dimensions be targeted in each treatment session whenever possible. This may seem unrealistic for one 30-min session, but we believe that it often is possible to incorporate all dimensions in a synergistic approach to treatment.

Table 12-3 summarizes several treatment principles and activities that facilitate addressing more than one goal area simultaneously. There are a few tasks that are specific to one goal (e.g., articulation drills). Unfortunately, space does not permit more detailed descriptions of the numerous treatment strategies we believe to benefit persons who clutter. Fortunately, clear and cogent descriptions of many strategies are available in the recent literature, including Daly[8,25,30,51] Daly and Burnett,[76] St. Louis and Myers,[77,78] Myers and Bradly,[79] Katz-Bernstein,[80] and Langevin and Boberg.[81] Although the prognosis for substantial improvement is better than previously suggested in the literature, the need for persistence and repetition in treatment cannot be overemphasized.

The following case example illustrates how a single therapy activity can have multiple treatment implications. A 9-year-old clutterer demonstrated the following impairments upon evaluation: misarticulations (primarily of /r/); excessive speech rate, which resulted in slurred, less precise articulation; disfluency characterized by excessive repetitions of words and phrases; poor language formulation and thought organization, word-finding difficulty, use of empty or filler words, and overuse of pronouns; difficulty with written language (content, penmanship, and spatial organization); reduced attention span; and poor self-monitoring and awareness. Additionally, this child had been diagnosed elsewhere as having a reading disability, and he was taking Ritalin three times daily to control hyperactivity.

In a typical 30-min session, each of the communication problems can be addressed. At the beginning of the session, the client names the two or three primary deficits he wishes to focus on in that session (awareness). He sets a timer for the length of time he believes that he can attend to one task during which the clinician tallies the number of times the client needs redirection (awareness and attention). Typically, for this individual, tasks include brief articulation drills, including tactile stimulation for lingual placement (speech articulation and oral-motor skills). Next, he may practice five to 10 statements utilizing the fluency techniques designed by Daly[30] (fluency, rate, prosody). This is followed by a verbal expression activity, such as describing objects or similarities and differences (thought

Table 12-3.   Suggestions for Treatment of Cluttering

Targeted Deficit Area	*Treatment Principles and Activities*
Awareness *It is important to address awareness as a whole and as it pertains to each deficit area.*	• Provide rationale for each task and goal in each session • Utilize video and audio recordings • Provide immediate, direct feedback with positive reinforcement for appropriate performance/behavior • Multisensory feedback; e.g., vibro-tactile feedback, pacing board • Negative practice
Self-Monitoring *Tasks for awareness also assist in improving self-monitoring and vice-versa. Impulsivity also improves.*	• Monitor number of times the client self-corrects (e.g., an articulation error, self-cues to reduce rate, etc.) • Use of Delayed Auditory Feedback • Self-rating for specific task performance (i.e., demonstrating ability to accurately judge correct or desirable performance) • Train awareness and accurate response to listener feedback
Attention Span	• Measure time on task (sustained attention) • Tally number of times redirection to task is required • Use timer or alarm to indicate task beginnings, endings • Listening for comprehension and details, following directions; selections of increasing duration • Auditory memory for increasingly longer series of numbers (forward or backward), words (related or unrelated)
Thought Organization/ Formulation *Note that each activity may actually address multiple target areas simultaneously*	• Naming attributes within given categories for specific objects • Categorization of items or objects • Detailed description of objects, increase use of descriptors/adjectives • Describe similarities and differences of two objects • Sequencing activities, such as naming steps to complete a task or giving directions • Story telling; structured with use of picture sequencing cards or unstructured narrative • Writing; same tasks as above with written responses
Semantics, Syntax, and Lexical Selection *The activities in the sections above as well as these can be targeted in verbal or written exercises*	• Unscramble words, sentences, paragraphs • Vocabulary building exercises • Naming activities, including confrontation naming and naming to description or category • Cloze activities at sentence or paragraph level • Sentence framing • Combining simple sentences into one complex sentence
Pragmatics/Social Skills	• Listening activities requiring careful follow-through; blind board activities • Training appropriate means of requesting clarification, questioning • Building awareness of specific behaviors through direct feedback (verbal, audio or video replay, role-playing) • Overt practice of social skills (greetings, introductions, salutations)

continued

Table 12-3. Continued

Targeted Deficit Area	Treatment Principles and Activities
Pragmatics/Social Skills (cont.)	• Topic-specific discussion; attempt to make all remarks pertain to one topic • Overt or exaggerated practice of acknowledging nonverbals (reading expressions, body language) • Practice of turn-taking in activities and conversation; move from highly structured to less structured tasks • Appropriately tell jokes (proper sequencing, timing)
Speech Production and Prosody *Many suggestions in this section address speech & motor abilities*	• Rate reduction programs; DAF; deliberate, exaggerated practice • Reduce repetitions via use of DAF, deliberate phonation, decreasing rate and increasing linguistic skills • Emphasize appropriate changes in inflection/intonation; stressing different words to change meaning, statements versus questions • Breathing modifications for better coordination with speaking and increased use of pauses; appropriate use of "verbal punctuation" • Overarticulation and exaggeration of mouth movements; articulation drills if necessary • Imitation or oral reading of nursery rhymes, poetry
Motor Skills	• Oral-motor skills training (e.g., Riley and Riley) • Recite tongue twisters • Address penmenship in written assignments • Practice various rhythmic patterns (tapped or verbalized)

organization, formulation, fluency, rate, prosody). Then, he uses picture sequencing cards to assist in generating a written narrative (language content, naming, thought organization and formulation, spatial organization, fine motor/penmanship). Throughout the session he is provided with direct, immediate feedback regarding performance. At the end of the session, the client is guided in self-assessment of his performance for that session (awareness, reinforcement).

It should be noted that this child has been in treatment for 2 years, receiving treatment in school as well as additional weekly sessions in a hospital-based program. At this point, he is significantly more aware of his communicative behaviors and its impact upon successful and unsuccessful communication interactions. Earlier in the treatment process, self-assessment followed each activity (and this is still required some of the time). As always, clinicians must exercise good clinical judgment so that some sessions may, in fact, focus more specifically on one or two activities. Times when this is likely to be appropriate include learning new skills or when the client appears to be more receptive to particular suggestions or specific strategies.

Another interesting issue in this case, as in others we have seen, was that initial work on this client's very rapid rate of speech did not result in functional improvement. He was able to slow his rate in structured therapy tasks after strategies were learned, but efforts to facilitate generalization were unsuccessful. Furthermore, reducing rate alone did not yield a significant improvement in fluency, articulation, or overall verbal expression. When rate reduction techniques were abandoned and the focus of treatment shifted to other deficits (especially language abilities) in a more synergistic approach, a positive effect on speaking rate was observed. Thus, rate reduction may have been a positive byproduct of the client's use of more appropriate formulation, pausing, and sentence framing techniques. Since these skills were easily practiced in conversational discourse, his rate in conversation was observed to become more normal.

Summary

This chapter presented a broad view of cluttering which conceptualized the disorder as an inability to successfully integrate and execute all of the necessary systems and skills required for effective communication. Cluttering was described as a complex of symptoms that vary within and among different individuals. Traditional perspectives about cluttering were reframed in this chapter, and a new definition was offered. The definition does not mandate the presence of a specific core or central features, but includes a concatenation of symptoms which may be present and contribute negatively to the individual's communication efforts. We believe that cluttering exists when an individual presents with one or more impairment(s) in each of five broad communicative dimensions reflecting cognitive, linguistic, pragmatic, speech, and motor abilities. This model acknowledges the variable presentations of cluttering symptoms while structuring a means for more consistent identification of cluttering.

Traditionally, cluttering has been viewed as a type of fluency disorder. It was depicted here as a broader communication disorder, encompassing a multitude of symptoms of which speech disfluency may be one. We are not yet convinced that cluttering and stuttering are distinguishable disorders with respect to etiology, but we are confident that they can be differentiated behaviorally. Cluttering and stuttering were presented as analogous disorder, with stuttering primarily affecting speech fluency and cluttering, more broadly, impacting linguistic fluency.

Tools for assessment and treatment planning were presented. The Checklist for Identification of Cluttering was designed to assist in the diagnosis of cluttering by providing a synopsis of frequently reported and observed symptoms and a means of ranking the severity of these features. Presently, we identify cluttering when there is at least one deficit in each of the five communicative dimensions.

The Profile Analysis for Planning Treatment with Cluttering Clients was redesigned to organize symptoms from the checklist and the theoretical model proposed and provide a visual display of the individual's speech pattern. The profile analysis facilitates a determination of whether or not a speaker exhibits deficits in each of the five dimensions and assists in differentiating cluttering from stuttering. Additionally, it assists in the formulation of individualized treatment objectives by displaying the client's relative strengths and weaknesses.

Three principles for guiding treatment were offered. These principles tend to focus on the metacognitive skills (awareness and self-monitoring) of the client, because these abilities are paramount to achieving durable change. The first principle involves frequent reiteration of goals and rationales to promote client awareness and understanding. The second principle states that immediate, direct, constructive feedback as well as positive reinforcement are essential to improve awareness and self-monitoring. The third principle cites the importance of direct, active involvement of parents and significant others in treatment programs to facilitate generalization. Treatment that addresses the multiple deficits individually and simultaneously to promote the client's ability to consistently and effectively orchestrate the various interrelated skills required for efficient and effective communication is most effective. Significant improvements in clutterers' communication abilities should occur when a multidimensional, synergistic treatment approach is utilized.

Suggested Readings

Daly DA: *The Clutterer*, in St. Louis KO (ed.): *The Atypical Stutterer: Principles and Practices of Rehabilitation*. New York, Academic Press, 1986.
> A comprehensive review of the various definitions and characteristics of cluttering by numerous investigators. Differentiations of stuttering and cluttering, as well as assessment and treatment procedures are presented.

Daly DA, Burnett ML: Cluttering: Assessment, treatment planning, and case study illustration. *J Fluency Dis* 1996, 21:239–248.
> Presents new methods for gathering and interpreting various information on clients suspected of cluttering. Case study analysis depicts strategies for successfully planning and treating cluttering.

Arnold GE, Luchsinger R: *Voice-Speech-Language, Clinical Communicology: Its Physiology and Pathology*. Belmont, CA, Wadsworth, 1965.
> This Herculean contribution by two physicians presents the most scholarly, in-depth analysis of cluttering (tachyphemia) up to that time. These authors present a thoughtful discussion of the possible relationship between disordered rhythm and disorders of music and motor ability.

Weiss DA: Cluttering. *Folia Phoniatr (Basel)* 1967; 19:233–263.
> This article is Weiss' most comprehensive description of cluttering as a central language imbalance. His theoretical framework is described and illustrated with figures and tables. Weiss' various features of cluttering are elaborated and faulty integration of language is highlighted as a main criterion of cluttering. A culmination of his most serious writings.

St. Louis KO, Myers FL: Management of Cluttering and Related Fluency Disorders, in Curlee RL, Siegel G (eds): *Nature and Treatment of Stuttering: New Directions*, 2nd ed, Boston, Allyn and Bacon, 1997.
> Up-to-date discussion of definitions of cluttering and descriptions of various characteristics. Conceptualizes cluttering from a synergistic framework. Treatment suggestions are highlighted.

References

1. Froeschels E: Contribution to the relationship between stuttering and cluttering. *Logopaedic Phoniatr* 1955; 4:1–6.
2. Weiss DA: *Cluttering*. Englewood Cliffs, NJ, Prentice-Hall, 1964.
3. Luchsinger R, Arnold GE: *Voice-Speech-Language, Clinical Communicology: Its Physiology and Pathology*. Belmont, CA, Wadsworth, 1965.
4. Tiger RJ, Irvine TL, Reis RP: Cluttering as a complex of learning disabilities. *Lang Speech Hear Serv Schools* 1981; 11:3–14.
5. St. Louis KO (ed): *The Atypical Stutterer: Principles and Practices of Rehabilitation*. New York, Academic Press, 1986.
6. Meyers FL: *Cluttering: A Synergistic Approach*. Paper presented at the Second International Oxford Dysfluency Conference, Oxford, England, 1988.
7. Diedrich WM: Cluttering: Its Diagnosis, in Winitz H (ed): *Treating Articulation Disorders: For Clinicians by Clinicians*. Baltimore, University Park Press, 1984.
8. Daly DA: The Clutterer, in St. Louis KO (ed): *The Atypical Stutterer: Principles and Practice of Rehabilitation*. New York, Academic Press, 1986.
9. Weiss DA: Similarities and differences between stuttering and cluttering. *Folia Phoniatr (Basel)* 1967; 19:98–104.
10. Luchsinger R: *Poltern*. Berlin-Charlottenberg, Manhold Verlag, 1963.
11. Weiss DA: Cluttering: Central language imbalance. *Pediatr Clin North Am* 1968; 15:705–720.

12. Burk K: Cluttering: A Rate Control Program. Presented at the annual convention of the American Speech–language, Hearing Association, Detroit, 1986.
13. Louis KO, Hinzman AR: A descriptive study of speech, language, and hearing characteristics of school-aged stutterers. *J Fluency Disord* 1988; 13:331–356.
14. Daly DA: Cluttering: A language-based syndrome. *Clin Connect* 1993, 6:4–7.
15. Dalton P, Hardcastle WJ: *Disorders of Fluency*. London, Whurr Publishers, 1989.
16. Myers FM, St. Louis KO: *Cluttering: A Clinical Perspective*. Kibworth, England, Fax Communications, 1992. Reissued by Singular Publishing Group, 1996.
17. St. Louis KO (ed): Research and opinion on cluttering: State of the art and science. *J Fluency Disord* 1996;2.
18. Gove PB (ed): *Webster's Third New International Dictionary*, Boston, Merriam, 1981.
19. *Terminology for Speech Disorders*. London, College of Speech Therapists, 1959.
20. St. Louis KO: On Defining Cluttering, in Meyers F, St. Louis KO (eds): *Cluttering: A Clinical Perspective*. Kibworth, England, Far Publications, 1992. Reissued by Singular Publishing Group, 1996.
21. de Hirsch K: Stuttering and cluttering: Developmental aspects of dysrhythmic speech. *Folia Phoniatr (Basel)* 1970; 22:311–324.
22. Freund H: Studies in the interrelationship between stuttering and cluttering. *Folia Phoniatr (Basel)* 1952; 4:146–168.
23. Froeschels E: Cluttering. *J Speech Disord* 1946; 11:31–36.
24. Op't Hof J, Uys IC: A clinical delineation of tachyphemia (cluttering). *S Afr Med J* 1974; 10:1624–1628.
25. Daly DA: Helping the Clutterer: Therapy Considerations, in Meyers F, St. Louis KO (eds): *Cluttering: A Clinical Perspective*. Kibworth, England, Far Communications, 1992. Reissued by Singular Publishing Group, 1996.
26. Perkins WH: *Human Perspectives in Speech and Language Disorders*. Mosby, St. Louis, 1978.
27. Van Riper C: Stuttering and cluttering: The differential diagnosis. *Folia Phoniatr (Basel)* 1970; 22:347–353.
28. Preus A: Cluttering and Stuttering: Related, Different, or Antagonistic Disorders, in Meyers F, St. Louis KO (eds): *Cluttering: A Clinical Perspective*. Kibworth, England, Far Communications, 1992.
29. Daly DA, Burnett-Stolnack M: Use of Cluttering Checklist and Profile Analysis in Planning Treatment for Cluttering Clients, in Starkweather CW, Peters HFM (eds): *Stuttering: Proceedings of the First World Congress on Fluency Disorders*. International Fluency Assoc., Nijmegen, The Netherlands: University Press, 1995.
30. Daly DA: *The Source for Stuttering and Cluttering*. East Moline, IL. LinguiSystems, Inc. 1996.
31. Pearson L: Studies in tachyphemia: V. Rhythm and dysrhythmia in cluttering associated with congenital language disability. *Logos* 1962; 5:51–59.
32. Daly DA, Ostreicher HJ, Jonassen SA, Darnton SW: Memory for Unrelated Sentences: A Normative Study of 480 Children. Presented at the annual convention of the International Neuropsychological Society, Atlanta, 1981.
33. Conture EG, Van Naerssen E: Reading abilities of school-age stutterers. *J Fluency Disord* 1977; 2:295–300.
34. Nippold MA, Schwartz IE: Reading disorders in stuttering children: Fact or fiction? *J Fluency Disord* 1990; 15:175–189.
35. Roman KG, Handwriting and speech. *Logos* 1959; 2:29.
36. Orton St: *Reading, Writing, Speech Problems in Children*. Norton, New York, 1937.
37. Spadino EJ: *Writing and Laterality Characteristics of Stuttering Children*. Teachers College, New York 1941.
38. Sheperd G: Studies in tachyphemia: II. Phonetic description of cluttered speech. *Logos* 1960; 3:73–81.
39. de Hirsch K: Studies in tachyphemia: IV. Diagnosis of developmental language disorders. *Logos* 1961; 4:3–9.
40. Roman-Goldzieher K: Studies in tachyphemia. VI. The interrelationship of graphologic and oral aspects of language behavior. *Logos* 1963; 6:41–58.
41. Teigland A: A study of pragmatic skills of clutterers and speakers. *J Fluency Disord* 1996; 21: 201–214.

42. Prutting C, Kirchner D: A clinical appraisal of the pragmatic aspects of language. *J Speech Hearing Disord* 1987; 52:105–119.
43. Myers FL: Cluttering: A matter of perspective. *J Fluency Disord* 1996, 21:175–185.
44. Martin R, Kroll R, O'Keefe B, Painter C: Cluttered Speech: Spectrographic Data. Presented at convention of the American Speech-Language-Hearing Association, Cincinnati, 1983.
45. Seeman M, Novak A: Ueber die Motorik bei Polteran. *Folia Phoniatr (Basel)* 1963; 15:170–176.
46. Seeman R: Relations between motorics of speech and general motor ability in clutterers. *Folia Phoniatr (Basel)* 1970; 22:376–378.
47. Wyatt GL: *Language Learning and Communication Disorders in Children.* The Free Press, New York, 1969.
48. Wohl MT: The treatment of the non-fluent utterance—A behavioral approach. *Br J Disord Commun* 1970; 5:66–76.
49. Bakwin RM, Bakwin H: Cluttering. *J Pediatr* 1952, 40:393–396.
50. Arnold GE: Studies in tachyphemia: I. Present concepts of etiologic factors. *Logos* 1960; 3: 24–45.
51. Daly DA: Cluttering: Another fluency syndrome, in Curlee, RF (ed): *Stuttering and Related Disorders of Fluency.* New York: Thieme Medical Publishers, Inc., 1993.
52. Bloodstein O: *A Handbook on Stuttering* (2nd ed). San Diego: Singular Publishing Group, 1995.
53. Frick JV: Evaluation of Motor Planning Techniques for the Treatment of Stuttering. US Department of Health, Education and Welfare, Office of Education Research Final Grant Report. 1965.
54. Grewel F: Cluttering and its problems. *Folia Phoniatr (Basel)* 1970; 22:301–310.
55. Hood SB: The Assessment of Fluency Disorders, in Singh S, Lynch J (eds): *Diagnostic Procedures in Hearing, Language, and Speech.* Baltimore, University Park Press, 1978.
56. Gregory HH, Hill D: Stuttering therapy for children. *Seminars Speech Lang Hear* 1980; 1:351–363.
57. Riley G, Riley J: Evaluation as a Basis for Intervention, in Prins D, Ingram RJ: *Treatment of Stuttering in Early Childhood.* San Diego, College-Hill Press, 1983.
58. Bloodstein O: Stuttering as Tension and Fragmentation, in Eisenson J (ed): *Stuttering: A Second Symposium.* New York, Harper & Row, 1975.
59. Blood GW, Seider R: The concomitant problems of young stutterers. *J Speech Hear Disord* 1981; 46:31–33.
60. Daly A: Considerations for Treating Stutterers with and without Concomitant Articulation Disorders. Presented at the annual convention of the American Speech-Language-Hearing Association, Toronto, 1982.
61. Nippold MA: Concomitant speech and language disorders in stuttering children: A critique of the literature. *J Speech Hear Disord* 1990; 55:51–60.
62. Preus A: The cluttering type of stutterer. *Scand J Logoped Phoniatr* 1987; 12:3–19.
63. Daly DA, Myers FL, St. Louis KO: Cluttering: A Pathology Lost but Found. Paper presented at the annual convention of the American Speech-Language-Hearing Assoc., San Antonia, 1992.
64. Freund H: Observations on tachylalia. *Folia Phoniatr (Basel)* 1970; 22:280–288.
65. Kidd KK: Genetic models of cluttering. *J Fluency Dis* 1980;5:187–202.
66. Seeman M: Speech Pathology in Czechoslovakia, in Rieber RW, Brubaker RS: *Speech Pathology: An International Study of the Science.* Philadelphia, JB Lippincott, 1966.
67. Van Riper C: Foreword, in Myers F, St. Louis KO (eds): *Cluttering: A Clinical Perspective.* Kinworth, Great Britain: Far Communications. 1992. Re-issued by Singular Publishing Group. 1996.
68. Woolf G: The assessment of stuttering as struggle, avoidance, and expectancy. *Br J Disord Commun* 1967; 2:158–171.
69. Daly DA, Oaks D, Breen K, et al.: Perceptions of Stuttering Inventory: Norms for Adolescent Stutterers and Nonstutterers. Presented at the annual convention of ASHA, 1981, Los Angeles.
70. Daly DA, Darnton SW: Intensive Fluency Shaping and Attitudinal Therapy with Stutterers. A Follow-up Study. Presented at the annual convention of the American Speech Language Hearing Assoc. Houston, 1976.
71. Fletcher SG: Time-by-count measurement of diadochokinetic syllable rate. *J Speech Hearing Res* 1972; 15: 763–770.
72. Riley G, Riley J: Oral motor discoordination among children who stutter. *J Fluency Dis* 1986; 11: 334–344.
73. Riley G, Riley J: *Oral Motor Assessment and Treatment: Improving Syllable Production.* Austin, TX, Pro-Ed, 1985.

74. Riley G, Riley J: Treatment Implications of Oral Motor Discoordination, in Peters HFM, Hulstijn W, Starkweather CW (eds): *Speech Motor Control and Stuttering*. Amsterdam, Elsevier Science Publishers, 1991.

75. Daly DA, Burnett-Stolnack M: Identification of and treatment planning for cluttering clients: Two practical tools. *Clin Connect* 1994; 8:1–5.

76. Daly DA, Burnett ML: Cluttering: assessment, treatment planning, and case study illustration. *J Fluency Disord* 1996; 21: 239–248.

77. St. Louis KO, Myers FL: Clinical management of cluttering. *Lang Speech Hearing Serv Schools* 1995, 26:187–195.

78. St. Louis KO, Myers FL: Management of Cluttering and Related Fluency Disorders, in Curlee RL, Siegel G (eds): *Nature and Treatment of Stuttering: New Directions*, 2nd ed. Boston, Allyn and Bacon, 1997.

79. Myers FL, Bradley CL: Clinical Management of Cluttering from a Synergistic Framework, in Myers FL, St. Louis KO (eds): *Cluttering: A Clinical Perspective*. Kibworth, England: Far Communications, 1992. Reissued by Singular Publishing Group, San Diego, CA, 1996.

80. Katz-Bernstein N: Psychological Emotional and Verbal Aspects of Speech Dysfluency: A Multidimensional Method of Treating Stuttering and Cluttering Children, in Starkweather CW, Peters HFM (eds): *Stuttering: Proceedings of the First World Congress on Fluency Disorders*. International Fluency Assoc., Nijmegen, The Netherlands: University Press, 1995.

81. Langevin M, Boberg E: Results of intensive stuttering therapy with adults who clutter and stutter. *J Fluency Dis* 1996; 21: 315–327.

Appendix A: Perceptions of Speech Communication

S _____	PSC Total
A _____	_____

Name _____   E _____

Address _____   Date _____

Directions

Here are 60 statements about speech behavior. Some of these may be characteristic of your speech. Read each item carefully and respond as in the example below.

Characteristic of me
□ Repeating sounds.

Put a check mark (✓ under characteristic of me if "repeating sounds" is part of your speech; if it is not characteristic, leave the box blank.

Characteristic of me refers only to what you do now, not to what was true of your speech in the past and which you no longer do; and not what you think you should or should not be doing. Even if the behavior described occurs only occasionally or only in some speaking situations, if you regard it as characteristic of your speech, check the box under characteristic of me. Be accurate in your judgments.

Characteristic of me
□ 1. Avoiding talking to people in authority (e.g., a teacher, employer, or clergyman).
□ 2. Feeling that interruptions in your speech (e.g., pauses, hesitations, or repetitions) will lead to speaking difficulty.
□ 3. Making the pitch of your voice higher or lower when you expect to get "stuck" on words.
□ 4. Having extra and unnecessary facial movements (e.g., flaring your nostrils during speech attempts).
□ 5. Using gestures as a substitute for speaking (e.g., nodding your head instead of saying "yes" or smiling to acknowlege a greeting).

☐ 6. Avoiding asking for information (e.g., asking for directions or inquiring about a train schedule).

☐ 7. Whispering words to yourself before saying them or practicing what you are planning to say long before you speak.

☐ 8. Choosing a job or hobby because little speaking would be required.

☐ 9. Adding an extra and unnecessary sound, word, or phrase to your speech (e.g., "uh," "well," or "let me see") to help yourself get started.

☐ 10. Replying briefly using the fewest words possible.

☐ 11. Making sudden jerky or forceful movements with your head, arms, or body during speech attempts (e.g., clenching your fist, jerking your head to one side).

☐ 12. Repeating a sound or word with effort.

☐ 13. Acting in a manner intended to keep you out of a conversation or discussion (e.g., being a good listener, pretending not to hear what was said, acting bored, or pretending to be in deep thought).

☐ 14. Avoiding making a purchase (e.g., going into a store or buying stamps in the post office).

☐ 15. Breathing noisily or with great effort while trying to speak.

☐ 16. Making your voice louder or softer when speaking difficulty is expected.

☐ 17. Prolonging a sound or word (e.g., m-m-m-m-my) while trying to push it out.

☐ 18. Helping yourself to get started talking by laughing, coughing, clearing your throat, gesturing, or some other body activity or movement.

☐ 19. Having general body tension during speech attempts (e.g., shaking, trembling, or feeling "knotted up" inside).

☐ 20. Paying particular attention to what you are going to say (e.g., the length of a word, or the position of a word in a sentence).

☐ 21. Feeling your face getting warm and red (as if you are blushing), as you are struggling to speak.

☐ 22. Saying words or phrases with force or effort.

☐ 23. Repeating a word or phase preceding the word on which speaking difficulty is expected.

☐ 24. Speaking so that no word or sound stands out (e.g., speaking in a singsong voice or in a monotone).

☐ 25. Avoiding making new acquaintances (e.g., not visiting with friends, not dating, or not joining social, civic, or church groups).

☐ 26. Making unusual noises with your teeth during speech attempts (e.g., grinding or clicking your teeth).

☐ 27. Avoiding introducing yourself, giving your name, or making introductions.

☐ 28. Expecting that certain sounds, letters, or words are going to be particularly "hard" to say (e.g., words beginning with the letter "s").

☐ 29. Giving excuses to avoid talking (e.g., pretending to be tired or pretending lack of interest in a topic).

☐ 30. "Running out of breath" while speaking.

☐ 31. Forcing out sounds.

☐ 32. Feeling that your periods of smooth speech are unusual, that they cannot last, and that sooner or later you will have speaking difficulty.

☐ 33. Concentrating on relaxing or not being tense before speaking.

☐ 34. Substituting a different word or phrase for the one you had intended to say.

☐ 35. Prolonging or emphasizing the sound preceding the one on which speaking difficulty is expected.

- [ ] 36. Avoiding speaking before an audience.
- [ ] 37. Straining to talk without being able to make a sound.
- [ ] 38. Coordinating or timing your speech with a rhythmic movement (e.g., tapping your foot or swinging your arm).
- [ ] 39. Rearranging what you had planned to say to avoid a "hard" sound or word.
- [ ] 40. "Putting on an act" when speaking (e.g., adopting an attitude of confidence or pretending to be antry).
- [ ] 41. Avoiding the use of the telephone.
- [ ] 42. Making forceful and strained movements with your lips, tongue, jaw, or throat (e.g., moving your jaw in an uncoordinated manner).
- [ ] 43. Omitting a word, part of a word, or phrase which you had planned to say (e.g., words with certain sounds or letters).
- [ ] 44. Making "uncontrollable" sounds while struggling to say a word.
- [ ] 45. Adopting a foreign accent, assuming a regional dialect, or imitating another person's speech.
- [ ] 46. Perspiring much more than usual while speaking (e.g., feeling the palms of your hands getting clammy).
- [ ] 47. Postponing speaking for a short time until you are certain you can use smooth speech (e.g., pausing before "hard words").
- [ ] 48. Having extra and unnecessary eye movements while speaking (e.g., blinking your eyes or shutting your eyes tightly).
- [ ] 49. Breathing forcefully while struggling to speak.
- [ ] 50. Avoiding talking to others of your own age group (your own or the opposite sex).
- [ ] 51. Giving up the speech attempt completely after getting "stuck" or if difficulty is anticipated.
- [ ] 52. Straining the muscles of your chest or abdomen during speech attempts.
- [ ] 53. Wondering whether you will have difficulty speaking and how it will it sound if you do.
- [ ] 54. Holding your lips, tongue, or jaw in a rigid position before speaking or when getting "stuck" on a word.
- [ ] 55. Avoiding talking to one or both of your parents.
- [ ] 56. Having another person speak for you in a difficult situation (e.g., having someone make a telephone call for you or order for you in a restaurant).
- [ ] 57. Holding your breath before speaking.
- [ ] 58. Saying words slowly or rapidly preceding the word on which speaking difficulty is expected.
- [ ] 59. Concentrating on how you are going to speak (e.g., thinking about where to put your tongue or how to breathe).
- [ ] 60. Using your speech difficulty as a reason to avoid a speaking activity.

The Perceptions of Stuttering Inventory (PSI) from which this inventory (PSC*) was adapted was developed by Dr. Gerald Woolf, currently at Montclair State College, Upper Montclair, New Jersey, and originally published in the *British Journal of Disorders of Communication* 1967; 2:158–177.

Do you now or have you ever had a speech problem?   Yes ☐   No ☐
If Yes, please specify.

Foreign dialect   Yes ☐   No ☐*

---

*PSC adapted by David A. Daly, University of Michigan, 1978.

Appendix B: Checklist for Identification of Cluttering—Revised (David A. Daly and Michelle L. Burnett, 1997)

Client's Name _____   Date _____

Instructions: Please respond to each descriptive statement below. Your answer should reflect how accurately you believe the statement is true for the client.

Statement True for Client	Not at all	Just a little	Pretty much	Very much
1. Repeats words or phrases	0	1	2	3
2. Started talking late; onset of words and sentences delayed	0	1	2	3
3. Never very fluent; fluency disruptions started early	0	1	2	3
4. Language is disorganized; confused wording	0	1	2	3
5. Silent gaps or hesitations common	0	1	2	3
6. Interjections; many filler words	0	1	2	3
7. Little or no tension observed during disfluencies	0	1	2	3
8. Rapid rate (tachylalia) or irregular rate; speaks in spurts	0	1	2	3
9. Compulsive talker; verbose or tangential	0	1	2	3
10. Respiratory dysrhythmia; jerky breathing pattern	0	1	2	3
11. Slurred articulation (deletes, adds or distorts speech sounds)	0	1	2	3
12. Speech better under pressure (during periods of heightened attention)	0	1	2	3
13. Difficulty following directions; impatient/disinterested listener	0	1	2	3
14. Distractible, attention span problems, poor concentration	0	1	2	3
15. Poor language formulation; storytelling difficulty; trouble sequencing ideas	0	1	2	3
16. Demonstrates word-finding difficulties resembling anomia	0	1	2	3
17. Inappropriate pronoun referents; overuse of pronouns	0	1	2	3
18. Improper linguistic structure; poor grammar and syntax	0	1	2	3
19. Clumsy and uncoordinated, motor activities accelerated or hasty, impulsive	0	1	2	3
20. Reading disorder or difficulty reported or noted	0	1	2	3
21. Disintegrated and fractionated writing; poor motor control	0	1	2	3
22. Writing shows omission or transposition of letters, syllables, or words	0	1	2	3

Statement True for Client	Not at all	Just a little	Pretty much	Very much
23. Initial loud voice, trails off to a murmur; mumbles	0	1	2	3
24. Seems to verbalize prior to adequate thought formulation	0	1	2	3
25. Above average in mathematical and abstract reasoning abilities	0	1	2	3
26. Poor rhythm, timing, or musical ability (may dislike singing)	0	1	2	3
27. Variable prosody; improper/irregular melody or stress patterns in speaking	0	1	2	3
28. Appears, acts or sounds younger than age; immature	0	1	2	3
29. Other family member(s) with similar speech problem(s)	0	1	2	3
30. Untidy, careless, or forgetful; impatient, superficial, short-tempered	0	1	2	3
31. Lack of awareness of self and/or communication disorder(s)	0	1	2	3
32. Inappropriate turn-taking	0	1	2	3
33. Inappropriate topic introduction/maintenance/termination	0	1	2	3
34. Poor recognition or acknowledgement of non-verbal signals	0	1	2	3
35. Telescopes or condenses words (omits or transposes syllables)	0	1	2	3
36. Lack of effective/sufficient self monitoring	0	1	2	3

DIAGNOSIS _____ TOTAL SCORE _____

Clinician _____

Appendix C: Profile Analysis for Planning Treatment With Cluttering Clients—Revised (David A. Daly and Michelle L. Burnett, 1997)

Client's Name _____ Date _____

	Undesirably different from normal		Normal or above
	−3	−2	−1	0

A. COGNITION and LANGUAGE

(12) Speech better under pressure (during periods of heightened attention)

(14) Distractible, attention span problems, poor concentration

	Undesirably different from normal		Normal or above
	−3	−2	−1	0

A. COGNITION and LANGUAGE (cont.)

(24) Seems to verbalize prior to adequate thought formulation

(25) Above average in mathematical and abstract reasoning abilities

(31) Lack of awareness of self and/or communication disorder(s)

(36) Lack of effective/sufficient self monitoring

(4) Language is disorganized; confused wording

(6) Interjections; many filler words

(13) Difficulty following directions; impatient/disinterested listener

(15) Poor language formulation; storytelling difficulty; trouble sequencing ideas

(16) Demonstrates word-finding difficulties resembling anomia

(17) Inappropriate pronoun referents; overuse of pronouns

(18) Improper linguistic structure; poor grammar and syntax

(20) Reading disorder or difficulty reported or noted

(22) Writing shows omission or transposition of letters, syllables, or words

B. PRAGMATICS

(9) Compulsive talker; verbose or tangential

(32) Inappropriate turn-taking

(33) Inappropriate topic introduction/maintenance/termination

(34) Poor recognition or acknowledgement of non-verbal signals

C. SPEECH and MOTOR

(1) Repeats words or phrases

(8) Rapid rate (tachylalia) or irregular rate; speaks in spurts

(11) Slurred articulation (deletes, adds or distorts speech sounds)

(23) Initial loud voice, trails off to a murmur; mumbles

(27) Variable prosody; improper/irregular melody or stress patterns in speaking

(35) Telescopes or condenses words (omits or transposes syllables)

(5) Silent gaps or hesitations common

(7) Little or no tension observed during disfluencies

(10) Respiratory dysrhythmia; jerky breathing pattern

(19) Clumsy and uncoordinated, motor activities accelerated or hasty, impulsive

(21) Disintegrated and fractionated writing; poor motor control

(26) Poor rhythm, timing, or musical ability (may dislike singing)

	Undesirably different from normal		Normal or above
	−3	−2 −1	0

D. DEVELOPMENT

  (2) Started talking late; onset of words and sentences delayed

  (3) Never very fluent; fluency disruptions started early

(28) Appears, acts or sounds younger than age; immature

(29) Other family member(s) with similar speech problem(s)

(30) Untidy, careless, or forgetful; impatient, superficial, short-tempered

Stuttering and Related Disorders of Fluency, 2nd edition.
Edited by Richard F. Curlee, Ph.D.
Thieme Medical Publishers, Inc., New York   1999.

13

Stuttering Associated with Acquired Neurological Disorders

Nancy Helm-Estabrooks

Introduction

Acquired Neurological Stuttering

Prior to 1978 references to onset of stuttering in association with some neurological event were sparse.[1] In that year, however, two papers describing a total of 17 cases were published. In one paper Rosenbek and colleagues[2] described seven brain-damaged patients who developed "cortical stuttering" after cerebral vascular accidents (CVAs). In the second paper two colleagues and I[3] described acquired stuttering in 10 adults, six of whom had CVAs and four with traumatic brain injury. Since these 1978 publications, over 60 additional cases of neurogenic stuttering have been described as associated with a variety of temporary, progressive, and nonprogressive neurological disorders. These include traumatic brain injury and strokes,[4] extrapyramidal diseases,[5,6] Alzheimer's Disease,[7] brain tumor,[8] encephalitis,[9] dialysis dementia,[10] drug toxicity,[11,12] and anorexia nervosa.[13] Thus, acquired stuttering may not be as rare as once thought. In fact, a national survey by Market and colleagues[14] found that 81% of more than 100 speech–language pathologists reported having seen patients with acquired stuttering.

In addition to those cases in which stuttering appeared for the first time in adulthood, several have been reported in which childhood stuttering worsened or reappeared with the onset of neurological disorders. For example, in their report of 16 cases of neurogenic stuttering, Mazzucchi et al.[4] described three adult patients whose mild developmental stuttering was exacerbated either by CVAs or head trauma. A fourth patient's childhood stuttering recurred with onset of a left temporal lobe stroke. Similarly, several colleagues and I reported on a 61-year-old, ambidextrous man who outgrew his childhood stuttering only to have it reappear after a stroke.[15] Recurrence of childhood stuttering was also the first symptom of an Alzheimer's-like dementia in a 62-year-old man described by Quinn and Andrews.[16] In this case, onset of stuttering occurred 7 months before the appearance of other neurological signs and was, therefore, a harbinger of the dementing disease. Thus, stuttering may occur, worsen, or recur in the presence of neurological dysfunction.

Defining and Delineating Neurogenic Stuttering

A crucial question regarding these reports of neurogenic stuttering is what behaviors are being labeled as "stuttering"? Classically, "stuttering" has been used to designate the signs and symptoms displayed by individuals whose speech becomes notably dysfluent* as children. Many clinicians, therefore, are not comfortable applying this label to the speech of adults having no history of childhood stuttering. The World Health Organization (WHO) definition of stuttering, however, makes no reference to when in life this phenomenon first appears. Instead, it focuses solely on speech behavior, defining stuttering as

> disorders in the rhythm of speech in which the individual knows precisely what he wishes to say but at the time is unable to say it because of an involuntary repetition, prolongation, or cessation of a sound.[17]

Two concepts in the WHO definition deserve special attention. The first is its use of "disorders." This implies that stuttering is *not* a unitary disorder, a view that seems to be true of developmental stuttering. For example, some forms of developmental stuttering persist into adulthood even though most disappear prior to puberty.[18] Some forms appear to be idiopathic, but others likely have a genetic component. Some forms are associated with phonological and other language problems, whereas others appear to be isolated motor speech phenomena.

Likewise, acquired stuttering appears not to be a unitary disorder.[19] Some forms of acquired stuttering are transient, but others are persistent. Some forms are associated with speech, language, and cognitive disorders; others are not. And, as mentioned above, neurogenic stuttering is associated with a variety of conditions affecting various areas of the brain, including the cerebral cortex, basal ganglia, cerebellum, and brain stem. Thus, acquired stuttering may result from damage to or involvement of the pyramidal, extra-pyramidal, corticobulbar, and cerebellar motor systems. In some studies, such as that by Ludlow and colleagues,[20] computed tomography (CT) scans were used to identify lesion sites in patients exhibiting this disorder. A more recent report[21] showed that SPECT studies may be more useful than CT or MRI in accurately determining sites of brain lesion.

The second concept in the WHO definition that deserves special attention is that "the individual knows precisely what he wishes to say ..." This implies that the dysfluency is not secondary to aphasic word-finding problems, which may pose diagnostic challenges because neurogenic stuttering has, indeed, been described in association with aphasia. According to Baumgartner and Duffy,[22] 35% of the neurogenic stuttering cases reported in the literature also had some degree of aphasia. In fact, Arnold and Luchsinger[23] discussed three varieties of acquired stuttering that accompany aphasia: aphasic stuttering, in which speech dysfluencies are a part of the language disorder; stuttering with aphasia, thought to reflect a psychological reaction to the aphasia; and dysarthric stuttering, which may occur during the recovery phase of any type of aphasia, especially expressive aphasia. It is important to note, however, that stuttering rarely accompanies aphasia which is a common sequelae of acquired brain damage. Furthermore, 65% of the cases of neurogenic stuttering reported did not have aphasia, so it would appear that although the two phenomenon may co-occur, they are not causally related. Still, in diagnosing acquired stuttering, it is crucial to rule out language problems as a basis for the dysfluency.

---

*In the neurogenic stuttering literature, the spelling "dysfluent" rather than "disfluent" is used most often.

To account for all cases of stuttering associated with acquired neurological disorders I propose the following definition:

> Stuttering associated with acquired neurological disorders (SAAND) is an acquired or reacquired disorder of fluency characterized by notable, involuntary repetitions or prolongations of speech that are not the result of language formulation or psychiatric problems.

Disappearance of Stuttering with Neurological Changes

Before discussing clinical evaluation of SAAND, I should mention that remission of developmental stuttering has occurred on occasion with changes in neurological status. Jones,[24] for example, described four males who stuttered prior to neurosurgical procedures (three for aneurysm, one for tumor). All had personal and family histories of left-handedness, and presurgical carotid amobarbital tests showed that all had bilateral representation of spoken language. Following surgery, all four ceased to stutter, and amobarbital testing now showed unilateral representation for speech.

Miller[25] described two male patients whose severe childhood stuttering continued into adulthood until they developed multiple sclerosis (MS) and their stuttering began to remit. As MS progressed, stuttering lessened until they no longer stuttered, although dysarthric speech had appeared. Both patients had clinical evidence of bilateral cerebellar disease.

Finally, I had an opportunity to work with an ambidextrous man whose severe developmental stuttering remitted following a head injury.[15] This young man sustained a right subdural hematoma and a loss of consciousness for 10 days. Upon awakening, he spoke at a slower rate than before, with signs of mild dysarthria but no stuttering. To quote Miller: "These cases serve to emphasize the complexity with which neurologic lesions can alter human speech, even result in a paradoxical improvement in oral communication."[25]

Diagnosis of SAAND

Neurogenic versus Psychogenic Stuttering

Compared to neurogenic stuttering, there are relatively few cases reported of adults diagnosed with psychogenic stuttering. According to Duffy,[26] however, 43 of 215 (20%) patients having acquired psychogenic speech or voice disorders also manifested stuttering-like dysfluencies. In a 1997 retrospective study, Baumgartner and Duffy[22] reviewed the characteristics of 69 patients, all of whom were diagnosed as having psychogenic stuttering by clinicians at the Mayo Clinic. Of these, 20 had confirmed neurologic impairments with closed-head injury and seizure disorders being the most common. Two claimed a history of mild aphasia which had resolved at the time of testing. After comparing the speech–language records of these psychogenic cases with those reported for cases of neurogenic stuttering, Baumgardner and Duffy concluded that the two groups could not be distinguished solely on the basis of the speech dysfluency. Features that did seem to distinguish the psychogenic patients, however, were as follows:

1. Rapid and favorable response to just one or two sessions of behavioral treatment.
2. Struggle behaviors and other signs of anxiety.
3. Intermittent or situational-specific episodes of stuttering.
4. Presence of unusual grammatical constructions, e.g., "Me get sick." and bizarre speech such as multiple repetitions of nearly all phonemes with simultaneous head bobbing, facial grimacing, and tremor-like arm movements.

As a word of caution vis à vis these patients' quick response to behavioral treatment, Duffy and Baumgartner point out that only about half received treatment and that the success rate reported may have been lower if all patients had been treated. As to the cause of psychogenic stuttering, Duffy and Baumgartner's cases were diagnosed most frequently as having a conversion reaction, anxiety neurosis, or depression. Some patients had no prior history of psychiatric problems.

My own experience with psychogenic stuttering[19] includes three cases, two patients of which were veterans of the armed services. Both had long histories of psychological problems and had repeatedly sought government compensation for stress they experienced while in the service. Their "stuttering" appeared suddenly, was not present in all situations, and disappeared after a few months without treatment. The third person's transient stuttering began during a severe anxiety attack and disappeared within a week.

I should mention also that onset of SAAND may coincide with psychologically traumatic events for persons with known neurological disease. For example, I once saw a man with Parkinson's disease who had a sudden worsening of speech problems and the onset of stuttering-like behaviors after his small car was sideswiped by a trailer truck on the highway. Although he received no apparent physical injuries, it was thought that the release of various neurochemicals in response to his great fright may have been responsible for the onset of stuttering in someone with an already compromised nervous system.

HANDEDNESS AND ACQUIRED STUTTERING

Interestingly, the man described just above had a lifelong history of ambidexterity which raised the long-standing issue of anomalous dominance for language in persons with either developmental or acquired stuttering.[15]

Unfortunately, handedness is seldom reported in cases of acquired stuttering. Without more thorough investigations of the handedness history of these patients and their families, the extent to which left-handed and ambidextrous people are at higher risk for SAAND remains uncertain. If anomalous language dominance does play a role in this disorder, then these patients might be expected to report a higher incidence of learning disabilities and other characteristics associated with left-handedness.[27]

The Case History

A detailed case history is of utmost importance in the differential diagnosis of SAAND. Information important for diagnosing SAAND includes the following:

1. Onset of current speech problem and any treatment received.
2. Handedness of individual and family members.
3. Individual's past history and treatment of speech, language, or learning problems.
4. Years of education and age when completed.
5. Employment history.
6. Family history of speech, language or learning problems.
7. Health history (with dates) to include the following:
   a. Neurologic disease
   b. Head trauma
   c. Periods of unconsciousness
   d. Seizures

e. Substance abuse
f. Prescriptive and nonprescriptive medications
g. Surgery and hospitalizations
h. Psychiatric problems and treatment

To underscore the importance of case history information, consider the following two cases whose primary diagnoses were psychogenic stuttering. In the first case, Deal[28] described a 28-year-old male who began to stutter after attempting suicide. The means employed in this suicide attempt were not reported, but the patient was in a methadone program at the time for drug abuse. At age 16 he had attempted suicide by cutting his throat and had stuttered for "approximately 7 or 8 days afterward." There was no mention of whether there was a loss of consciousness with either attempt. Furthermore, he had a history of arrests for car theft and other behaviors that placed him in a group at high risk for head trauma. Lastly, he was "well known" to the psychiatry service, which suggests that he may have been receiving antidepressive or antipsychotic drugs. Clearly, this case presents a difficult diagnosis because of the documented history of psychiatric, and possible neurologic, problems. The fact that he was dysfluent across speech tasks and showed no anxiety or secondary behaviors suggest a neurogenic basis for his stuttering. The fact that he showed good response to a month of treatment to delayed auditory feedback (DAF) does not help solve this diagnostic dilemma, because DAF has been used successfully with neurogenic cases.

A second case thought to be "psychogenic in onset" was described by Attanasio,[29] who also acknowledged that there was a "possible neurologic base" for the stuttering. The problem began in an adult male who was having marital difficulties and whose stuttering worsened until it became "full blown" at the time of the divorce a few years later. Attanasio went on to say that "what cannot be ignored is the fact that he had epilepsy." His first seizure occurred at age 11, and he was taking premedian (Mysoline) and phenobarbital at time of his speech evaluation at age 36. His last "grand mal" seizure was at age 33. Thus, one must rule out that his stuttering was unrelated to epilepsy or his medications and was, indeed, psychogenic in nature.

The Speech and Language Exam

Distinguishing Features of SAAND

The diagnosing label of SAAND indicates that an individual currently evidences or has a history of a neurological problem. If a patient demonstrates the features that Baumgartner and Duffy[22] identified for psychogenic stuttering, however, a diagnosis of psychogenic stuttering may be made even in the presence of a neurologic disorder.

The first step in a differential diagnosis of SAAND is to rule out aphasia as basis for the patient's dysfluencies, using a standardized exam. My choice is the Aphasia Diagnostic Profiles (ADP),[30] which can be administered in about a half hour and has norms for both aphasic and nonaphasic individuals. These norms will be helpful in determining whether language formulation problems are present. If they are, then it is important to note the loci of the sound and syllable repetitions and prolongations vis à vis word-finding pauses. This can be accomplished by analyzing the three taped samples of narrative speech obtained for ADP scoring.

Once aphasia has been ruled out, attention can be focused on the speech dysfluencies.

Several features are commonly described for neurogenic stuttering[2,31] and help to distinguish it from both psychogenic and developmental stuttering in adults. These are as follows:

1. Dysfluencies occur on grammatical words nearly as frequently as on substantive words.
2. The speaker may be annoyed but does not appear anxious.
3. Repetitions, prolongations, and blocks do not occur only on initial syllables of words and utterances.
4. Secondary symptoms such as facial grimacing, eye blinking, or fist clenching are not associated with moments of dysfluency.
5. There is no adaptation effect.
6. Stuttering occurs relatively consistently across various types of speech tasks.

Analysis of the taped ADP narrative samples can be used to determine the presence of the first four distinguishing features. Ideally, videotapes should be used to record any accessory behaviors, such as facial grimacing, eye blinking, or fist clenching, that may accompany instances of stuttering. But in the absence of videotaping, clinicians should watch for these behaviors, note their presence, and describe their nature.

Another important step in the diagnosis of SAAND is to establish if the patient displays an adaptation effect with fewer and fewer dysfluencies on repeated readings of a passage. To determine the presence of adaptation, a standard passage such as "The Rainbow Passage"[32] which contain all the sounds in the English language is recommended.

Finally, the clinician needs to determine whether the person suspected of SAAND produces dysfluencies on highly automatized speech tasks such as counting to 30; reciting the months of the year, "The Lord's Prayer," or "The Pledge of Allegiance", and singing popular songs.

Thus, the following speech and language tasks are recommended for diagnosing SAAND:

1. Aphasia Diagnostic Profiles[31]
2. "The Rainbow Passage"[32]
3. Automatized recitations:
   Counting to 30.
   Months of the year.
   "The Pledge of Allegiance" or "The Lord's Prayer."
4. Singing familiar songs.

In some cases, SAAND may need to be distinguished from the neurological speech disorder, palilalia. In this disorder, whole words and phrases, rather than individual sounds, are repeated, often with increasing speed and decreasing distinctness. Palilalia is most often associated with diseases affecting the basal ganglia, particularly postencephalitic Parkinson's disease. For example, I reported on such a patient who, when asked his name, repeated, "My name, my name, my name ..." over 30 times.[33]

OTHER TESTS SOMETIMES NEEDED FOR OPTIMAL MANAGEMENT OF SAAND

Individuals who have SAAND, by definition, also suffer from some neurological disorder. Depending on the nature, site of lesion, and extent of brain involvement, this neurological disorder may give rise to problems other than stuttering which are important to treatment decisions. Consider, for example, that some patients with dementia develop SAAND, but also commonly experience memory problems from the earliest stages of the disease. Similarly, head trauma, probably the most common cause of SAAND, may be associated with memory loss. Closed head injury, in particular, often results in the shearing of neuronal axons and swelling of brain tissue, causing complex behavioral sequelae and cognitive deficits that affect memory and initiation skills. Obviously, memory problems will interfere with learning new strategies for speaking, and initiation problems may result in the patient's failure to use communication aids such as a pacing board.[34] Depending on the etiology of SAAND, therefore, the speech–language pathologist may need to probe other skill areas with such tests as the Arizona Battery for Communication Disorders in Dementia,[35] the Brief Test of Head Injury,[36] or the Scales of Cognitive Ability for Traumatic Brain Injury.[37] In addition, reports of neuropsychological and neurological examinations may be crucial in selecting patients for treatment of SAAND and in choosing appropriate management techniques.

Criteria for Case Management Decisions

In foregoing sections I stressed the importance of obtaining thorough case histories and formal test results in diagnosing SAAND and identifying any coexisting language and cognitive deficits. Based on the information gleaned from these findings, decisions can be made whether or not a particular patient is a candidate for therapeutic intervention and, if so, what specific approaches may produce the best results.

Probably, the first question in selecting SAAND patients for therapeutic intervention is, "Does stuttering present a communication handicap?" In some cases the patient's dysfluencies are so mild that, although noticeable, they do not interfere appreciably with communication. In other cases, stuttering may be part of a larger communication problem which must take precedence in the rehabilitation program. If stuttering is judged to be a significant speech handicap, then the next question is the following: "Is the individual motivated to work on this problem?" One of the behavioral features of SAAND is that patients may be somewhat annoyed, but not highly anxious, about the stuttering. Probably depending on the neuropathology of their disorders, other patients may show total indifference to their dysfluencies, making them poor candidates for any therapeutic program that involves behavior modification. Similarly, patients with initiation problems often fail to implement newly learned strategies and techniques when left to their own devices. For example, one highly dysfluent patient I saw could speak without repeating sounds and words when using a pacing board but he never initiated its use. This did not deter us from giving him the board[34] and training him to pace his speech, but we also had to train caretakers to place it in his hands and encourage him to use it when talking.

Another question regarding a patient's candidacy for SAAND treatment is: "Does the patient have a rapidly progressing neurological disorder?" If so, then even severe stuttering may be only a minor problem in the overall scheme of life. For example, two studies[10,38] described adult-onset stuttering in patients with dialysis dementia. These patients had been given extensive dialysis therapy for kidney disease when stuttering appeared along with early signs of confusion and dementia. As their conditions worsened, the patients became mute and finally died. Because of the severe and progressive nature of their disease, these patients probably were not candidates for speech therapy. Similarly, I examined a patient who developed severe stuttering 3 weeks after the first neurological signs of an inoperable brain tumor.[8] Although there was time to perform a speech and language examination, it was mutually agreed that his remaining time was too short to spend it in speech therapy.

Sometimes patients may be candidates for drug therapy, which requires interdisciplinary cooperation between a speech–language pathologist and a neurologist. For example, Baratz and Mesulam[39] described a 42-year-old woman who developed seizures and began to stutter following a closed head injury. When her seizures were brought under control with phenytoin (Dilantin), her speech dysfluencies diminished.

Thus, selection of SAAND patients for various therapeutic interventions depends on the overall health status of each individual as well as the etiology of the stuttering, its neuropathological correlates, its persistence, and the presence of concomitant behavioral disorders.

CLINICAL MANAGEMENT OF SAAND

Treatment Goals.   Because SAAND is a speech problem of adults, each patient should take an active role in setting treatment goals to the extent he or she is capable. These goals will be determined, in part, by each individual's life-style, work status, age, general health, prognosis, etc. For example, a salesperson with relatively infrequent, mild dysfluencies may consider his or her stuttering to be a significant handicap. In contrast, a bedridden person who is able to communicate basic needs may not consider himself or herself significantly handicapped by the stuttering. In some cases, however, memory and other cognitive deficits can prevent patients from participating in the goal-setting process. In such cases, clinicians, family members, and other caregivers will determine the extent to which stuttering interferes with the communicative needs of the individual patient. The next step following a clinical evaluation, therefore, is to establish the level of handicap by document-ing the situations in which communication suffers as a result of stuttering. This information, which may be obtained using a formal questionnaire, can be used to establish treatment goals. Readministration of the questionnaire also can serve as one measure of treatment effectiveness.

Treatment Procedures.   The literature indicates that SAAND has been treated with sur-gery, various pharmacological agents, thalamic stimulation, transcutaneous nerve stimula-tion (TNS), delayed auditory feedback and auditory masking, biofeedback and relaxation, and speech-pacing techniques. In the following sections, each of these treatments will be considered, beginning with surgery.

Surgical Intervention.   In 1979 Donnan[40] described a 65-year-old woman who developed stuttering concurrently with an episode of cerebral ischemia. He described her stuttering as "rapid, easy repetition of the initial sound syllable of every other word" and reported that she displayed no sound blocks or facial grimacing, agnosia, or apraxia. Slight word-finding problems were present. A carotid angiogram showed left carotid stenosis with elevated plaques due to hemorrhaging beneath them. An endarterectomy was performed, and upon recovering from the anesthesia, the woman "was found to be completely free from stutter." A postsurgical angiogram showed uninterrupted left carotid blood flow. In such cases the role of the speech clinician is limited to documenting the nature and severity of stuttering associated with carotid artery disease and its status following surgery.

Another treatment for SAAND that must be provided by physicians, with the speech clinician only documenting the effectiveness of the intervention, involves the use of pharmacological agents.

Pharmacological Agents. There is evidence to suggest that drugs may have either a negative or positive effect on speech fluency. Earlier, I cited Baratz and Mesulam's case[39] whose stuttering, associated with head injury and seizures, diminished when the seizures were brought under control with phenytoin. In contrast, McClean and McClean[41] reported that a patient with post-head injury seizures stuttered when he was treated with phenytoin. When he was switched to carbamazepine, stuttering was reduced. These cases indicate that, when stuttering occurs in patients with documented or suspected seizures, the choice of antiepileptic agents should be carefully explored.

Stuttering also has been associated with administration of dopamine receptor-blocking drugs like phenothiazine. Nurnberg and Greenwald[11] described two patients with chronic schizophrenia who developed severe stuttering when phenothiazine levels were high enough to eliminate psychosis. The investigators had to find a dosage that would manage both the psychosis and stuttering at acceptable levels for daily living.

Quader[42] described two patients whose stuttering was associated with the administration of amitriptyline, a tricyclic antidepressant. In both cases, speech returned to normal when the drug was discontinued. Similarly, Elliott and Thomas[43] reported onset of stuttering in a 22-year-old woman who was treated with alprazolam for anxiety and depression. A double-blind, placebo-controlled study verified the negative effect of alprazolam on speech fluency. This drug is thought to have some pharmacological effects which are similar to those of tricyclics.

Together, these reports indicate that SAAND may result from or be eliminated by administration of various pharmacological agents. In such cases the speech clinician works in consultation with a physician to achieve optimal management of a patient's stuttering in relation to other medical or psychological disorders.

Thalamic Stimulation. In a unique report, Bhantnagar and Andy[44] described a 61-year-old man whose stuttering was associated with a long history of trigeminal pain. Over an 18-year period he was treated with various medications and bilateral, trigeminal ganglion blocks. Methysergide maleate (Sansert) was the only drug that reduced speech dysfluencies, but it had adverse affects on kidney function. There were no co-occurring aphasia or memory problems, and the patient showed no adaptation effect, anxiety, or secondary features. A surgical procedure was used to implant a chorionic stimulation electrode in his left centromedian thalamic nucleus to relieve his chronic pain. Using a battery-operated stimulator, the patient self-stimulated three or four times a day for 20-min periods, which resulted in remarkable improvements in speech fluency as well as in reduction of pain.

Transcutaneous Nerve Stimulation. In 1977 Butler and I described the case of a 68-year-old woman who had a series of minor strokes to both cerebral hemispheres.[45] Severe stuttering occurred after the fifth stroke with transient left hemiparesis. The woman was left-handed but had been converted to use her right hand for writing. Her language skills remained essentially intact, but she had mild dysarthria and markedly dysfluent speech with severe blocking and prolongations of initial and medial syllables, especially consonant blends. Trials with a speech-pacing board increased her dysfluency when she tried to speak in a deliberate, syllable-by-syllable manner. But when an electrolarynx was vibrated against her left hand, moments of stuttering during an oral reading task decreased from 38 to eight. We wondered if the noise produced by the electrolarynx was acting as a masking device, so to test this possibility, we applied a TNS unit to the bicipital groove eof her left arm. This unit, originally developed for pain control, was also successful in reducing this woman's speech dysfluencies.

Auditory Masking and Delayed Auditory Feedback.   There is some evidence that patients with SAAND may show positive responses to auditory masking. In 1984 Rentschler and colleagues[46] described a 41-year-old man who began stuttering following a drug overdose with chlorazepate dipotassium (Tranxene), and possibly chlordiazepoxide hydrochloride (Labrum). Binaural white noise masking at 95 db resulted in fluent speech; with reduced levels of noise intensity, however, stuttering returned. I have used the Edinburgh masker[47] to reduce dysfluency in some patients with SAAND.

Marshall and Starch[48] used DAF with success to treat a 32-year-old man who developed SAAND after a closed head injury. The DAF procedures were introduced 4 years after the injury, and were consistent with the protocol used by Curlee and Perkins[49] with developmental stutterers. Earlier, Downie and associates[50] reported that DAF was effective with two Parkinson's patients with speech disorders, one of whom had stuttering-like hesitations.

Biofeedback and Relaxation.   Biofeedback techniques similar to those employed with developmental stuttering have been used for treating SAAND. One such patient's onset of moderately severe stuttering began after a series of small strokes.[19] His articulation and grammar were normal, and he showed no evidence of oral apraxia. Using an electromyographic (EMG) biofeedback unit, an integrated baseline of masseter tension level was obtained for 5 min of conversation, followed by 5 min of relaxation techniques. Then the patient was asked to maintain a lower tension level, by observing and responding to biofeedback for 5 more min of conversation. After a 4-month, twice-weekly course of such biofeedback/relaxation therapy and home relaxation exercises, he was discharged with only mild stuttering. Likewise, Rubow and colleagues[51] reported using EMG biofeedback and relaxation training to successfully treat a man with SAAND following a stroke.

Speech Pacing.   Some patients with SAAND may respond to pacing techniques that involve slowing speech rate and speaking one syllable at a time.[52] Often, however, patients do not respond to instructions for producing slower, paced speech because of an underlying neurological drive to speak at faster rates. This appears to be especially true of individuals with Parkinson's disease, for whom a pacing board may be required. The pacing device I first described in 1979[33] had six multicolored squares with raised dividers. A patient was encouraged to tap his or her forefinger from square to square while speaking in a syllable-by-syllable manner.

Both a large pacing board and a smaller, more portable, pocket-size board[34] are now available for those patients who can manage finer finger movements; however, other, even smaller pacing devices may prove as effective as a pacing board. For example, one of my Parkinson's patients with SAAND was able to control his speech rate and stuttering by pacing himself with a toggle switch mounted on a piece of wood. A 1984 article[46] described another small device that fits over the patient's forefinger. Holes are punched in Kayo-splint material which then is molded over the finger. The patient paces his or her speech by moving the thumb from hole to hole. I have found that some patients progress from using a pacing instrument to tapping the table, then tapping their thigh, eliminating the need for a device.

According to the survey conducted by Market et al.[14] clinicians most commonly use slow speech rate techniques, easy voice onset approaches, or a combination of the two for treating SAAND. Although 82.2% reported positive results, no specific descriptions of the therapy protocols were provided.

Expected Outcomes

Given the many approaches described for treating SAAND, one might expect that there is an effective form of therapy for any individual whose stuttering is associated with acquired neurological disorder. But as I stressed elsewhere in this chapter, SAAND is not a unitary disorder, nor is it typically unidimensional. It is, therefore, not possible to predict with accuracy how well a specific patient will respond to a specific therapeutic intervention. Sometimes, clinicians and patients must make compromises, such as when a certain drug is best for alleviating neurological or psychiatric symptoms but also results in speech dysfluency. Parkinson's patients with SAAND seem to respond well to a variety of techniques, whereas stroke patients with SAAND seem harder to treat. Fortunately, in many of the latter cases, stuttering is a transient phenomenon. SAAND is not uncommon following closed head injury and may be associated with seizure activity. Control of the seizures also may result in control of stuttering. Patients with rapidly progressing disorders, such as tumors, probably are not candidates for formal treatment, although short-term recommendations for improving communication along with supportive counseling may be helpful.

Thus, a blanket statement about SAAND patients and response to treatment cannot be made. Instead, one should consider each patient individually, beginning with the case history, progressing through the clinical evaluation, and finally choosing what appears to be the best initial approach to management and treatment.

Conclusion

SAAND is one of the more interesting, puzzling, and challenging speech problems of adults referred to speech–language pathologists. There is mounting evidence that a variety of transient, static, and progressive neurological disorders result in dysfluent speech patterns labeled "stuttering" by clinicians, family members, and patients themselves. In fact, the evidence is so compelling, clinicians should consider adult onset of stuttering as a symptom of possible neurological dysfunction. Fluent speaking is, perhaps, the most refined motor act performed by humans, requiring complex coordination of many different muscle groups. It can be sensitive, therefore, to even small changes in neurological status, which may be why stuttering occurs in a wide range of neurological disorders, from Parkinson's disease to closed head injury. If this fact is ignored, clinicians may be overlooking an important early indicator of neurological disease. For example, a man was referred to me with sudden onset of mildly dysfluent speech. The admitting physician having found "no positive neurological signs," sent him to the psychiatry unit of the hospital. The man, however, had a long history of good mental health, and the psychiatrists found no psychiatric basis for his speech problem. When he was evaluated by me, about a week later, I detected a slight right facial weakness. A few months later he died of a brain tumor. The lesson to be learned is that adult onset of stuttering should be considered a potentially positive neurological sign. Early diagnosis of SAAND may lead to successful treatment of either a neurological disorder causing stuttering or the communication disorder itself.

Acknowledgments.   I would like to thank Richard Curlee for his helpful comments on this chapter. My work is supported, in part, by the National Institute for Deafness and Communication Disorders Grant number DC01409 to the National Center for Neurogenic Communication Disorders at the University of Arizona.

Suggested Readings

Baumgartner J, Duffy JR: Psychogenic stuttering in adults with and without neurologic disease. *J Med Speech-Lang Path* 1997; 5(2):75–95.

This is a retrospective study of 69 individuals (49 without and 20 with neurologic disease) identified as having pyschogenic stuttering by clinicians at the Mayo Clinic. The authors provide guidelines for the differential diagnosis of this disorder versus neurogenic stuttering. The most distinguishing characteristic of psychogenic stuttering was quick response to one or two sessions of behavioral therapy, but others were found as well.

Helm NA, Butler RB, Benson DF: Acquiring stuttering. *Neurology* 1978; 28:1159–1165.

This report of 10 patients with acquired stuttering was the first to describe specific neuropathological, neuropsychological, and language correlates of transient and persistent forms of this disorder. It is widely cited and its findings have been used as reference points for comparing cases examined in subsequent reports.

Ludlow C, Rosenberg M, Salazar A, Grafman I, Smutok A: Site of penetrating brain lesions causing chronic acquired stuttering. *Ann Neurol* 1987; 21:60–66.

In this well-controlled and scientific study of acquired stuttering, Ludlow and her colleagues compared test performance and CT scans of 10 men who developed stuttering after penetrating missile wounds with those of other head-injured and normal subjects. Their findings indicate that acquired stuttering is a motor control disorder most commonly associated with unilateral subcortical and extrapyramidal system lesions in this form of brain damage.

Ringo CC, Dietrich S: Neurogenic stuttering: An analysis and critique. *J Med Speech-Lang Path* 1995; 3(2):111–122.

In this review of all cases of neurogenic stuttering published through 1993, the authors examine the value of seven features identified as characteristic of this disorder. Five of the seven features were reported in the majority of cases, which were tested as guidelines for distinguishing neurogenic stuttering from developmental stuttering.

References

1. Arend R, Handzel L, Weiss B: Dysphatic stuttering. *Folia Phoniatrica* 1962; 14:55–66.
2. Rosenbek JC, Messert B, Collins M, Wertz RT: Stuttering following brain damage. *Brain Lang*, 1978; 5(6):82–96.
3. Helm NA, Butler RB, Benson DF: Acquired stuttering. *Neurology* 1978; 28:1159–1165.
4. Mazzuchi A, Moretti G, Carpeggiani P, Parma M, Paini P: Clinical observations on acquired stuttering. *Br J Dis Commun* 1981; 16:19–30.
5. Koller WC: Dysfluency (stuttering) in extrapyramidal disease. *Arch Neurol* 1983; 40:175–177.
6. Lebrun Y, Devreau F, Rousseau J-J: Language and speech in patient with a clinical diagnosis of progressive supranuclear palsy. *Brain Lang* 1986; 27:247–256.
7. Lebrun Y, Leleux C, Retif J: Neurogenic stuttering. *Acta Neuorchirur* 1987; 85:103–109.
8. Helm NA, Butler RB, Canter GJ: Neurogenic acquired stuttering. *J Fluency Disord* 1980; 5:269–279.
9. Chen W-H, Peng M-C: Acquired stuttering in a patient with encephalitis. *Kaoshiung J Med Sci* 1993; 9:183–185.
10. Rosenbek J, McNeil MR, Lemme ML, Prescott TE, Alfrey AC: Speech and language findings in a chronic hemodialysis patient: A case report. *J Speech Hear Disord* 1978; 40:245–252.
11. Nurnberg HG, Greenwald B: Stuttering: An unusual side effect of phenothiazines. *Am J Psych* 1981; 138:386–387.
12. Rosenfield DB, McCarthy M, McKinney K, Viswanath NS, Nudelman HB: Stuttering induced by theophylline. *Ear Nose Throat J* 1994; 73:918–920.
13. Byrne A, Byrne MK, Zibin TO: Transient neurogenic stuttering. *Int J Eat Disord* 1993; 14:511–514.
14. Market KE, Montague JC, Buffalo MD, Drummond SA: Acquired stuttering: Descriptive data and treatment outcomes. *J Fluency Disord* 1990; 15:21–33.
15. Helm-Estabrooks N, Yeo R, Geschwind N, Freedman M, Weinstein C: Stuttering: Disappearance and reappearance with acquired brain lesions. *Neurology* 1986; 36:1109–1112.

16. Quinn PT, Andrews G: Neurologic stuttering: A clinical entity? *J Neurol Neurosurg Psych* 1977; 40:699–701.
17. *Manual of the International Statistical Classification of Diseases Injuries and Causes of Death*, vol. 1. Geneva, World Health Organization, 1977.
18. Andrews G, Craig A, Feyer A, Hoddinott S, Howie R, Neilson M: Stuttering: A review of research findings and theories circa 1982. *J Speech Hear Disord* 1982; 47:226–246.
19. Helm-Estabrooks N: Diagnosis and Management of Neurogenic Stuttering in Adults, in St. Louis KO (ed): *The Atypical Stutterer: Principles and Practices of Rehabilitation*. New York, Academic Press, 1986.
20. Ludlow C, Rosenberg M, Salazar A, Grafman J, Smutok A: Site of penetrating brain lesions causing chronic acquired stuttering. *Ann Neurol* 1987; 21:60–66.
21. Heuer RJ, Sataloff RT, Mandel S, Travers N: Neurogenic stuttering: Further corroboration of site of lesion. *Ear Nose Throat J* 1996; 75(3):161–168.
22. Baumgartner J, Duffy JR: Psychogenic stuttering in adults with and without neurologic disease. *J Med Speech-Lang Path* 1997; 5(2):75–95.
23. Arnold GE, Luchsinger R: *Voice-Speech-Language Clinical Communicology: Its Physiology and Pathology*. Belmont, CA, Wadsworth, 1965.
24. Jones RK: Observations on stammering after localized cerebral injury. *J Neurol Neurosurg Psych* 1966; 29:192–195.
25. Miller AE: Cessation of stuttering with progressive multiple sclerosis. *Neurology* 1986; 35:1341–1343.
26. Duffy JR: *Motor Speech Disorders: Substrates, Differential Diagnosis, and Management*. St. Louis, MO, Mosby-Year Book, 1995.
27. Geschwind N, Behan P: Left-handedness: Association with immune disease, migraine and developmental learning disorder. *Proc Natl Acad Sci USA* 1982; 79:5097–5100.
28. Deal J: Sudden onset of stuttering: A case report. *J Speech Hear Disord* 1982; 47:301–304.
29. Attanasio JS: A case of late-onset or acquired stuttering in adult life. *J Fluency Disord* 1987; 12:287–290.
30. Helm-Estabrooks N: *Aphasia Diagnostic Profiles*. Chicago, Applied Symbolix, 1992.
31. Ringo CC, Dietrich S: Neurogenic stuttering: An analysis and critique. *J Med Speech-Lang Path:* 1995; 3(2):111–122.
32. Fairbanks G: *Voice and Articulation Drill Book*. New York, Harper, 1960.
33. Helm NA: Management of palilalia with a pacing board. *J Speech Hear Disord* 1979; 44:350–353.
34. Helm-Estabrooks N, Kaplan E: *Boston Simulus Boards*. Chicago, Applied Symbolix, 1989.
35. Bayles K, Tomoeda C: *Arizona Battery for Communication Disorders in Dementia*. Tuscon, AZ, Canyonlands Press, 1991.
36. Helm-Estabrooks N, Hotz G: *Brief Test of Head Injury*. Chicago, Applied Symbolix, 1991.
37. Adamovich B, Henderson J: *Scales of Cognitive Ability for Traumatic Brain Injury*. Chicago, Applied Symbolix, 1991.
38. Madison D, Baeher E, Bazell M, Hartman K, Mahurkar S, Dunea G: Communicative and cognitive deterioration in dialysis dementia: Two case studies. *J Speech Hear Disord* 1977; 42:238–246.
39. Baratz R, Mesulam M: Adult-onset stuttering treated with anticonvulsants. *Arch Neurol* 1981; 38:132–133.
40. Donnan GA: Stuttering as a manifestation of stroke. *Med J Aust* 1979; 1:44–45.
41. McClean MD, McClean A: Case report of stuttering acquired in association with phenytoin use for post-head-injury seizures. *J Fluency Disord* 1985; 10:241–255.
42. Quader SE: Dysarthria: An unusual side effect of trycyclic antidepressants. *Br Med J* 1977; 9:97.
43. Elliott RL, Thomas BJ: A case report of alprazolam-induced stuttering. *J Clin Psychopharmacol* 1985; 5:159–160.
44. Bhantnagar SC, Andy OJ: Alleviation of acquired stuttering with human centremedian thalamic stimulation. *J Neurol Neurosurg Psych* 1989; 52:1182–1184.
45. Helm NA, Butler RB: Transcutaneous nerve stimulation in acquired speech disorder. *Lancet* 1977; 2:1177–1178.
46. Rentschler GI, Driver LE, Callaway EA: The onset of stuttering following drug overdose. *J Fluency Disord* 1984; 9:265–284.

47. Dewar A, Dewar AD, Austin WTS, Brash HM: The long term use of an automatically triggered auditory feedback masking device in the treatment of stammering. *Br J Disord Commun* 1976; 14:219–229.

48. Marshall RC, Starch SA: Behavioral treatment of acquired stuttering. *Aust J Commun Disord* 1984; 12:87–92.

49. Curlee RF, Perkins WH: Conversational rate control therapy for stuttering. *J Speech Hear Disord* 1969; 34:245–250.

50. Downie AW, Low JM, Linsay DD: Speech disorders in parkinsonism: Use of delayed auditory feedback in selected cases. *J Neurol Neurosurg Psych* 1981; 44:852–853.

51. Rubow RT, Rosenbek JC, Schumaker JG: Stress management in the treatment of neurogenic stuttering. *Biofeedback Self Regul* 1986; 11:77–78.

52. Pacing devices developed. *ASHA* 1983; 25(4):16.

Stuttering and Related Disorders of Fluency, 2nd edition.
Edited by Richard F. Curlee, Ph.D.
Thieme Medical Publishers, Inc., New York © 1999.

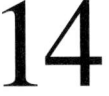

Acquired Psychogenic Stuttering

John M. Baumgartner

This chapter deals with the provision of clinical services to individuals who have acquired, as adults, a fluency disorder that is thought to be psychogenic. Throughout the chapter, the term *psychogenic stuttering* will be used to refer to this speech disorder. Use of the term *stuttering* in this context is not meant to imply that the speech impairment in this population is the same as that seen in developmental stuttering. It is used in the interest of brevity. It is also the most commonly used term to refer to the dysfluent speech (instances of stuttering) and the disorder (stuttering). Other terminology such as "stuttering-like" speech could also be used.

Of more significance, though, is the use of the etiologic term *psychogenic*. In a recent technical paper[1] on terminology it has been suggested that "psychogenic stuttering" should be used to refer only to people in whom psychopathology is verifiable. The material I will present in this chapter is not consistent with that suggestion. In many, but not necessarily all cases, a psychiatric evaluation should be sought; however, my own belief is that a diagnosis of psychopathology is not required for the speech–language pathologist (SLP) to determine that the speech disorder is psychogenic. My position on this issue is that impaired speech fluency, like other speech and voice disorders, can be caused by psychologic distress or disequilibrium (Aronson's[2] term). In addition, the reality is that some patients do not follow a recommendation for obtaining a psychiatric evaluation and others are unable to obtain one. In such cases a "verified" psychiatric diagnosis is not possible. Nevertheless, by comparing findings on a given patient to the characteristics of known acquired speech disorders, obtaining a comprehensive interview/history, and trial therapy (when needed); the SLP can determine that the patient's disorder differs from any known neurogenic speech disorder but does compare favorably with characteristics of psychogenic speech disorders. This clearly must be done carefully and with full recognition that diagnostic decisions can be made with varying degrees of certainty, and the degree of diagnostic certainty should be made clear by the clinician. Diagnosing specific psychopathology is clearly not within the province of the SLP, but placing an acquired speech disorder into an etiologic category is critical to participation in the diagnostic process. It also plays a crucial role in management planning, statements of prognosis, and communicating with other professionals involved in the case.

Clinicians are repeatedly encouraged by literature in our field to view speech and voice changes as sensitive indicators of both psychologic and neurologic well being. This is also true of the diagnostic teaching medical students and residents receive. The SLP who conducts an evaluation is expected, for example, to report dysarthria and its type when thought to be present. This, by definition, is a statement that the speech findings are indicative of neuropathology. If a neurologic diagnosis has not yet been made in such a patient, the diagnosis of the SLP helps determine not only the presence of neuropathology but also the site(s) of lesion. This, in turn, contributes to determination of specific neurologic diagnosis. Clinicians who evaluate voice patients are expected to recognize those in whom the overall pattern of findings is not consistent with a known organic voice disorder but is indicative of a "functional" voice disorder. This, too, is an etiologic statement, and it does not depend on neurologic or laryngologic exam. Various medical examinations may occur before the SLP sees the patient, but in other cases, the findings of the SLP, especially trial therapy, will be of considerable help in determining the medical specialties that need (or don't need) to be involved in the case. It may be that no medical evaluations are needed; that is, diagnosis and successful management can be carried out by the SLP. When an SLP examines a patient and finds a pattern of results that are consistent with aphasia, it is the clinician's responsibility to report the presence of aphasia (and, therefore, neurogenicity) whether neuropathology has been "verified" or not. Primary progressive aphasia, for example, is defined by progressing focal aphasia in the absence of known neuropathology.[3] It is the power of speech and language disorders to assist with diagnostic decisions regarding someone's overall health that makes our input of considerable value. If we cannot use the term *psychogenic*, then our value as clinicians is greatly reduced. Again, it is important not to confuse statements of etiologic category with diagnosis of specific psychiatric illness.

It seems markedly inconsistent to me to suggest that acquired psychogenic stuttering is so different from other acquired speech disorders that SLPs must first receive "verification." Evaluation by other professionals may or may not serve to confirm our stated opinion, but the absence of this information should not render us "opinionless." I feel just as strongly that it is our right and responsibility to disagree, when we do, with the stated opinions of other professionals. Clearly, professionals do not always agree. Giving no opinion seems to me to be more detrimental to the advancement of our field than giving carefully considered ones and participating in the differential diagnostic process. Again, careful clinical work should lead to a stated diagnosis and the level of certainty with which it is made. It may follow other diagnoses (psychiatric, for example) but it may, on the other hand, be instrumental in helping to determine that other evaluations are needed and in one way or another arriving at an accurate diagnosis. In this chapter, acquired stuttering is considered in the same context as other acquired speech disorders and, therefore, the same decision-making strategies apply. So, too, does the ability and responsibility of the SLP to comment on etiology and thus pursue an appropriate and useful role in the differential diagnostic process.

Differential diagnosis of acquired speech disorders involves making a decision as to whether the disorder is organic, psychogenic, or idiopathic. In the case of acquired stuttering, "organic" means neurogenic. The material to follow will hopefully be of benefit in the task of distinguishing neurogenic from psychogenic stuttering. We know that neuropathology can cause stuttering (see chapter 13 for coverage of this material), but, complaints that raise suspicion about the presence of neuropathology are found in many patients with psychogenic speech disorders. Even when neuropathology has been diagnosed and acquired stuttering is present, it is not necessarily neurogenic. It could be, but acquired stuttering in the presence of neuropathology is not the same as acquired neurogenic stuttering. A recent report[4] described a retrospective study in which 20 of 69 cases of acquired psychogenic stuttering also showed demonstrable neuropathology. Other authors have described similar co-occurrence of neuropathology and stuttering thought to be psychogenic.[5,6] Duffy[7] and others[8] have discussed this comorbidity at some length with respect to a number of acquired speech disorders, including stuttering, and detailed coverage of this material, as it pertains to voice disorders, is provided in Aronson's text.[2] It is also true that patients with acquired speech disorders often have complaints that raise strong suspicions of neuropathology, but none can be found, or what is found has no relationship to neurologic control of speech production. In our retrospective study[4] 49 subjects had complaints raising suspicions of neuropathology. In a recent paper[9] I presented a number of cases in which the specific speech symptoms varied but all were psychogenic and had been diagnosed as such based on similar patterns of findings. Several of these cases presented with acquired stuttering and in all cases there was some reason to suspect neuropathology.

The purpose of these comments is to make clear the point that neither suspicion nor presence of neuropathology is sufficient to place any acquired speech disorder, including stuttering, into the neurogenic category. The clinical process I will describe has been helpful in the past with the very important task of evaluating these kinds of patients and has been shaped, in many ways, by the clinical environment in which these patients are most often seen. Because they most often present with multiple complaints, they are usually seen first by one or more physicians. In turn, they are referred to the SLP. The point in their overall diagnostic work-up at which they were seen by the SLP can vary considerably. They are most often seen in multidisciplinary medical settings, often while hospitalized. Though not "common," these patients do appear frequently enough to comprise a significant portion of the speech pathology caseload. In one review[7] of cases seen over a 4-year period, it was reported that 215 patients received a speech–language diagnosis of acquired psychogenic speech or voice disorder, and 20% of these were acquired stuttering. When patients are in a medical setting, the need to be thorough must be tempered by the reality that one must be efficient in today's managed care environment. Priority is given to "high-yield" procedures. Procedures that may be informative but not demonstrably necessary for clinical decisions are discouraged. Therefore, you should keep in mind that the clinical procedures I will describe are "high yield" in terms of clinical utility, yet efficient enough to be carried out in a busy, day-to-day patient care setting. There are no clinical procedures that "might be of interest," or that are done just because they can be. There are many unanswered questions regarding this clinical population, and additional procedures shown by prospective studies to be of clinical utility would be welcome additions to those mentioned here. The clinical approach I use is not drawn primarily from what is known about or usually done with developmental stuttering. My belief is that these cases are best placed in the context of what we know about acquired speech and voice disorders.

Evaluations Needed

Key Case History Information

Obtaining a clear and thorough history in cases of acquired speech disorders requires a very careful, systematic conversation with the individual being evaluated. The interview and attainment of the case history is crucial and adequate time must be devoted to it. It requires knowledge about the salient characteristics of acquired speech disorders and indications from the history that are relevant to etiology. Accurate identification of psychogenic cases requires more than a passing knowledge of the primary types of psychologic distress (acute or chronic) and, in more severe cases, of the psychopathologies that are known to be associated with speech changes. Several recent references do an admirable job of covering this material,[2,5,7] and a recent edited text by a group from Great Britain[10] is devoted entirely to this area. The examiner should attempt to obtain information which can be tied together in chronologic order, as much as this is possible. Because psychogenicity should be suspected until it is ruled out, the interviewer should seek information not only about various aspects of the patient's speech difficulty, but also any current or past organic illnesses and life stressors, keeping in mind that illness is a life stressor.

Acquisition of specific information is most important; however, it must be done in a way that achieves another, different goal, one that is both diagnostic and therapeutic. The history must be obtained in a way that encourages, supports, and gives repeated opportunities for a patient to go beyond presentation of objective facts and descriptions in response to a list of specific, fact-seeking questions. This represents "psychologic interviewing,"[2] which is both a science and an art. Such an interview not only seeks to acquire information, but also to lay the groundwork for and initiate the counseling process. Psychologic interviewing and counseling are recognized as important to competent provision of services in our field,[11–13] and identification and management of psychogenic communicative disorders depends heavily on this kind of clinical activity. The skilled interviewer creates an atmosphere that encourages and supports discussions of feelings, fears, and information not previously disclosed (very possibly to anyone). It is not enough to find out what has happened in an individual's life. The truly successful interview explores how people feel about these things, how they have dealt with them, and whether they would "really like" to do something else about them. The clinician deliberately, yet subtly, steers the patient through a combination of fact finding and emotional disclosure. Such disclosures get at psychogenic issues, if there are any, to a much greater degree than do objective recitations of answers to questions about specific events in the patient's life. Conducting successful psychologic interviews and counseling, in general, require clinicians to possess certain attributes and pay careful attention to their own behavior. There seems to be little disagreement on what these attributes are, and they are described briefly, but very well, in at least two sources.[2,11] Another recent text[14] presents a well-organized chapter on psychological approaches used in speech pathology as it is practiced in Great Britain.

If a clinician can successfully create an environment in which both facts and feelings are discussed, then the opportunity exists for the patient's presenting speech symptoms to change noticeably, either in the direction of becoming worse or lessening in severity. Occasionally, they may disappear altogether. Symptom resolution, or a marked reduction in severity, during disclosure of emotionally sensitive information is powerful evidence in support of psychogenicity and argues strongly against organicity. This concept has been presented most often with respect to voice disorders,[2,15,16] but it is also relevant to other acquired speech disorders, including acquired stuttering.[4,7,8] Speech symptoms that change in character (not necessarily for the better) during such an interview are also difficult to explain on a neurologic basis which argues for a psychologic etiology.

I am not suggesting that the SLP should attempt to arrive at a psychiatric diagnosis or that this kind of interview is psychotherapy. The goal is to determine if signs of psychogenicity exist and, in so doing, perhaps bring about dramatic speech improvement. Certainly, if an SLP does not understand that psychogenicity is a valid diagnosis for some acquired speech disorders, then that SLP will not identify psychogenic cases as such. The real dilemma, in my opinion, is how SLPs can best be trained in this area, not whether it is part of their clinical domain.

If the history and interview is obtained in a systematic manner, and if the clinician recognizes the importance of relating speech-specific information to the patient's life (e.g. relationships, work, school, social activities, and degree of satisfaction with these things), then key pieces of information can be identified. A patient's description of the speech disorder and its effect on day-to-day function, onset, and course up to the time of the evaluation are all significant. Descriptions of other complaints, their diagnoses, and management, if any, of each should be obtained. The temporal relationships between a patient's speech disturbance, complaints of other problems (if any), and fluctuations in speech and/or other complaints should be explored. Of particular importance is a careful search for evidence of CNS disease or impairment and, if present, its onset and course in comparison to that of the speech problem, and the degree to which medical/surgical management has been successful. Inquiry into the presence of non-CNS illness, neurologic or otherwise, and its temporal relationship to the speech problem is equally important.

Psychologically stressful events or periods of time, acute psychologic trauma, and the degree to which these have been "resolved," should be detailed. It is often useful to determine the temporal relationships between these episodes as well as the patient's opinion as to whether speech is "connected" to them. The same is true of patients' beliefs regarding a "connection" between speech and an apparent or diagnosed illness. The clinician is looking here for a pattern of repeated, perhaps, variable unexplained problems in either the recent or distant past. Behavioral descriptions of previous communication difficulties and their similarity to the current problem should be discussed thoroughly. The clinician should attempt to obtain objective, behavioral descriptions rather than labels. It may be helpful to obtain past records even though they should be viewed with caution; many patients with psychogenic speech disorders have received previous, organic diagnoses.

Finally, the clinician should inquire about the patient's reasons for seeking an evaluation at this time. Throughout the interview particular attention should be given to the apparent concern, or lack thereof, shown by a patient. Many remain apparently unconcerned in the face of multiple medical complaints and serious difficulty using speech to communicate. Others are very aware of and concerned about speech and any other difficulties they are experiencing. When a patient notes or "complains of" a problem, it does not mean he or she is truly bothered by it. Some patients, in fact, report that others are concerned (e.g., family, health care providers) but they are not.

The order in which case history information is obtained is less important than the way in which it is obtained. The clinician needs to be organized and systematic but at the same time flexible. Categories of information should probably be pursued one at a time in order to help both the clinician and patient stay on track. Some clinicians prefer to use a case history "form"; others, like myself, prefer not to. It should be noted, however, that the case history forms commonly used in communicative disorders do not include guidelines for the exploration of potential psychologic issues.

Observations and Tests Used

Evaluation of all patients with acquired speech disorders should include a motor speech examination, which should include assessment of both physical and speech components. The speech portion should include tasks ranging from those that place minimal demands on motor capacity, such as vowel prolongation, to connected speech. It is best if these tasks are arranged in an approximate order of difficulty. In my experience, the perceptually based approach to motor speech testing, first developed and used by the Speech Pathology service at the Mayo Clinic[17] and more recently discussed in detail by Duffy,[7] is efficient to administer and successfully identifies a motor speech impairment, if one is present. Task protocols appropriate to a search for apraxia of speech and oral, nonverbal apraxia should be administered if there is reason to suspect either of these disorders. Similarly, if the possibility of dysphagia is apparent, the clinician should be prepared to arrange for follow-up evaluation of this area. The clinician should also be prepared to at least sample both language and cognitive performance if signs of potential impairments in these areas are evident during the interview or in prior records, and in-depth testing should be done when appropriate. In addition to providing evidence of cognitive/language status, the interview provides a speech sample.

The purpose of these procedures is to determine whether acquired stuttering is accompanied by a known, identifiable communication and/or swallowing disorder. The clinician should make every attempt to differentiate between structurally based and neurogenic disorders because structural disorders would not be expected to directly cause dysfluent speech. Indeed, I am not aware of any case reports in which a structural abnormality has even been suggested to produce stuttering, or stuttering-like speech. With respect to neurogenic disorders, it is worth repeating that clinicians should look for examination and history findings that fit with the salient characteristics of a known neurogenic disorder. The diagnosis of neurogenicity must be based on specific findings that fit with a known neurogenic communication disorder. Characteristics of various neurogenic communication disorders are described in detail in numerous publications and clinicians need to be thoroughly familiar with this material. The presence or absence of a coexisting neurogenic communication disorder is a significant variable to consider when attempting to differentiate between acquired neurogenic and psychogenic stuttering.

There are a number of observations that are of value in evaluating the fluency disorder itself. Type(s) of dysfluencies should be specified. The literature does not suggest, however, that frequency counts of dysfluencies help with this differential diagnosis. The number of dysfluencies or the percent words stuttered, however defined, is an indication of severity, but not etiology. Types of dysfluency can be described utilizing the same categories used commonly in the evaluation of developmental stuttering.

Variability of stuttering should also be described. The issue is whether stuttering varies at all and, if so, does it vary in ways that are consistent with what would be expected if caused by neurologic impairment. Situational variability, marked differences between conversation and reading, periods of time during which there is no stuttering, and a worsening of symptoms during the performance of less difficult tasks are examples of the variability suggestive of psychogenicity. Adequate information can usually be obtained from the patient's motor speech performance, speech during conversation/interview, and descriptions of the onset and course of stuttering. Presence or absence of "accessory," "struggle," or "adjustive" behaviors should be noted also, along with their variability, if present. Of particular interest is the degree to which these behaviors appear "bizarre." Patients with acquired neurogenic speech impairments may demonstrate "struggle" behaviors that look compensatory or appear to reflect the effortful nature of their speech attempts, but "bizarre" movements unrelated to speech production are not characteristic of these disorders. One exception may be the "bizarre" appearing movements that are sometimes part of the movement disorders that produce hyperkinetic dysarthria. In these cases, though, the motor speech examination should identify them as such. Clinicians should also look for speech that is telegraphic-like or agrammatic in the absence of a nonfluent aphasia.

If further evidence is needed in order to arrive at a differential diagnosis, other procedures in which manner of speech and/or task difficulty are systematically varied may be utilized. I may use such procedures as paced or rhythmic speech, whispered speech, an adaptation sequence, or similar procedures drawn from the literature on developmental stuttering. Improved fluency during these tasks is not necessarily incompatible with psychogenicity, even though a clear pattern of improved fluency when demands on the speech control system are decreased, is, by itself, more consistent with neurogenic than psychogenic stuttering (chapter 13 also contains information pertinent to this issue). There is, however, a pattern of performance on such tasks that is highly suggestive of psychogenicity—increasingly dysfluent speech as task difficulty is reduced. Therefore, if the clinician decides to utilize these additional tasks, improved fluency is of only limited value, but an increase in dysfluencies and/or struggle behavior is strongly suggestive of psychogenicity. Again, these procedures are optional. Sufficient information on patterns of variability that are of diagnostic significance can usually be obtained through conversation, the motor speech examination, and information obtained during the interview.

Finally, and very importantly, direct symptomatic therapy, done in a counseling-like manner, should be attempted if there is other evidence of psychogenicity. Acquired psychogenic speech and voice disorders may respond rapidly and dramatically to direct therapy conducted during an initial evaluation. There may be complete or near complete resolution of symptoms. Such "symptom reversibility,"[8] when achieved, is dramatic evidence in support of a psychogenic etiology, and two recent publications[4,5] describe its prominence in acquired, psychogenic stuttering.

Acquired psychogenic stuttering has not received nearly as much attention as neurogenic stuttering. Most published reports include only one case, although a few include more than one.[4,5,18] There is, therefore, a lack of specific data on which to base diagnostic decisions. Cases of psychogenic stuttering cannot be identified on the basis of a numeric score or the frequency of certain behaviors. In addition, there is no single profile of characteristics that fit the population of individuals who acquire psychogenic stuttering. A recent[4] review of the demographic characteristics of these patients revealed certain trends, but clearly they comprise a very heterogeneous population. Comparison of reported cases[5,18–21] in which there was no evidence of coexisting neuropathology with case reports in which there was neurologic disease evident[6,22–24] does reveal a pattern of findings that are repeatedly reported, but every patient does not fit every aspect of the pattern. Nevertheless, multiple findings that do fit the pattern, in conjunction with lack of support for neurogenicity, will usually allow clinicians to make a diagnosis.

Accurate identification of these cases does not involve extensive testing. History and interview, the limited examination procedures just described, and trial symptomatic therapy are usually sufficient. The real work is conceptual rather than procedural. Clinicians must look for a pattern rather than individual findings, in the same way that dysarthria, for example, is identified and typed on the basis of findings that comprise a "cluster."[7,17]

The variables on which to base a diagnostic decision include onset, course, and relationship of stuttering to identified psychologic stressors; absence of symptoms that characterize known neurogenic disorders; performance on fluency-enhancing tasks, if employed; presence, type, and variability of "struggle" behavior; and response to direct symptomatic therapy. Evidence of a diagnosed psychopathology or neuropathology may be helpful; however, such information must be considered carefully. The presence of neuropathology does not mean the patient's stuttering is neurogenic, and the presence of psychopathology may not mean it is psychogenic. Neurogenic and psychogenic disorders often coexist, and the presence of one does not render a patient immune to the other. The following discussion is based on published case studies and, especially, the results of a large, retrospective study of 69 cases.[4]

There is considerable heterogeneity in age at onset, but onset occurs most often before age 60. It is not a transient disorder and may be present anywhere from days to years. It is similarly prevalent in both sexes. There are no apparent differences between these patients as a group and the general population with respect to either education or handedness.

Most people with psychogenic stuttering have multiple complaints, including their speech difficulty, but stuttering is very likely to be their only or primary complaint, regarding communication. Other complaints usually refer to symptoms that raise suspicions about a CNS pathology. Evaluation of such complaints may delay their speech evaluation, but evidence confirming a neuropathology often is not found. These patients' records frequently document a pattern of repeated physician visits and evaluations and patient complaints that are variable. In other cases, however, the results of neurologic evaluations are positive. In our series[4] of cases, the most common complaint without a neurologic explanation was headache. In patients with demonstrable CNS disease, the most frequent diagnoses were, interestingly, degenerative diseases, closed head injury, and seizure disorder. In these cases it is certainly reasonable to suspect that stuttering is neurogenic; however, other findings from the history and motor speech examination, along with response to symptomatic therapy, led us to the conclusion that the stuttering was psychogenic. CNS pathology that produces ongoing impairment and disability and requires repeated visits to health care professionals may be a variable that serves to heighten the suspicion that any speech changes that develop may be psychogenic.

Another variable that should heighten suspicion of a psychogenic etiology is the absence of a coexisting neurogenic communication disorder. Aphasia, dysarthria, or apraxia of speech were seldom present in the cases of psychogenic stuttering described in the previously cited literature; however, the literature on neurogenic stuttering indicates that more than half present with unambiguous, coexisting aphasia, dysarthria or both. Apraxia of speech is not mentioned as frequently. Clearly, there is some overlap between the two types of stuttering with respect to comorbidity. Some psychogenic cases present with a history or current evidence of a coexisting neurogenic communication disorder, and some cases of neurogenic stuttering have no coexisting neurogenic communication disorder. This suggests that, at times, acquired stuttering may be a sign of neurologic disease which has not yet been diagnosed. In spite of the overlap, the absence of a known neurogenic communication disorder is most often associated with psychogenic stuttering and its presence is most often associated with neurogenic stuttering. In some cases, however, determining the etiology of acquired stuttering on the basis of type of neuropathology or presence of dysarthria, in particular, may be especially difficult. One neuropathology that overlaps to about the same degree in psychogenic and neurogenic cases is closed head injury. Similarly, use of medications and possible toxic blood levels resulting from their use is not associated to a greater extent with either type of acquired stuttering. Lastly, it is especially difficult to distinguish acquired stuttering from the dysfluent speech that often may reflect a hypokinetic dysarthria. The problem here is not so much one of identifying etiology, which can be determined by looking at other findings, but determining whether or not two, separate speech disorders are present. Thus, Parkinson's disease may be an exception to the finding that progressive neurologic diseases co-occur more often in psychogenic than in neurogenic stuttering in light of the fact that hypokinetic dysarthria occurs commonly in Parkinson's disease.

Type of dysfluency does not seem to differentiate the two types of stuttering; sound and syllable repetitions are the most common type reported. Other types have been reported but do not appear to assist in making the differential diagnosis. However, an important indicator of likely psychogenicity is struggle behavior, especially if it appears completely unrelated to speech production and, thus, appears "bizarre" to the clinician. There is overlap with respect to this variable, like others, but the literature suggests that struggle is much more common in psychogenic cases, and our[4] data certainly is consistent with this notion.

Variability of stuttering does not seem to be a distinguishing characteristic of either type of acquired stuttering; some variability is common in both types. As was mentioned previously, however, stuttering that is highly intermittent or unpredictable, that varies with the situation, person, time of day, or that differs substantially between reading and conversation, is not consistent with what is typical of a neurogenic speech disorder. Although some cases in each diagnostic category show an adaptation effect, most often it is not seen in either population.[4,25] Occasionally, however, a clinician may carry out the adaptation procedure to see if stuttering worsens. If found, then this strongly suggests psychogenicity. Likewise, stuttering that worsens, with easier tasks or is unvarying throughout various portions of the motor speech examination (e.g., conversation versus vowel prolongation, or alternate motion rate [AMRs]) is showing strong signs of psychogenicity.

Of obvious interest is the role that psychiatric diagnosis plays in identifying acquired psychogenic stuttering. Certainly, it may serve as a confirmatory sign, but careful attention to other findings that can be obtained through an evaluation by an SLP can also yield a diagnosis of psychogenicity. This allows the SLP to continue with the provision of services which stem from a belief that the etiology is psychogenic and which need not be delayed while the SLP awaits a psychiatric diagnosis. This is a crucial point, because trial therapy during the initial evaluation and continued therapy, if necessary, depends on the clinician's belief that the disorder is not organic and the degree to which the patient can look at the disorder from this perspective.

It is also important that SLPs consider a referral for psychiatric or psychologic evaluation if this has not already been done, recognizing that such evaluations may not occur. When these patients do receive psychiatric evaluations, evidence of prior, similar or different psychiatric symptoms may be found but many patients do not present evidence of earlier psychiatric difficulties. In our retrospective study,[4] all of the patients seen for psychiatric evaluations received a diagnosis, but this does not mean that all such cases suffer from some form of psychopathology. Conversion reaction, anxiety, and/or depression were the most frequent diagnoses found in our study, but diagnoses of reactive depression, personality disorder, drug dependence, and posttraumatic neurosis were also made. Some patients received more than one diagnosis. Other literature supports these findings; the most common psychiatric diagnoses in these cases are conversion reaction, anxiety, and some form of depression.[5,8] It should also be noted that, at least in the cases we reviewed, neurologic and/or psychiatric evaluation results always agreed with the SLP decision that stuttering was psychogenic. There were no instances of disagreement. The course of patients' psychologic difficulties at the time of stuttering onset is variable, but most begin at the same time. In some cases, onset of stuttering coincided with worsening psychologic difficulty, but onset occurred in only a minority of cases when psychologic status was reported to be stable.

Psychopathology need not always be present for stuttering to be psychogenic. Reports of distress or of stress as a normal reaction to life events, or anticipation of them, may precipitate stuttering just as they are commonly said to precipitate dysphonia or aphonia. Aronson's[2] concept of psychologic disequilibrium is a helpful way to consider the relationship between psychologic issues and impaired behavior such as acquired stuttering. In this context, information uncovered in the interview showing a temporal relationship between signs of psychologic disequilibrium and the speech disorder should alert the clinician. When further findings continue to suggest psychogenicity, a speech diagnosis need not await a positive psychiatric diagnosis.

The interview may also uncover two other signs of psychogenicity. The report of prior, transient episodes of stuttering, when combined with an absence of findings for neurologic disease, is one of these signs. This is especially true if prior episodes were linked temporally to periods of psychologic distress or diagnosed psychopathology. Second, dramatic improvement in fluency or a return to normal speech during the expression of emotionally sensitive material is a signal to consider seriously a psychogenic etiology. Indeed, if the interviewer creates an atmosphere that encourages disclosure of sensitive information, and the patient is willing and possesses sufficient insight to disclose that information, speech may return to normal and stay that way.

The final and most convincing support for a psychogenic diagnosis is the patient's response to behavioral treatment. In our study, 70% of treated patients returned to normal or near-normal speech in one or two sessions. A number of cases, as was mentioned previously, returned to normal during the psychosocial interview. Such dramatic, rapid improvement in response to direct behavioral suggestions is not consistent with any known neurogenic speech or language disorder. The presence or absence of a coexisting neuropathology does not appear to affect the likelihood that a patient will show such a positive response. This kind of response to short-term treatment has been noted in several other publications[5,6,20] and is also consistent with what has been reported for cases of psychogenic voice disorders.[2,26,27] Absence of a rapid and dramatic response to therapy does not necessarily rule out psychogenicity; there are reports of psychogenic patients who do well with longer periods of therapy.

Management

Treatment Goals

Treatment goals, of necessity, are somewhat general for at least two reasons. First, the specific behaviors presented varies from individual-to-individual. Second, in this population, assessment procedures may be therapeutic. Some patients draw conclusions and gain insight, especially during a thorough psychosocial interview. The speech of some changes markedly or returns to normal during the evaluation, especially the interview. In such cases, the clinician builds on what has already begun. In other cases, when insight appears to be lacking and the patient's speech does not improve as initial evaluation tasks are conducted, speech change may require targeting of multiple behavioral changes in a very systematic manner. It is important, therefore, that a clinician keep treatment goals in mind during the evaluation. Thus, the SLP should recognize from the beginning that acquired speech disorders such as stuttering can be psychogenic and that an evaluation should set the stage for a transition to treatment. Progress toward "treatment goals" can be greatly facilitated when kept in mind as the evaluation is conducted.

Two early and essential treatment goals are an explanation of the evaluation's findings and the creation of an atmosphere in which a patient becomes receptive to the idea that these findings are good news and indicate that a total resolution of symptoms is possible. This does not require that patients understand exactly how stuttering developed. It is more important that they accept that stuttering is not due to a serious medical or neurologic illness and that there is a good chance that they can change the way they produce speech. The need to achieve this kind of goal through behavioral counseling in cases of nonorganic voice disorders was discussed in a recent report[28] and is equally applicable to cases of acquired psychogenic stuttering.

If significant speech improvement does not occur spontaneously during the evaluation and if the clinician suspects psychogenicity, then a direct, organized presentation of findings is the first step in dealing with the commonly held belief by these patients that their speech disorder is organic. If symptom resolution has occurred during the psychosocial interview, then the absence of stuttering can be made evident to the patient at that time. The goal in either case is to focus on acknowledging that a speech disorder exists in the absence of findings of organic disease. A "cognitive set" must be achieved so that the lack of organicity is perceived in a positive light by the patient, as is the clinician's belief that this is a reasonable, not unexpected finding. If this is not achieved, a patient may have received indirectly the message that the clinician is surprised or that the findings are, somehow, mysterious. Worse yet would be the message that a lack of organicity indicates that there is not a real problem. In my opinion, a prerequisite for patients achieving such a cognitive set is the clinician's belief that psychogenicity is a valid concept and that findings pointing to such a diagnosis are reasonable and not uncommon.

When patients' speech improves markedly during the examination, the goals of presenting findings and developing a confident atmosphere are easily achieved and can be followed immediately by the goal of approximating normal conversational speech. This includes reinforcing the concept that there are no physical barriers to improved, normal speech production. The opportunity to experience sustained fluency should follow as soon as possible, the patient's initial production of normal or near-normal speech. This needs to be done carefully, without any sense of "rushing." The recognition by patients that they are producing normal or much improved speech and what this means for prognosis is more important than repeated opportunities to speak. Motor practice is important, but even more important is this crucial change in the patient's belief system.

For those patients whose speech does not begin to change during the examination, the presentation of findings, including the absence of organic disease, should be followed by tasks whose goals are to identify and reduce struggle behavior. Initial targets would include any abnormal movements that do not involve the speech production mechanism, for example, movements of one or more limbs, the torso, or the head. Other more unusual, or "bizarre," examples might include such behaviors as keeping the eyes closed, attempting speech only when lying down or holding an object, or darkening the room to prevent light from causing "spasms" that interfere with speech. Reduction of these kinds of behavior reduces the effort or extraneous muscle tension accompanying speech attempts. The reduction or elimination of extraneous motor activity also changes patients' thinking; they no longer believe that such movements are needed or helpful. Procedures for achieving these goals will be described in the next section.

If excess, extraneous, or bizarre motor activity indicative of excessive effort or muscle tension associated with speech attempts can be markedly reduced or eliminated, then the next goal is identifying dysfluencies and reducing their frequency. Procedures that may be helpful here are not markedly different from techniques used to manage developmental stuttering; "modified stuttering," "fluency shaping," or an "integration" of these approaches.

My comments on early treatment goals reflect the belief that speech which is as near normal as can be achieved should be the target of the first session. The pursuit of dramatic speech changes, in an upbeat, positive context is more important, initially, than are discussions of specific stressors and how they may have played a role in the patient's acquisition of disordered speech. Once a clinician suspects psychogenicity, attempts aimed at speech change will yield results that either help confirm or question the diagnosis. If an initial session does not yield normal or near-normal speech then a second and third session, if necessary, should be scheduled as soon as possible devoted to achieving positive speech change (i.e., direct symptomatic therapy).

Discussions of the role played by specific stressors or the nature of psychogenic speech disorders, in general, are probably best deferred until after significant changes in speech have been sought. It should be remembered that the most common psychiatric diagnosis in these patients is a conversion reaction, which—by definition—results in an involuntary loss of control over speech production. The patient is not deliberately producing abnormal speech. Rather, the loss of speech control happens to the patient as a result of psychologic conflict. Many patients, at least initially, deny the possibility that psychologic issues are a problem or that they play any role in their disordered speech. Some degree of secondary "gain" may also be present. Expending time and energy attempting to refine what is known about a given patient's psychodynamics or "convincing" the patient that complex psychologic mechanisms are at work may not be successful in my experience and may delay work in obtaining the most convincing evidence a clinician can have: symptom resolution. Nevertheless, exploration of specific psychologic factors and the extent to which they appear to be resolved or ongoing definitely should be a goal of the SLP during the first or one of the early sessions. Several goals may be achieved by this kind of discussion.

One important goal is determining whether a psychologic or psychiatric referral should be made. If the SLP can successfully develop an atmosphere in which the patient discusses sensitive psychologic information, then it is seldom a problem to determine if relevant psychologic variables are at work. When this is combined with a patient's acquisition and use of normal speech at the conversation level, there may be no need for referral. On the other hand, when ongoing stressors are apparent or the patient requests assistance in dealing with psychologic issues, a prompt referral should be made. In such cases, however, the need to attend to a patient's speech symptoms is probably not going to be met very well when psychiatrists or psychologists are responsible for such monitoring. Certainly, the management of disordered speech, if needed, is better carried out by SLPs than mental health professionals. If patients are referred for a psychiatric evaluation too early, it may have the effect of driving them away from help for their speech unless they are willing to consider psychologic factors as central to their speech difficulty. If speech change comes rapidly, another goal is to convince patients that they are welcome to see the SLP again if there is a return of speech difficulty and that this does not in any way reflect a "failure" on their part. Repeated visits to the SLP, especially if a return of speech to normalcy results, may set the stage for a patient's eventual acceptance of the need for psychiatric evaluation and management.

If resolution of a patient's speech symptoms cannot be achieved, especially if psychologic issues are clearly ongoing, then a psychiatric referral should be made. The goal in making this referral is to assist in initiating therapy (pharmacologic, cognitive-behavioral, or both) that may be a necessary precursor to improved speech. This should not be a first management choice. The professionals best trained to bring about speech change are SLPs. There are, however, patients whose denial, lack of insight, severity of psychiatric illness, or some combination of them, make benefit from working with an SLP unlikely. In these cases, I believe that the SLP should consider recommending conjoint therapy. Treatment of psychogenic voice disorders within a framework of cognitive–behavior therapy is discussed in detail in a recent text,[14] and examples of conjoint approaches to stuttering are included in this material also. If normalization of speech does not occur rapidly but the patient appears motivated and seemingly free of severe psychopathology, I think that continued speech therapy with the goal of establishing normal speech is still warranted. The literature does provide some evidence supporting continued attempts to establish normal speech in patients with psychogenic speech disorders who do not respond rapidly.[6,18,19,23]

Generalization and maintenance of normalized speech is a long-term goal which has received, unfortunately, very little systematic study. Case reports documenting the return to normal speech have not included follow-up data. Clearly, this should be a goal, but there are a number of variables that make long-term follow-up difficult if not impossible. Patients seen in a medical setting are unlikely to return unless there is a resumption of their speech symptoms; however, an absence of patient-initiated return for services is extremely weak evidence for supporting the long-term efficacy of patients' management. It should be recognized that stabilization of normal speech is an especially complex issue in these patients and certainly reflects more than just the efficacy of speech pathology services. These are patients whose speech impairments result from psychogenic issues, and the return of their psychologic disequilibrium or psychopathology may bring with it a return of speech symptoms. Thus, resumption of psychogenic stuttering may be a more valid indicator of a patient's psychologic imbalance than the adequacy of initial speech pathology services. Unlike developmental disorders, the long-term status of these acquired disorders is intimately tied to issues of etiology, few of which are under the control of SLPs.

Treatment Procedures

Useful treatment procedures are based to a significant extent on individual patient characteristics and specific clinical scenarios. The following discussion, therefore, should be viewed as providing general guidelines which should be modified to fit individual circumstances.

I stated in an earlier section that assessment, itself, can be therapeutic and that clinicians should be aware of early treatment goals while conducting an evaluation. My early and essential treatment goals include careful explanations of findings and development of a positive atmosphere. The first procedural implication of my approach to treatment is that the clinician should seek to draw the patient's attention to findings that do not support organicity and conduct the evaluation in a way that should reveal support for psychogenicity if it is there. One procedure that I find helpful is to ask the patient what they've been told regarding prior medical evaluations. Alternatively, I might briefly review the patient's prior findings and mention that when acquired stuttering is organic it is associated with various abnormalities of the brain, which would show up on clinical, radiologic, neurophysiologic, or laboratory studies. Thus, negative neurologic findings can be placed in the context that makes possible another diagnosis and that this is a very "encouraging" possibility. Clinicians should be careful not to equate psychogenicity with psychopathology, stating simply that the ups and downs of everyday life and certainly chronic or recurring sources of distress can interfere with speech, just as they can produce other common physical symptoms. The speech examination, then, can be introduced as a series of tasks that will identify either a neurologically based pattern of findings or one that is more consistent with the absence of neurologic findings. Both possibilities should be presented as perfectly reasonable, with the latter possibility offering the potential of a return to normal speech. Further comments could note that this often occurs during the evaluation session itself. Clinicians must also be careful not to imply that the absence of support for organicity makes the problem less significant. Commenting specifically that the patient clearly has a significant problem with speech can help express empathy, which can then be tied to a statement of optimism regarding the absence of findings for organicity.

The psychosocial interview can be therapeutic, and the clinician should be attentive to signs that the patient is willing to discuss psychologically stressful issues. Sometimes a clinician may only note findings that are suggestive of distress but, if the patient appears receptive, direct inquiry can be made about feelings and reactions to issues or events. Often times, an unambiguous willingness on the part of the clinician to investigate these issues will help bring patients to the point where feelings are brought to the surface and emotional "venting" and disclosure will occur. This, in turn, may lead to a resolution of speech symptoms, either as a function of emotional disclosure and related conflict resolution and/or as a function of the reduced musculoskeletal tension that accompanies the release obtained by discussing difficult or suppressed issues. It must be remembered, however, that an interview that involves only the recitation of facts is unlikely to produce symptom resolution. The ability to create an open, supportive, and trusting atmosphere is necessary for this kind of interview to be successful. Clinician attributes that are helpful in this kind of atmosphere have been described previously in the literature.[2,12]

If symptom resolution does occur during the initial interview, the clinician should point this out, emphasizing that it is a very positive sign. It must be made clear to the patient that this is perfectly reasonable and fits a pattern with which the clinician is familiar. Clearly, these suggestions indicate that the clinician is providing a patient with an acceptable "explanation" for the resolution of symptoms. This does not mean, however, that psychogenic stuttering is the same as malingering and that these patients need to be given an acceptable way to drop their deception. Rather, the clinician is creating a road that the patient can feel free to follow. After pointing out that a patient is speaking fluently, the clinician can move to nonpropositional speech tasks, such as counting and reciting days of the week and months of the year. These tasks can be followed by the recitation of automatic, overlearned responses such as the patient's name, address, phone number, date of birth, and other biographic information. This needs to be done slowly, with careful attention not to rush the patient, and with verbal reinforcement not just for fluency but for the fact that this behavior fits a known, expected pattern and that there is no physical barrier to the patient's continued success. Comments regarding the absence of a physical barrier and genuinely supportive statements that things are going well and as expected should be repeated frequently. From automatic, overlearned utterances the clinician can move to questions requiring only brief answers, reading of single sentences, reading groups of sentences, then to longer periods of reading and conversation. There is no definitive continuum of tasks; the idea is to move the patient without rushing into increasingly lengthy and complex interactions that approximate normal conversation.

If resolution of a patient's speech symptoms does not occur spontaneously, the clinician's task is somewhat more difficult, but complete resolution of the speech problem is still possible. Symptomatic treatment should be introduced in a positive manner, accompanied by statements to the effect that rapid improvement is possible if the patient will attempt what is asked. First, the patient should be asked if he/she is willing to participate. If the answer is no or the patient is otherwise resistant, the reason(s) for this should be explored. In my experience, however, this is a negative prognostic sign; such patients are not likely to do well in symptomatic therapy, or will be unwilling to try it. Either possibility often leads to the conclusion that psychiatric evaluation and management may be necessary before any benefit will be derived from therapy for speech-related behaviors. On the other hand, if the patient shows a willingness to proceed, this should be met with confident reinforcement and an immediate move to symptom modification (e.g., "good, then let's get started right away").

In general, my approach shares much in common with the symptomatic modification of psychogenic voice disorders and with procedures for reducing the struggle behavior and effort that is targeted in adults with developmental stuttering (see, especially chapter 9 for a discussion of these approaches). An initial step is to identify behaviors that are not related directly to speech production and that reflect excessive effort or the perceived, irrational need to meet certain conditions before speech can be produced. The clinician may comment that the patient appears to be having considerable difficulty but that, in fact, some of the extra motor activity may not really be needed because there does not appear to be a clear physical barrier to speech production. In addition, any conditions that the patient feels must be met in order to speak need to be identified, one at a time, and removed, starting with those that are least related to speech production. It is important to reinforce any changes made. The fact that this is hard work and may be uncomfortable should be acknowledged repeatedly. In many cases, early portions of this therapy move more slowly than do later portions, which also should be made known to the patient. It seems as if a certain amount of momentum must first be achieved, after which continued change becomes less difficult. It is important to keep in mind that there really is no physical barrier to fluency in these cases and this should be reflected continually by the clinician's attitude that with continued work significant progress can be made. The goal, here, is not fluency but the removal of extraneous, effortful motor activity and the belief that certain unusual conditions must be met for speech. Once this has been achieved, fluent speech can be targeted.

The following case illustrates this. The patient was a male in his 20s who believed that his speech difficulty was probably due to tetanus, resulting from a cut he'd received. He'd been told at one point that his effortful, "spasm-like" attempts to produce speech could be treated effectively with injections of botulin toxin. He sought a second opinion at another medical center. His neurologic workup was negative, and a diagnosis of possible conversion disorder was made. The specific neurologic diagnosis ruled out a hyperkinetic movement disorder. The patient was hospitalized on the neurology floor and, at the outset of my initial speech session I found him lying in bed with eyes closed, lights out, and the shades drawn. When asked if he could sit up and talk for awhile he shook his head "no." When asked if he needed to remain reclined, he attempted to say "yes" but was unable to produce any voice. His attempts to produce this word were accompanied by facial grimacing, head bobbing, and erratic opening and closing of the eyes. He did manage to produce /s/. At this point, I began work on the first "stage" of therapy. I suggested that, even though it may be uncomfortable, he could probably tolerate having the blinds open if the lights were left off and he kept his eyes closed. The blinds were opened and I placed my hand on his shoulder. As is true with many voice patients, physical contact often helps to identify and then reduce muscle tension. I told him not to attempt any speech but rather to remain quiet and try to relax. After a few minutes I suggested that he would be able to tolerate the lights being turned on. All he had to do was relax. The lights were turned on but he remained reclined with his eyes closed with my hand on his shoulder. The next step was to suggest that he was able to open his eyes but that no speech would be required. At this point, he readily opened his eyes, which was followed by rapid eye blinking. I encouraged him to relax and look at the ceiling, even though this appeared to be difficult for him. He did so, which was followed by verbal reinforcement of his efforts and a brief review of the progress he had already made. His eye blinking stopped and both of us simply waited in silence. After a minute or two I suggested that speech production might be easier if he sat up than if he remained lying down. I provided both verbal and physical encouragement in order to help him assume a sitting posture on the bed but not to attempt speech. He did this without apparent difficulty, at which point it was suggested that sitting on the chair next to the bed was no different than sitting on the bed. He was encouraged to move to the chair, and he did. This move was followed by my acknowledgment of how difficult this was and that his progress was very encouraging. At this point the patient is sitting up, out of bed, eyes open, lights on, and ready to move to the next "stage."

When moving to speech production, it is important to focus on an area of the body that appears to reflect excessive effort or tension. It is helpful if this area can be touched and even manipulated in an effort to reduce musculoskeletal tension. In this case, the patient had particular difficulty initiating phonation. I pointed this out to him and palpated his laryngeal area, which did reveal excessive musculoskeletal tension. The area was manipulated and shortly after starting this I asked him to produce a humming sound. Though strained, it was not accompanied by the struggle behavior that was evident earlier. As soon as humming could be sustained, I asked him to add a sustained vowel to the end. This progression is, of course, very similar to that utilized with musculoskeletal tension voice disorders. Humming plus the vowel was followed by the vowel in isolation and then nonpropositional single words. When single-word production is achieved, the patient is in a similar position to those patients who achieve fluency during the psychosocial interview. In the example I have been describing, I reinforced both fluency and lack of struggle and repeated that he was doing very well and there were no physical obstacles to continued improvement. I moved on to short, nonpropositional utterances such as his name, address, city, and state in which he lived, roads he drove to the hospital, and the like. Each utterance was followed by verbal encouragement and a repetition of how well he was doing and that there were no apparent obstacles to successful completion of the next task. Once the patient is able to answer simple, rather nonpropositional questions, I move directly to conversation in which I ask for increasingly more complex answers. I make very frequent reference to how well the patient is doing, how sure I am that continued progress can be made, and I specifically mention the relaxed, "easy" way in which he is producing speech. In the case I have been describing, the patient was participating in conversation, while sitting, with normal speech, after approximately 30 min. I then moved away from him but stayed in the room and asked him to increase volume. He did not encounter any difficulty in doing so.

In some cases, multiple behaviors may need to be targeted, and this would proceed in the same general way just described. A behavior is identified, an explanation for the value of modifying it is given, and muscle tension is monitored, by touch if possible. Any modification is accepted, and the behavior is shaped toward normalcy. It does appear that, once progress begins, additional progress occurs more readily. This is another reason to move toward symptom modification rapidly and continue once progress has begun. If additional sessions are needed, I believe that they should be scheduled as soon as can be arranged. It has been my experience that patients with acquired psychogenic stuttering usually present with a wider variety of effortful movements that are associated with speech than do voice patients. This is consistent with our[4] finding that many of these patients showed considerable struggle behavior. In addition, they may need more attempts at modifying dysfluencies than is typical of voice patients who are attempting to modify or only vocalize. Once progress begins, however, it often accelerates, so that the time necessary to modify each type of behavior is reduced as one moves from one behavior to the next.

In the section on treatment goals, I stated that discussion of psychologic stressors can be deferred until symptom reduction has been attempted. This may be done by reviewing with the patient those psychologic stressors mentioned in the interview and asking how they have been dealt with, whether they are ongoing, and the extent to which they still affect the patient. If they are still active, the way in which they affect the patient's life needs to be explored. This is not an attempt to conduct psychotherapy or alleviate distress, although discussion may lead to this. Rather, it is an effort to determine if a psychiatric or psychologic referral is indicated. If the patient's symptoms can be alleviated and there are no apparent ongoing stressors, a referral may not be needed.[2,7] Of course, the presence of ongoing stressors or a request by the patient for psychologic assistance should always lead to referral. So, too, should a patient's refusal to participate in symptomatic therapy or in the psychosocial interview. These patients, however, are not likely to be helped by the referral, if indeed they even pursue it.

If symptom resolution is not achieved within a few sessions, therapy should be continued, because there is some evidence that long-term therapy can be helpful. Several of these references[6,18,19] have been reviewed by Duffy.[7]

Expected Outcomes

The most common outcome in these patients is a complete resolution of symptoms over a short period of time. Others may require a longer term of therapy. A significant number of those who respond well to symptomatic therapy do not show a current need for psychiatric referral. Those who do, or about whom there is a question, should be referred. In the meantime, therapy with an SLP should be pursued. Unfortunately, some patients do not do well. Some are unwilling to participate in symptomatic therapy, do not cooperate with the psychosocial interview, or steadfastly deny that a speech problem exists. In these cases, the clinician should document why the speech problem is thought to be psychogenic and terminate pursuit of symptomatic therapy.

Conclusions

Acquired psychogenic stuttering can be identified from a combination of psychosocial factors and patterns of speech difficulty that do not fit any predictable findings associated with known neurogenic speech disorders. It can occur in the presence of neuropathology and is a good example of the fact that neurogenic and psychogenic disorders commonly coexist. The presence of neuropathology, alone, should not exclude psychogenicity from differential diagnostic considerations.

In this chapter I have suggested that, although these patients' speech symptoms are different, the principles of clinical services for these patients are the same as those used with other psychogenic speech disorders, especially disorders of voice. Most of these patients respond very rapidly to therapy and produce normal or near-normal speech within one or two sessions, regardless of whether their stuttering is accompanied by neurologic disease or not. Psychiatric referral is not always necessary. The SLP does not need a psychiatric diagnosis to make a diagnosis of psychogenicity, and these patients often can be managed successfully by an SLP alone.

Little is known about these patients' outcomes. It is not readily apparent that their speech disorder, or some other disorder, would necessarily return if successful psychotherapy is not accomplished. On the other hand, some of these patients may be "predisposed" somehow to respond to life's stresses with physical symptoms and, having happened once, it may happen again.

Information regarding speech and voice signs that are indicative of various kinds of psychologic difficulty is available in the literature. Similarly, speech and voice characteristics of various organic illnesses are well described in the literature. Speech pathologists have, therefore, not only the ability to become familiar with this literature, but the responsibility to do so. Without such familiarity, acquired speech disorders cannot be dealt with confidently, and it is the confidence that is based on a firm mastery of this knowledge base that clinicians need to project in order to work successfully with these patients.

Suggested Readings

Aronson AE: *Clinical Voice Disorders*, 3rd ed. New York, Thieme, 1990.
   This text, and especially the chapter on psychologic interviewing, presents comprehensive coverage of clinical issues in psychogenic voice disorders. There are also multiple case studies included in the text.
Baumgartner J, Duffy JR: Psychogenic stuttering in adults with and without neurologic disease. *J Medical Speech–Language Pathology* 1997; 5:75–95.
   This recent article presents a retrospective review of findings on a large number of patients with psychogenic stuttering. It also contains an extensive review of the literature. The findings and clinical implications included in this article form much of the basis for the clinical material in the current chapter.
Duffy JR: *Motor Speech Disorders: Substrates, Differential Diagnosis and Management*. St. Louis, Mosby, 1995.
   This comprehensive text includes a chapter on differential diagnosis of psychogenic disorders and another chapter on management. It also includes extensive references. The material in the current chapter is consistent with Duffy's text. I highly recommend the entire text. There are, as in Aronson's text, multiple case studies.

Crowe TA (ed.): *Applications of Counseling in Speech–Language Pathology and Audiology*. Baltimore, Williams and Wilkins, 1997.
This edited text includes a review of the foundations of counseling, counseling approaches, and the use of counseling with selected communicative disorders. It highlights the necessary role the SLP must play in counseling and gives suggestions about how to go about it. Crowe also carefully covers the issue of psychotherapy vs. counseling, and how they are similar, yet different.

References

1. Terminology Pertaining to Fluency and Fluency Disorders. Technical paper prepared for Special Interest Division 4, American Speech Language and Hearing Association, 1997.
2. Aronson AE: *Clinical Voice Disorders*, 3rd ed. New York, Thieme, 1990.
3. Duffy JR, Petersen DC: Primary progressive aphasia. *Aphasiology* 1992; 6:1–15.
4. Baumgartner J, Duffy JR: Psychogenic stuttering in adults with and without neurologic disease. *J Med Speech-Language Pathology* 1997; 5:75–95.
5. Roth ER, Aronson AE, Davis LJ: Clinical studies in psychogenic stuttering of adult onset. *J Speech Hearing Dis* 1989; 54:634–646.
6. Tippett DC, Siebens AA: Distinguishing psychogenic from neurogenic dysfluency when neurologic and psychologic factors coexist. *J Fluency Dis* 1991; 16:3–12.
7. Duffy JR: *Motor Speech Disorders: Substrates, Differential Diagnosis and Management*. St. Louis, Mosby, 1995.
8. Sapir S, Aronson AE: The relationship between psychopathology and speech and language disorders in neurologic patients. *J Speech Hearing Dis* 1990; 55:503–509.
9. Baumgartner JM: Speech Disorders that Look Neurogenic but Aren't: Case Studies. Paper presented at the convention of the American Speech-Language-Hearing Association, San Francisco, 1996.
10. Gravell R, France J (eds): *Speech and Communication Problems in Psychiatry*. San Diego, Singular Publishers, 1992.
11. Crowe TA: Counseling: Definition, History, Rationale, in Crowe TA (ed): *Applications of Counseling in Speech-Language Pathology and Audiology*. Baltimore, Williams and Wilkins, 1997.
12. Luterman DM: *Counseling the Communicatively Impaired and Their Families*, 2nd ed. Austin, Pro-Ed, 1991.
13. Shipley KG: *Interviewing and Counseling in Communicative Disorders: Principles and Procedures*. New York, Merrill, 1992.
14. Butcher P, Elias A, Raven R: *Psychogenic Voice Disorders and Cognitive-Behavior Therapy*. San Diego, Singular Publishers, 1993.
15. Boone DR, McFarlane SC: *The Voice and Voice Therapy*, 5th ed. Englewood Cliffs, Prentice-Hall, 1994.
16. Murphy AT: *Functional Voice Disorders*. Englewood Cliffs, Prentice-Hall, 1964.
17. Darley FL, Aronson AE, Brown JR: *Motor Speech Disorders*. Philadelphia, Saunders, 1975.
18. Mahr G, Leith W: Psychogenic stuttering of adult onset. *J Speech Hearing Res* 1992; 35:283–286.
19. Deal JL: Sudden onset of stuttering: A case report. *J Speech Hearing Dis* 1982; 47:301–304.
20. Duffy JR: A Puzzling Case of Adult Onset Stuttering, in Helm-Estabrooks N, Aten JL (eds): *Difficult Diagnosis in Communication Disorders*, Boston, College-Hill, 1989.
21. Wallen V: Primary stuttering in a 28-year-old adult. *J Speech Hearing Dis* 1961; 26:394–395.
22. Attanascio JS: A case of late-onset or acquired stuttering in adult life. *J Fluency Dis* 1987; 12:287–290.
23. Brookshire RH: A Dramatic Response to Behavior Modification by a Patient with a Rapid Onset of Dysfluent Speech, in Helm-Estabrooks N, Aten JL (eds.): *Difficult Diagnoses in Communication Disorders*, Boston, College-Hill, 1989.
24. Deal JL, Doro JM: Episodic hysterical stuttering. *J Speech Hearing Dis* 1987; 52:299–300.
25. Ringo CC, Dietrich S: Neurogenic stuttering: An analysis and critique. *J Med Speech-Language Pathology* 1995; 2:111–122.

26. Sapir S, Aronson AE: Coexisting psychogenic and neurogenic dysphonia: A source of diagnostic confusion. *Br J Dis Commun* 1987; 20:73–80.

27. Sapir S, Aronson AE: Aphonia after closed head injury: Aetiologic considerations. *Br J Dis Commun* 1985; 20:289–296.

28. Stone RE: Behavioral Counseling in Voice Disorders, in Crowe TA (ed): *Applications of Counseling in Speech-Language Pathology and Audiology*. Baltimore, Williams and Wilkins, 1997.

Stuttering and Related Disorders of Fluency, 2nd edition.
Edited by Richard F. Curlee, Ph.D.
Thieme Medical Publishers, Inc., New York © 1999.

15

Principles and Practices of Current Stuttering Therapy

Gerald M. Siegel
Conrad Gold

In preparing this concluding chapter we have assumed that the contents of this text can be viewed as a microcosm of the approaches to stuttering therapy that are currently being used in the field. In the preceding chapters, the authors described their approaches to the assessment and remediation of stuttering. To varying extent they also provided the rationale for their methods. We assume that by examining the general principles and practices of current stuttering therapy as they are exemplified in this book, it will be possible to characterize areas of agreement and disagreement and point to some of the unresolved issues in the delivery of service to adults and children who stutter.

Applications of Theory

There are two generalizations that can be drawn concerning the relationship between theory and therapy. The first is that, after many decades in which theories of stuttering were primarily environmental and it was assumed that stuttering was learned, the pendulum has swung and most authorities once again believe that the cause of stuttering is organic and probably includes a genetic component.[1] Although the exact nature of this constitutional etiology has not yet been determined, many candidates have been proposed as the potential source of the organic breakdown, including, once again, disturbed cortical dominance,[2] the speech motor system,[3–5] (and Kully and Langevin, this volume, chapter 8), the respiratory and laryngeal systems,[6] or some complex interaction among systems.[7] The words "motor speech disorder" seem to roll most trippingly off the tongue, even among therapists with a strong behavioral tradition.[5] It is the rare contemporary writer who would suggest that stuttering is "learned behavior," although it is generally acknowledged that learning plays a role in the elaboration of the original condition.[4]

The second generalization is that most authorities writing about treatment of stuttering seem unconcerned about theories.* Rarely do they justify their approach or methods in

---

*Prins's (1997)[25] application of cognitive learning theory to therapy is an exception.

terms of an explicit theory, nor do they seem to be constrained in any formal way by existing theory. This is not to say that they do not hold any beliefs about stuttering, but rather that these beliefs tend to exist outside the framework of a formal theory. For example, Manning (this volume, chapter 9) believes that cognitive and affective aspects of stuttering deserve at least as much attention as the surface speech behaviors of the person who stutters, a view endorsed by many other experts. Such a belief will surely influence a clinician's approach to therapy, but it hardly defines a theory of stuttering.

Similarly, a number of the writers in the current volume describe procedures that were developed out of the operant analysis of behavior (chapter 4, Harrison and Onslow; chapter 5, J.C. Ingham; and chapter 11, R.J. Ingham), but they do not seem to subscribe to any particular theory of stuttering other than that it involves behaviors that can be modified by consequences. Furthermore, such concepts as reinforcement, extinction, punishment, and successive approximations are by now familiar to most clinicians, irrespective of their knowledge of learning theory. The techniques that emerged from the learning laboratories and were adopted by behavior modifiers have become detached from the theory that originally generated them.

Current clinical practice seems less concerned with ideology than with designing therapy that is intuitively sensible and achieves satisfactory results. It is undoubtedly true that clinical practice has always been influenced by pragmatic considerations, but the current times are especially besieged by political and social demands for accountability, especially the demonstration of efficacy.[9,10]

This pragmatic, atheoretical focus is infused with its own problems. Clinicians are presented with conflicting recommendations about which aspects of the disorder should be targeted in therapy. For example, both Ingham and Cordes (1997)[11] and Manning (this volume, chapter 9) suggest that therapy should be directed at the stutterer's handicap, but for Manning stuttering behaviors are only a small part of the handicap, while for Ingham and Cordes (1997, p. 414)[11] "the handicapping effects of stuttering lie at the level of speech output and the effects of that output on communicative interaction." If one agrees with Manning that the stutterings are only the tip of the iceberg, one must still decide whether that "tip" should be the focus of therapy, or whether therapy should be directed at the more murky aspects that are less available to observation and measurement.

Tied up with these concerns is the question of how to decide when treatment has succeeded, when there is no more that can be done in formal therapy, when the goals of therapy have been realized. Using the terminology that Manning favors, behaviorally oriented clinicians are suspicious that focusing on cognitive and affective aspects of the "handicap" may stem from an unwillingness to tackle the difficult problem of ameliorating stuttering behaviors—that clinicians may be content to produce well-adjusted stutterers. Alternatively, cognitively oriented therapists believe that behaviorists focus on superficial aspects of the "disability" and fail to recognize the profound and handicapping effects of stuttering on the person who stutters. A pragmatic, outcome-based approach to stuttering therapy cannot resolve these differences. The clinician and the client, it seems, are left to resolve them on their own.

Incurability of Stuttering Among Adults

In speech–language pathology, as in all helping professions, it is unethical to guarantee a cure. Some of the authors in the current volume, and in the profession at large, go to the other extreme. For example, Kully and Langevin write, "We want to ensure the client and family understand that there is no cure for stuttering." A similar admonition is expressed by Neilson and Andrews (1993)[12] in the first edition of the book and Neilson in the current volume (chapter 10).

The assertion that it is not only difficult, but essentially impossible to cure stuttering among adults represents a significant change in professional attitude. Johnson,[13] we suspect, would have subjected "cure" to a semantic analysis, and would surely have pointed out that the very term implies a deep-seated condition, an implication that he would have rejected. One does not "cure" maladaptive attitudes or semantic habits, any more than one is cured of bigotry or racial stereotyping. "Cure," we suspect, would not have been admissible in Johnson's lexicon of stuttering.

It is entirely appropriate and professionally responsible to tell clients that it is very difficult to treat stuttering in adults. This information could be offered while, at the same time, acknowledging that the cause and development of stuttering are not yet understood, but that there are ways of managing the problem and diminishing its handicapping consequences. Clinicians who tell their clients that there is no cure for stuttering undoubtedly wish to shield them from false hopes or expectations, but this information at the same time presumes the outcome of therapy and appears to be an indication of the pervasive, almost unquestioned belief in the underlying organicity of the condition. It might be more useful and accurate to admit the limits of current knowledge without implying that the cause of stuttering is, in fact, known.

Approaches to Stuttering in Young Children

In general, the authors are far more confident of success with children than with adults. Gregory and Gregory (this volume, chapter 3) indicate that therapy is very successful if the children are treated within 6 months of onset of stuttering. Although Curlee's chapter (chapter 1) is primarily concerned with identification of stuttering, he too expresses confidence about stuttering therapy for young children. At least two of the programs set very high expectations for their clients. Harrison and Onslow (this volume, chapter 4) indicate that the goal of the Lidcombe program is nothing less than to "eliminate stuttering from all speaking situations and to maintain this for at least 12 months." Similarly, for J.C. Ingham (this volume, chapter 5), "The goal of this treatment is that its beneficiaries become normal speakers."

It is interesting that children are thought to be so amenable to therapy despite the general belief that stuttering is a physiologically based disorder. Apparently, whatever the underlying condition may be, it is susceptible to very different approaches. The methods described by J.C. Ingham are modeled on single-subject research. An individual child is the focus of controlled procedures, including collection of extensive objective data on percentage of stuttering and word rate. Therapy is built around contingent responses to the child's speech behavior, dispensing approval and rewards for fluent utterances and disapproval for stuttering. The parents are not asked to alter their speaking or discourse style. The focus is kept on the child's speech.

In the Lidcombe program, presented by Harrison and Onslow, parents carry out therapy, rate their child's severity of stuttering, and collect performance data at home and other extra-clinic environments. Information and counseling are provided as required but, as with J.C. Ingham's approach, there is no attempt to have the parents modify their own speech and discourse patterns.

A very different approach is exemplified in the chapter in this volume by Louko,

Conture, and Edwards (chapter 7) for children who have both stuttering and phonological problems. They attempt to change the child's communication environment in the interest of reducing the "demands" component of the Demands and Capacities equation. Parents are taught to alter their style of discourse, speak more slowly, use more pauses, and avoid interrupting the child. The child may be taught general pragmatic skills in a setting with other children, but stuttering is not called to the child's attention and no attempt is made to modify speech disfluencies.

The therapy described by Gregory and Hill (this volume, chapter 2) also emphasizes teaching parents to reduce communicative stress. While the parent observes, the clinician models speaking in a relaxed manner, giving the child plenty of time to respond, reducing direct questioning, etc. When these strategies are not sufficient, the clinician also teaches the child the methods of "slower easy relaxed speech" through modeling and imitation at an appropriate level of speech difficulty, with reinforcement for achieving the desired speech style. Counseling parents is an integral aspect of this approach to treatment. Successful therapy, it is believed, involves consideration of the attitudes, thoughts and feelings of the child and the parents.

Not all of the chapters in the book can be fit neatly into one or the other camp. Runyan and Runyan (this volume, chapter 6) describe a set of very practical exercises that are framed in ways that should appeal to children. Through a variety of imaginative games the children are taught such rules as speak slowly, use speech breathing, start Mr. Voice Box running smoothly, etc. Although not described in behavioral terms, the focus of this program is on modifying speech. There is no discussion of parent or child counseling. To that extent, the approach seems more behavioral than cognitive.

It is evident from this brief overview that there are large differences in treatment approaches to young children who stutter. As with adults, some of the approaches focus very directly on the child's speech, but neither J.C. Ingham nor Onslow and Harrison "teach" the child how to be fluent. They do not provide instruction on how to modify or avoid stuttering. Basically, they control the complexity of the speech task, provide a great deal of support and encouragement for speech behaviors, and provide feedback concerning performance. The children draw on their own repertoire of speech skills to produce the fluent utterances that are then acknowledged and praised by the parent or clinician. It is not at all clear how these procedures might help to overcome an underlying condition, such as a motor speech disorder. Rather, it seems that the child uses the practice and feedback in a supportive environment to fortify skills that are already available.

As we analyze the indirect approach, it seems to be built on a chain of important, though implicit, assumptions.

1. *The parents of children who stutter are using a speech and discourse style that is not optimal for promoting normal speech development in the child.* If this were not so, there would be little justification to ask parents to change their natural style of interacting with the child.

2. *The parents can be taught to use a new, optimal style in the clinic and at home.* If parents cannot carry out this part of the program, then the critical feature of therapy is eliminated.

3. *When successfully adopted by the parents, the new style will encourage the child to change his own discourse and speech style.* This is the basis for making the therapy *indirect*. By working on the parents, the child is changed.

4. *The changes the child makes will reduce stuttering behaviors and protect the child from developing maladaptive attitudes concerning speech and communication.* This is the endpoint of the therapy chain. It cannot be reached if the earlier assumptions, 2 and 3, are not realized.

These are large assumptions that have been only partly supported by research.[14,15] If assumptions 2 and 3 are false, then it would seem that the rest of the program is meaningless.

Similarly, in the Lidcombe direct therapy program described by Harrison and Onslow, if the parents do not fulfill their roles as agents of therapy outside of the clinic, there is, in essence, no therapy program, or at least no therapy as it is envisioned by the authors. In the case of both the direct and indirect therapy, however, there is as yet little information to show that the parents accomplish the critical role they presumably play in implementing the respective therapies.

In summary, diametrically different approaches to therapy for young children claim considerable success, but in neither instance do we have a firm understanding of why the approach is successful. Perhaps there is some more general level at which the approaches are more similar than they currently appear, but if that is the case, it has not yet been elucidated.

Behavioral and Integrative Approaches

R. Ingham describes in elaborate detail the procedures used in his program to achieve and maintain fluency in adults who stutter. There is no discussion in his chapter of the stutterer's inner emotions, feelings, or cognitions. The focus of therapy is clearly on giving the stutterer the tools to eliminate stuttering and maintain fluency once formal therapy is ended. Manning characterizes this approach to therapy as dealing only with the tip of the iceberg because, in his view, it fails to account for the depth of the client's handicap and the features of stuttering that occur under the surface.

These disparate approaches to therapy reveal profound disagreement concerning the primary goals of therapy and how those goals should be accomplished. Behaviorally oriented therapists view the elimination of stuttering as the goal and the experimental laboratory as the model for achieving that goal. Within the behavioral model, the efficacy of therapy is determined by making precise and reliable measurements of such indices as the frequency of stutterings, the rate of speech, and the judged naturalness of the speech. A major effort is allocated to devising reliable, objective measures of speech performance and to modeling therapy on the principles of scientific method.

Cognitively oriented therapists fear that "eliminating" stuttering is really another form of hiding it. Authorities who were schooled in the therapies developed by Johnson, Van Riper, or Sheehan feel that any approach to therapy is incomplete or even misguided if it fails to acknowledge the deep-seated fears and the powerful motivation to hide stuttering which form the emotional substrate of the disorder. The aspects of the disorder that are of central concern to the cognitively oriented therapist are by their very nature subjective and difficult to quantify. Authorities who promote these methods seem less preoccupied with precise measurement and are more open to clinical experience and intuition rather than laboratory designs in the formulation and conduct of therapy.

It is an old disagreement. Kully and Langevin (chapter 8) respond by using features of both approaches. They describe systems for collection of objective data that are fully consistent with those of the staunchest behaviorally oriented clinicians, but also include measures of attitudes and feelings as cautious supplements to speech measures. This will not be satisfactory to the more committed advocates of one or the other philosophy, and there is no blueprint concerning how to reconcile discrepancies when, for example, clients register high levels of satisfaction with their current status but objective measures indicate that their speech behavior is grossly abnormal. The client is the final arbiter of the success of therapy, but the behaviorally oriented clinician may reasonably be suspicious of subjective measures when such marked discrepancies appear.

The most elaborate example of a program that integrates cognitive and behavioral approaches in conscious and explicit ways is described in this volume by Neilson. She incorporates research and theory from several disciplines, and the program is packed with measures of internal and external behaviors and with procedures that are directed at all aspects of the cognitive, affective, and behavioral dimensions of stuttering. It is interesting that Neilson's program has its roots in the same early intervention program that gave rise to Ingham's approach,[16] and retains some of the same features, although, as is evident in this book, the programs have veered in very different directions as Neilson has increasingly made the stutterer's subjective experience an integral part of therapy.

Related Disorders Section

We were struck by the inclusion of three chapters devoted to topics that, in earlier times, would have received only passing notice in a book on stuttering. Chapter 12 (Cluttering by Daly and Burnett) is one of these. For many years cluttering was ignored in most textbooks on stuttering.[17] Although cluttering is receiving renewed attention by speech–language pathologists, Daly and Burnett in this present volume suggest that fluency is only one aspect of this complex and multilayered disorder. Cluttering does receive some brief attention in Bloodstein's (1995)[18] *Handbook*, but mostly as a potential contributor to the development of stuttering.

Similarly, stuttering associated with neurogenic (chapter 13) and psychogenic (chapter 14) diagnoses has received scant attention in past books on stuttering. Helm-Estabrooks (1993)[19] had a chapter on neurogenics in the first as well as the current edition, but psychogenic stuttering was not treated in the earlier text. These variants of stuttering receive brief notice in Bloodstein (1995),[18] and Johnson (1956)[13] flatly stated that, despite any superficial resemblances, neurogenic and psychogenic conditions are not stuttering and should not be called by that name.

The inclusion of these three chapters in the current book suggests that current authorities may not be as concerned—or as certain—about the precise nature of stuttering as was true in earlier eras, possibly because current theories or models tend to focus on rather limited aspects of the problem of stuttering. For example, a modern psycholinguistic theory that has attracted a good deal of attention[20] is the "covert repair hypothesis."[21–23] It assumes that "stuttering constitutes a covert repair reaction to some flaw in the normal speech plan,"[22,p.190] but it makes no claims concerning why some children develop this flaw. Thus, almost any condition that affects phonological processing, including a neurogenic or psychological disturbance (or perhaps even fatigue or inebriation), could produce behaviors that the theory would label as "stuttering." Similarly, the Demands and Capacities Model[4,24] has proven to be quite utilitarian, but, as Starkweather[4] acknowledges, it is not a theory of the cause or the nature of stuttering and it too provides no guidance about how to distinguish stuttering from other fluency disorders.*

On the other hand, Johnson's (1956)[13] diagnosogenic theory attempted to account not only for the development of stuttering, but also for the variables that affect stuttering in

---

*See Neilson, this volume (chapter 10), for an example of how the model can be applied in justifying a therapy system, and Ingham and Cordes (1997)[11] for a critique of the logic of the model.

daily experience. His theory served as a template. For example, disordered disfluency in the absence of anticipation and fear was simply not stuttering in his scheme. Furthermore, his theory explicitly excluded psychological or neurological conditions as causes of stuttering. Current models or theories do not seem sufficiently elaborated to serve as filters in the same way.

Summary and Final Comments

In summary, there appears to be a consensus that the prospects are very good for treating young stutterers; however, it is perplexing that authorities disagree so fundamentally on how therapy for these children should be designed and that very discrepant approaches are nonetheless reported to be effective. Obviously, we still do not have a good grasp of the early development of stuttering or a satisfactory explanation for the success that is achieved through therapy.

The promise of this apparent success in treating young children who stutter is that in time it should be possible to eliminate stuttering in the population by educating the public so that parents and other professionals will seek help early enough. This optimistic outlook presumes that resources are adequate so that there is no outcry about including some children who might have developed normal fluency even without therapy. Something like this optimistic outcome was also promised by Johnson's diagnosogenic theory with its focus on widespread parent education. It remains to be seen whether these new optimistic prospects will be realized.

The prognosis for adults who stutter is not nearly as positive. Many authorities now seem comfortable informing these adults that there is no known cure for stuttering, but that they can become much more effective communicators and learn strategies to cope with their stuttering if they are willing to devote the considerable attention and energy that is required. There continues to be disagreement concerning the extent to which therapy should be directed at eliminating the nonfluent behaviors versus the maladaptive emotions and attitudes that accompany a lifetime of stuttering, although programs such as Neilson's (chapter 10) attempt to integrate the two orientations fully at the outset. Some of the therapy programs described in this chapter are directly linked to the single-subject research model that was so fundamental to operant conditioning and its clinical application in behavior modification. Others seem more indebted to approaches originally developed by Johnson, Van Riper, Sheehan, and others, who concentrated on eliminating avoidance and the fears associated with stuttering. The difference in approach is reflected also in the kinds of measures taken and in discrepant outcome goals. To the extent that the approaches also specify different goals and, therefore, different criteria, it is virtually impossible to compare their relative effectiveness.

Although all of the authorities necessarily operated according to some implicit beliefs concerning the nature of stuttering and the dimensions that should be targeted in therapy, there was little reference to formal theory. We had the impression that for many, therapy is governed by common sense, agreement and negotiation with the client, and pragmatic performance measures.

Manning suggested that the most important therapeutic ingredient is the relationship between the client and the therapist, a view which suggests that therapy is more art than science. Others in the book, particularly those with strong behavioral leanings, would surely prefer to elevate the scientific aspect of the therapy process, both as a source of therapy procedures and as a model for the design and conduct of therapy. Starkweather and Givens-Ackerman[26] included an appendix in their new textbook that summarizes the "best practices" position paper developed by ASHA's special interest division of fluency and fluency disorders, and ultimately by ASHA. These are useful guidelines, but at this point in the development of treatment methods, there are a number of approaches to therapy that meet the guidelines and yet are quite discrepant in methods and goals. It is up to the clients to find the program that seems most suited to their requirements. It is equally urgent that clinicians test the assumptions and the outcomes of their various approaches to stuttering therapy, either by collecting and publishing results in their own right, or in concert with the research community. Such collaboration will not only serve the needs of the public in assuring adequate clinical service, it will also advance our knowledge of the nature and mutability of this complex human behavior.

References

1. Felsenfeld S: Epidemiology and Genetics of Stuttering, in Curlee RF, Siegel GM (eds): *Nature and Treatment of Stuttering: New Directions*, 2nd ed. Boston, Allyn and Bacon, 1997.
2. Watson BC, Freeman FJ: Brain Imaging Contributions, in Curlee RF, Siegel GM (eds): *Nature and Treatment of Stuttering: New Directions*, 2nd ed. Boston, Allyn and Bacon, 1997.
3. Zimmerman GN: Stuttering: A disorder of movement. *J Speech Hear Res* 1980; 23:122–136.
4. Starkweather CW: Learning and Its Role in Stuttering Development, in Curlee RF, Siegel GM (eds): *Nature and Treatment of Stuttering: New Directions*, 2nd ed. Boston, Allyn and Bacon, 1997.
5. Onslow M: *Behavioral Management of Stuttering*. San Diego, California, Singular Publishers, 1996.
6. Denny M, Smith M: Respiratory and Laryngeal Control in Stuttering, in Curlee RF, Siegel GM (eds): *Nature and Treatment of Stuttering: New Directions*, 2nd ed. Boston, Allyn and Bacon, 1997.
7. Smith A, Kelly E: Stuttering: A Dynamic, Multifactorial Model, in Curlee RF, Siegel GM (eds): *Nature and Treatment of Stuttering: New Directions*, 2nd ed. Boston, Allyn and Bacon, 1997.
8. Bloodstein O: Stuttering as an Anticipatory Struggle Reaction, in Curlee RF, Siegel GM (eds): *Nature and Treatment of Stuttering: New Directions*, 2nd ed. Boston, Allyn and Bacon, 1997.
9. Olswang LB, Thompson CK, Warren SF, Minghetti N (eds): *Treatment Efficacy Research in Communication Disorders*. Rockville, MD, American Speech-Language-Hearing Foundation, 1990.
10. Prins D: Models for treatment efficacy studies of adult stutterers. *J Fluency Disord* 1993; 18: 333–349.
11. Ingham RJ, Cordes AK: Self-measurement and Evaluating Stuttering Treatment Efficacy, in Curlee RF, Siegel GM (eds): *Nature and Treatment of Stuttering: New Directions*, 2nd ed. Boston, Allyn and Bacon, 1997.
12. Neilson M, Andrews G: Intensive Fluency Training of Chronic Stutterers, in Curlee RF (ed): *Stuttering and Related Disorders of Fluency*. New York, Thieme, 1993.
13. Johnson W: Stuttering, in Johnson W, Brown SJ, Curtis, JJ, Edney CW, Keaster J: *Speech Handicapped School Children*, rev. ed. New York, Harper & Bros., 1956.
14. Bernstein Ratner N: Measurable outcomes of instructions to modify normal parent–child verbal interactions: Implications for indirect stuttering therapy. *J Speech Hear Res* 1992; 35:14–20.
15. Bernstein Ratner N: Parents, children, and stuttering. *Semin Speech Lang* 1993; 14:238–250.
16. Ingham RJ, Andrews G: Details of a token economy stuttering therapy program for adults. *Australian J Human Commun Disord* 1973; 1:13–20.
17. St. Louis KO, Myers FL: Management of Cluttering and Related Fluency Disorders, in Curlee RF, Siegel GM (eds): *Nature and Treatment of Stuttering: New Directions*, 2nd ed. Boston, Allyn and Bacon, 1997.
18. Bloodstein O: *A Handbook on Stuttering* (5th ed). San Diego, Singular Publishing, 1995.

19. Helm-Estabrooks N: Stuttering Associated with Acquired Neurological Disorders, in Curlee RF (ed): *Stuttering and Related Disorders of Fluency.* New York, Thieme, 1993.
20. Bernstein Ratner N: Stuttering: A Psycholinguistic Perspective, in Curlee RF, Siegel GM (eds): *Nature and Treatment of Stuttering: New Directions,* 2nd ed. Boston, Allyn and Bacon, 1997.
21. Kolk HHJ: Is Stuttering a Symptom of Adaptation or of Impairment? in Peters HFM, Hulstijn W, Starkweather CW (eds): *Speech Motor Control and Stuttering.* Amsterdam, Elsevier, 1991.
22. Kolk HHJ, Postma A: Stuttering as a Covert Repair Phenomenon, in Curlee RF, Siegel GM (eds): *Nature and Treatment of Stuttering: New Directions,* 2nd ed. Boston, Allyn and Bacon, 1997.
23. Postma A, Kolk HHJ: The covert repair hypothesis: Prearticulatory repair processes in normal and stuttered disfluencies. *J Speech Hear Res* 1993; 36:472–487.
24. Starkweather CW: *Fluency and Stuttering.* Englewood Cliffs, NJ, Prentice Hall, 1987.
25. Prins D: Modifying Stuttering—The Stutterer's Reactive Behavior: Perspectives on Past, Present, and Future, in Curlee RF, Siegel GM (eds): *Nature and Treatment of Stuttering: New Directions,* 2nd ed. Boston, Allyn and Bacon, 1997.
26. Starkweather CW, Givens-Ackerman J: *Stuttering.* Austin, TX, Pro-Ed, 1997.

This page is blank

Index

Note: Page numbers followed by f indicate figures; those followed by t indicate tables.